D1518953

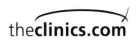

VETERINARY CLINICS

OF NORTH AMERICA

Small Animal Practice

Wound Management

GUEST EDITORS
Steven F. Swaim, DVM, MS
D.J. Krahwinkel, DVM, MS

July 2006 • Volume 36 • Number 4

SAUNDERS

An Imprint of Elsevier, Inc.
PHILADELPHIA   LONDON   TORONTO   MONTREAL   SYDNEY   TOKYO

W.B. SAUNDERS COMPANY
A Division of Elsevier Inc.

Elsevier, Inc., 1600 John F. Kennedy Blvd., Suite 1800, Philadelphia, PA 19103-2899

http://www.vetsmall.theclinics.com

VETERINARY CLINICS OF NORTH AMERICA:	**Volume 36, Number 4**
SMALL ANIMAL PRACTICE	**ISSN 0195-5616**
July 2006	**ISBN 1-4160-3827-2**

Editor: John Vassallo

Veterinary Clinics of North America: Small Animal Practice (ISSN 0195-5616) is published bimonthly (For Post Office use only: volume 36 issue 4 of 6) by W.B. Saunders, 360 Park Avenue South, New York, NY 10010-1710. Months of publication are January, March, May, July, September, and November. Business and Editorial offices: 1600 John F. Kennedy Blvd., Suite 1800, Philadelphia, PA 19103-2899. Accounting and circulation offices: 6277 Sea Harbor Drive, Orlando, FL 32887-4800. Periodicals postage paid at New York, NY and additional mailing offices. Subscription prices are $170.00 per year for US individuals, $275.00 per year for US institutions, $85.00 per year for US students and residents, $225.00 per year for Canadian individuals, $345.00 per year for Canadian institutions, $235.00 per year for international individuals, $345.00 per year for international institutions, and $115.00 per year for Canadian and foreign students/residents. To receive student/resident rate, orders must be accompanied by name of affiliated institution, date of term, and the *signature* of program/residency coordinator on institution letterhead. Orders will be billed at individual rate until proof of status is received. Foreign air speed delivery is included in all *Clinics* subscription prices. All prices are subject to change without notice. **POSTMASTER**: Send address changes to *Veterinary Clinics of North America: Small Animal Practice*, Elsevier Periodicals Customer Service, 6277 Sea Harbor Drive, Orlando, FL 32887-4800, USA; phone: 1-800-654-2452 [toll free number for US customers], or (+1)(407) 345-4000 [customers outside US]; fax: (+1)(407) 363-1354; email: usjcs@elsevier.com.

Veterinary Clinics of North America: Small Animal Practice is also published in Japanese by Inter Zoo Publishing Co., Ltd., Aoyama Crystal-Bldg 5F, 3-5-12 Kitaaoyama, Minato-ku, Tokyo 107-0061, Japan.

Reprints: For copies of 100 or more, of articles in this publication, please contact the Commercial Reprints Department, Elsevier Inc., 360 Park Avenue South, New York, New York 10010-1710. Tel. (212) 633-3813 Fax: (212) 462-1935, email: reprints@elsevier.com

Veterinary Clinics of North America: Small Animal Practice is covered in *Current Contents/Agriculture, Biology and Environmental Sciences, Science Citation Index, ASCA, Index Medicus, Excerpta Medica, and BIOSIS*.

Printed in the United States of America.

ELSEVIER
SAUNDERS

VETERINARY CLINICS
SMALL ANIMAL PRACTICE

Wound Management

GUEST EDITORS

STEVEN F. SWAIM, DVM, MS, Professor Emeritus, Scott-Richey Research Center and
Department of Clinical Sciences, College of Veterinary Medicine, Auburn
University, Alabama

D.J. KRAHWINKEL, DVM, MS, Diplomate, American College of Veterinary Surgeons;
Diplomate, American College of Veterinary Anesthesiologists; Diplomate,
American College of Veterinary Emergency and Critical Care; Professor
of Surgery, Department of Small Animal Clinical Sciences, The University
of Tennessee College of Veterinary Medicine, Knoxville, Tennessee

CONTRIBUTORS

TANNAZ AMALSADVALA, DVM, MS, Clinical Instructor, Department of Clinical
Sciences, College of Veterinary Medicine, Auburn University, Auburn, Alabama

JAMIE R. BELLAH, DVM, Diplomate, American College of Veterinary Surgeons;
Professor of Small Animal Surgery, Department of Clinical Sciences, College
of Veterinary Medicine, Auburn University, Auburn, Alabama

MARK W. BOHLING, DVM, Diplomate, American College of Veterinary Surgeons;
Assistant Professor of Surgery, Department of Small Animal Clinical Sciences,
College of Veterinary Medicine, University of Tennessee, Knoxville, Tennessee

HARRY W. BOOTHE, Jr, DVM, MS, Diplomate, American College of Veterinary
Surgeons; Professor of Surgery, Department of Clinical Sciences, College of
Veterinary Medicine, Auburn University, Auburn, Alabama

BONNIE GRAMBOW CAMPBELL, DVM, PhD, Diplomate, American College of
Veterinary Surgeons; Assistant Professor of Small Animal Soft Tissue Surgery,
Department of Veterinary Clinical Sciences, College of Veterinary Medicine,
Washington State University, Pullman, Washington

WILLIAM S. DERNELL, DVM, MS, Diplomate, American College of Veterinary
Surgeons; Associate Professor, Surgical Oncology, Animal Cancer Center,
Colorado State University, Fort Collins, Colorado

DAVID FOWLER, DVM, MVetSc, Diplomate, American College of Veterinary
Surgeons; Western Veterinary Specialist Centre, Calgary, Alberta, Canada

CHERYL S. HEDLUND, DVM, MS, Diplomate, American College of Veterinary Surgeons; Professor of Surgery, Veterinary Clinical Sciences, School of Veterinary Medicine, Louisiana State University, Baton Rouge, Louisiana

RALPH A. HENDERSON, DVM, MS, Professor of Surgery and Oncology, Department of Clinical Sciences, College of Veterinary Medicine, Auburn University, Auburn, Alabama

GISELLE HOSGOOD, BVSc, MS, PhD, Fellow, Australian College of Veterinary Scientists; Diplomate, American College of Veterinary Surgeons; Professor, Veterinary Surgery, Veterinary Clinical Sciences, School of Veterinary Medicine, Louisiana State University, Baton Rouge, Louisiana

D.J. KRAHWINKEL, DVM, MS, Diplomate, American College of Veterinary Surgeons; Diplomate, American College of Veterinary Anesthesiologists; Diplomate, American College of Veterinary Emergency and Critical Care; Professor of Surgery, Department of Small Animal Clinical Sciences, The University of Tennessee College of Veterinary Medicine, Knoxville, Tennessee

MICHAEL M. PAVLETIC, DVM, Diplomate, American College of Veterinary Surgeons; Director of Surgical Services, Angell Animal Medical Center, Boston, Massachusetts

ERIC R. POPE, DVM, MS, Diplomate, American College of Veterinary Surgeons; Associate Professor, College of Veterinary Medicine, University of Missouri, Columbia, Missouri

STEVEN F. SWAIM, DVM, MS, Professor Emeritus, Scott-Richey Research Center and Department of Clinical Sciences, College of Veterinary Medicine, Auburn University, Alabama

NICHOLAS J. TROUT, VetMB, Diplomate, American College of Veterinary Surgeons; Diplomate, European College of Veterinary Surgeons; Staff Surgeon, Angell Animal Medical Center, Boston, Massachusetts

RICHARD A.S. WHITE, BVetMed, PhD, DSAS, DVR, FRCVS, Diplomate, American College of Veterinary Surgeons; Diplomate, European College of Veterinary Surgeons; Dick White Referrals, The Six Mile Bottom Veterinary Specialist Centre, Six Mile Bottom, Newmarket, England

ELSEVIER
SAUNDERS

VETERINARY CLINICS
SMALL ANIMAL PRACTICE

Wound Management

CONTENTS
VOLUME 36 • NUMBER 4 • JULY 2006

Wound healing describes the host mechanisms involved in the process
of restoring the continuity of tissues after injury. Wound healing progresses through a continuum of overlapping stages characterized by
macroscopic, microscopic, and biochemical events. An understanding
of the relation between these events can enhance clinicians' skills in
wound management.

Regardless of the species involved, wound healing follows a predictable
course of overlapping phases. In spite of these commonalities, significant species differences in cutaneous wound healing have been uncovered in the Equidae and, more recently, between the dog and cat. It has
also recently been shown that the subcutaneous tissues play an important supporting role in cutaneous wound healing, which may help to explain healing differences between cats and dogs. These discoveries may
improve veterinarians' understanding of problem wound healing in the
cat and, hopefully, lead to better strategies for wound management in
this sometimes troublesome species.

Some wounds do not heal normally and present the practitioner with
a challenge. These can be thought of as hard-to-heal wounds. There
are numerous causes of such wounds, and when they occur, the veterinarian should consider all factors associated with the wound. When
diagnostic tests are indicated, they should be performed. Finally,
appropriate measures should be taken to correct the underlying cause
of the hard-to-heal wound.

be repaired using basic reconstructive surgery procedures. The excellent blood supply in this area and the availability of local tissues provide many options for repairing most wounds. This article describes the indications and techniques for reconstructing wounds in this area.

David Fowler

Distal limb reconstruction is complicated by the paucity of local tissues and the frequent association of orthopedic injury with cutaneous loss. Second-intention healing or skin stretching techniques are used for wounds involving less than a 30% circumference of the limb. Skin grafts are recommended for reconstruction of larger superficial wounds after establishing a bed of granulation tissue or for immediate reconstruction of clean wounds overlying healthy muscle. Wounds complicated by orthopedic injury benefit from early reconstruction using vascularized tissue. Weight-bearing surface reconstruction and management of partial amputation injuries are functionally difficult because of the environmental stress placed on the paw pads. Paw pad grafts, paw pad transposition techniques, centralization of digits, and microvascular free tissue transfer of paw pads can be considered for weight-bearing surface reconstruction. Definitive guidelines describing when each of these techniques should be used have not been established.

Cheryl S. Hedlund

Management of large trunk wounds begins with good wound management and bandaging. When a healthy wound bed exists and adequate tissue is present, the wound is closed. Fortunately, there is an abundance of loose trunk skin in most animals, and wound closure can be accomplished by simple reconstructive techniques, such as undermining and tension or "walking sutures." Nevertheless, some wounds and areas of the torso may require more advanced tension-relieving techniques, skin stretching, and tissue implants or flaps to achieve tension-free closure and successful wound healing. Use of these techniques allows wound closure and good cosmetic results for even those wounds that initially may seem foreboding.

Michael M. Pavletic and Nicholas J. Trout

Veterinarians are frequently presented with bullet, bite, or burn trauma patients. Injuries can vary from simple minor penetrating skin wounds to major life-threatening soft and hard tissue damage with concurrent complex metabolic ramifications. This article reviews the diagnostic and therapeutic options for each type of injury.

GOAL STATEMENT

The goal of the *Veterinary Clinics of North America: Small Animal Practice* is to keep practicing veterinarians up to date with current clinical practice in small animal medicine by providing timely articles reviewing the state of the art in small animal care.

ACCREDITATION

The *Veterinary Clinics of North America: Small Animal Practice* offers continuing education credits, awarded by Cummings School of Veterinary Medicine at Tufts University, Office of Continuing Education.

Cummings School of Veterinary Medicine at Tufts University is a designated provider of continuing veterinary medical education. Veterinarians participating in this learning activity may earn up to 6 credits per issue up to a maximum of 36 credits per year. Credits awarded may not apply toward license renewal in all states. It is the responsibility of each participant to verify the requirements of their state licensing board.

Credit can be earned by reading the text material, taking the examination online at *http://www.theclinics.com/home/cme*, and completing the program evaluation. Following your completion of the test and program evaluation, and review of any and all incorrect answers, you may print your certificate.

TO ENROLL

To enroll in the *Veterinary Clinics of North America: Small Animal Practice* Continuing Veterinary Medical Education Program, call customer service at 1-800-654-2452 or sign up online at *http://www.theclinics.com/home/cme*. The CVME program is now available at a special introductory rate of $99.95 for a year's subscription.

VETERINARY CLINICS
SMALL ANIMAL PRACTICE

FORTHCOMING ISSUES

September 2006

Pharmacology and Therapeutics
Dawn M. Boothe, DVM, PhD
Guest Editor

November 2006

Dietary Management and Nutrition
Claudia A. Kirk, DVM, PhD
and Joseph W. Bartges, DVM, PhD
Guest Editors

January 2007

Effective Communication in Veterinary Practice
Karen Cornell, DVM, PhD
Jennifer Brandt, PhD, MSW
Kathleen A. Bonvicini, MPH
Guest Editors

RECENT ISSUES

May 2006

Pediatrics
Autumn P. Davidson, DVM, MS
Guest Editor

March 2006

Practice Management
David E. Lee, DVM, MBA
Guest Editor

January 2006

Updates in Dermatology
Karen L. Campbell, DVM, MS
Guest Editor

THE CLINICS ARE NOW AVAILABLE ONLINE!

Access your subscription at:
http://www.theclinics.com

Vet Clin Small Anim 36 (2006) xi–xiii

VETERINARY CLINICS
SMALL ANIMAL PRACTICE

PREFACE

Wound Management

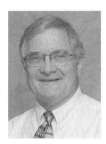 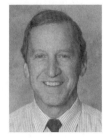

Steven F. Swaim, DVM, MS
D.J. Krahwinkel, DVM, MS

Guest Editors

HISTORY

The management of wounds has been a topic of interest over the ages. As part of wound management, man has an instinct to pour things into wounds. It has been stated, "...wounds are still lathered, bathed, and sprayed with notions, potions, and lotions." [1] As a reflection of this, a compilation of some of the things that have been described over the ages for placement in wounds and their proposed mechanism of action was published [2]. The materials ranged from those that are accepted by the medical community (eg, silver sulfadiazine, Dakin's solution) at one end of the spectrum to the more bizarre materials at the other end of the spectrum, (eg, dung and beer for their ammonia and alcohol content, respectively).

As early as 3000 BC, the Egyptians were using grease, resin, honey, lint, and meat as topical dressings. In 200 AD, Galen tended gladiators using the "laudable pus" theory, whereby uninfected wounds were inoculated with a dressing to induce infections. The practice persisted for more than a thousand years [3].

In the sixteenth century, wounds were scalded with boiling oil. However, in the battle of Turin, there was no oil; thus, Ambrose Paré, a French army barber-surgeon, used a potion of eggs, turpentine, and oil of roses as a vulnerary in wound therapy. With this treatment, fewer soldiers died, their wounds healed faster, and they experienced less pain. He coined the term, "I dressed the wound, and God healed him" [3].

The concept of moist wound healing began to be accepted in the 1970s and 1980s. It is only in the last 10 to 20 years that there has been a virtual explosion

0195-5616/06/$ – see front matter
doi:10.1016/j.cvsm.2006.05.004

in wound care knowledge, technology, and products. The discovery of growth factors essential for wound healing and the crucial concept of moist wound healing are just two examples of the recent advances in wound care. With the current knowledge of antimicrobial medications, the practice of wound debridement, the application of growth factor technology, the concept of moist wound healing, and the preservation of wound perfusion and oxygenation, modern wound care continues to be advanced.

Simultaneous with the improvement in topical wound care, veterinary surgeons have developed advanced skills in surgical wound closure with the use of skin flaps and skin grafts. These skills, along with the development of microvascular surgical techniques for skin grafting, have truly brought veterinary wound care into the 21st century.

VETERINARY WOUND MANAGEMENT SOCIETY

We would like to inform the reader about the recently founded Veterinary Wound Management Society (VWMS). The VWMS was established as an interest organization for veterinarians, veterinary students, interns, residents, and technicians, as well as personnel involved in the veterinary wound care industry. The mission of the VWMS is to advance the art and science of animal wound management, thus promoting excellence in the field.

Activities of the VWMS include encouragement of research and scientific progress relating to the prevention, diagnosis, and therapy of animal wounds, to include comparative medicine studies. The society also promotes education by the communication and dissemination of knowledge related to wound management. The VWMS strives to provide service to the public using current wound management medications, materials, and techniques.

Those interested in joining the VWMS can visit the VWMS Web site, www.vwms.org, to learn more about the society and apply for membership online.

Steven F. Swaim, DVM, MS
Scott-Ritchey Research Center and
Department of Clinical Sciences
College of Veterinary Medicine
Wire Road
Auburn University, AL 36849, USA

E-mail address: swaimsf@auburn.edu

D.J. Krahwinkel, DVM, MS
Department of Small Animal Clinical Sciences
C247 Veterinary Teaching Hospital
University of Tennessee
Knoxville, TN 37996-4544, USA

E-mail address: djk@utk.edu

References

[1] Miller SH. Chronic problem wounds (review). Plast Reconst Surg 1983;67:131.
[2] Rudolph R. Wound treatments, nostrums, and hokums. In: Rudolph R, Noe JM, editors. Chronic problem wounds. Boston: Little Brown and Co.; 1983. p. 47–51.
[3] Lee BY, DaSilba CE. Historical aspects of wound healing. In: Lee BY, editor. The wound management manual. New York: McGraw-Hill; 2005. p. 72–9.

Vet Clin Small Anim 36 (2006) 667–685

VETERINARY CLINICS
SMALL ANIMAL PRACTICE

Stages of Wound Healing and Their Clinical Relevance

Giselle Hosgood, BVSc, MS, PhD

Department of Veterinary Clinical Sciences, School of Veterinary Medicine,
Louisiana State University, South Stadium Drive, Baton Rouge, LA 70803, USA

STAGES OF WOUND HEALING

The stages of wound healing based on microscopic characteristics are well described [1–7]. It is important to understand that these microscopic events are initiated, mediated, and sustained by biochemical mediators known as cytokines and growth factors (Table 1) [5]. The biochemical events of wound healing are complex. The platelet initiates wound healing through the release of cytokines and certain essential growth factors. The events of healing are then amplified, sustained, and modified by wound macrophages, endothelial cells, and fibroblasts. The wound matrix that is formed also sustains and modifies wound healing.

Immediate Wound Reaction and Initiation of Wound Healing

Blood and lymph from damaged blood vessels and lymphatics fill the wound and cleanse the wound surface [1–7]. Almost immediately, vasoactive compounds, including catecholamines, serotonin, bradykinin, and histamine, mediate vasoconstriction of damaged blood vessels to minimize blood loss. Vasoconstriction lasts only 5 to 10 minutes. The blood vessels then vasodilate, and intravascular cells and fluid pass through the vessel walls into the extravascular space. The activated platelet, in combination with the blood and fluid, forms a blood clot in the wound defect (Fig. 1).

The blood clot incorporates trapped blood proteins and other molecules that facilitate cellular entry into the wound site. Fibronectin dimers within the clot, in the presence of activated factor XIII, become covalently cross-linked to fibrin and to themselves, forming a provisional extracellular matrix (ECM). This provisional ECM has many binding sites for adhesive molecules on the surface of migrating neutrophils, macrophages, and connective tissue cells. Thus, the clot provides a hemostatic plug and an immediate barrier to infection and fluid loss as well as a substrate for early organization of the wound. The clot stabilizes the wound edges and fibrin within the clot and provides minimal wound strength.

E-mail address: ghosgood@vetmed.lsu.edu

0195-5616/06/$ – see front matter
doi:10.1016/j.cvsm.2006.02.006

Table 1
Mediators of wound healing

Mediator	Source	Functions
Colony-stimulating factors (CSFs) [39]	Multiple cells	Induce differentiation and proliferation of granulocytes, modulate monocytes and macrophage function
Connective tissue growth factor (CTGF) [40]	Endothelial cells, and fibroblasts	Chemotactic and mitogenic for various connective tissue cells
Epidermal growth factor (EGF) [41]	Platelets, macrophages, saliva, urine, milk, and plasma	Mitogenic for epithelial cells and fibroblasts Stimulates epithelial cell migration and granulation tissue formation
Fibroblast growth factor (FGF) [42]	Macrophages, mast cells, T lymphocytes, endothelial cells, fibroblasts, and many tissues	Chemotactic for fibroblasts Mitogenic for fibroblasts and epithelial cells Stimulates epithelial cell migration, angiogenesis, wound contraction, and matrix deposition
Insulin-like growth factor-1 (IGF-1) [41]	Macrophages, fibroblasts, liver, and other tissue	Stimulates synthesis of sulfated proteoglycans, collagen, epithelial cell migration and fibroblast proliferation Has endocrine effects similar to growth hormone
Interferons (e.g., IFNα)	Lymphocytes and fibroblasts	Activate macrophages Inhibit fibroblast proliferation and synthesis of MMPs Regulate other cytokines
Interleukins (IL-1,4,6, and 8)	Macrophages, mast cells, epithelial cells, lymphocytes, and many tissues	Chemotactic for leukocytes (IL-1) and fibroblasts (IL-4) Stimulate MMP-1 synthesis (IL-1), angiogenesis (IL-1 and 8), and TIMP synthesis (IL-6) Regulate other cytokines
Keratinocyte growth factor (KGF, also called FGF-7)	Fibroblasts	Stimulates epithelial cell migration, proliferation, and differentiation
Matrix metalloproteinases (MMPs) [34,43]	Multiple families, including collagenases, gelatinases, and stromelysins; numerous cell sources within the ECM, including macrophages, epithelial cells, endothelial cells, and fibroblasts	Activate other MMPs, and degrade cell basement membranes, collagen, and other proteins Important in cell migration and collagen remodeling

Nerve growth factor (NGF)	Neural and glial cells	Neurotrophic factor that modulates neuronal cell survival by positive and negative regulation; may alter VEGF expression [44]
Platelet-derived growth factor (including isoforms PDGF-AA, AB, and BB) [45]	Platelets, macrophages, endothelial cells, epithelial cells, and smooth muscle cells	Chemotactic for leukocytes, macrophages, fibroblasts, and smooth muscle cells Activates leukocytes, macrophages, and fibroblasts Mitogenic for fibroblasts, endothelial cell, and smooth muscle cells Stimulates production of MMPs, fibronectin, and hyaluronic acid Stimulates angiogenesis and wound contraction and remodeling Inhibits platelet aggregation
Tissue inhibitor's of matrix metalloproteinases (TIMP-1,2,3, and 4) [46,47]	Fibroblasts, macrophages, and endothelial cells	Regulates integrin expression Inhibit MMPs; important for balance between collagen deposition and removal in ECM remodeling; involved in vascular smooth muscle migration and apoptosis
Transforming growth factor-α (TGFα) [41]	T lymphocytes, macrophages, epithelial cells, and many tissues	Similar to EGF
Transforming growth factor-β (including isoforms TGF-β1, -β2, and -β3) [48]	Platelets, T lymphocytes, macrophages, endothelial cells, epithelial cells, smooth muscle cells, and fibroblasts	Chemotactic for leukocytes, macrophages, lymphocytes, fibroblasts, and smooth muscle cells Stimulates TIMP synthesis, epithelial cell migration, angiogenesis, and fibroplasia Inhibits production of MMPs and epithelial cell proliferation Regulates integrin expression and other cytokines Induces TGFβ production
Tumor necrosis factor (TNF)	Macrophages, mast cells, and T lymphocytes	Activates macrophages Mitogenic for fibroblasts Stimulates angiogenesis Regulates other cytokines
Vascular endothelial cell growth factor (VEGF) [49]	Epithelial cells	Increases vascular permeability Mitogenic for endothelial cells

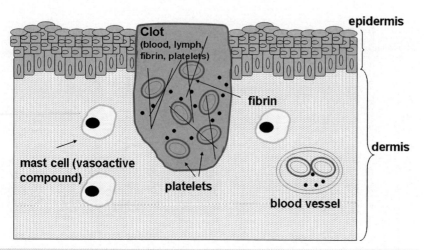

Fig. 1. Blood and lymph from damaged vessels and lymphatics fill the wound immediately after injury. Vasoactive compounds released from local tissue mast cells cause the vessels to vasoconstrict immediately. The platelet, in combination with the blood, fluid, and fibrin, causes a blood clot to form in the wound defect.

The blood clot dries and forms a scab that protects the wound, prevents further hemorrhage, and allows the healing process to continue underneath. The scab does not provide any wound strength and eventually sloughs, along with dead inflammatory cells and dead bacteria, as wound healing progresses underneath it.

Inflammation and Debridement

The inflammation that occurs is characterized by migration of leukocytes into the wound, which happens within 6 hours of injury (Fig. 2) [1–7]. Mediators in the provisional ECM promote the margination, adhesion, and extravasation of neutrophils to the wound. The conversion of fibrinogen into fibrin releases fibrinopeptides, which are potent chemoattractants for neutrophils. Proteinases released by neutrophils as they degrade necrotic tissue attract more neutrophils. The neutrophil phagocytizes bacteria and extracellular debris, removing them from the wound. In addition, release of toxic oxygen species from the neutrophil kills bacteria and degrades bacterial macromolecules, denatured ECM, and damaged cells. Note that neutrophils may be present in a sterile wound also. The neutrophil is, however, not essential for wound healing. The combination of wound fluid, degrading neutrophils, and denatured tissue constitutes the wound exudate commonly referred to as pus. The presence of wound exudate gives the wound a mistakenly unhealthy appearance but is, in fact, vital to the healing process.

Monocytes migrate into the wound with neutrophils in the same proportion as peripheral blood. Neutrophils predominate in early inflammation; however, because neutrophils are short-lived, monocytes predominate in older wounds.

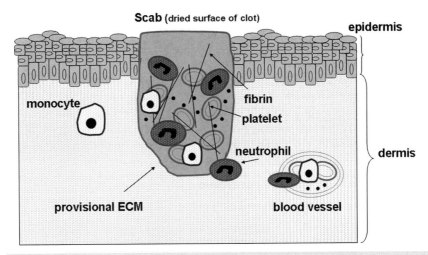

Fig. 2. Inflammation is characterized by migration of leukocytes into the wound soon after injury. Tissue damage releases mediators that are potent chemoattractants for neutrophils. Monocytes also migrate into the wound. The dried surface of the blood clot may form a scab.

Cytokines released from activated neutrophils and the degradation products from the provisional ECM and inflammatory proteins attract circulating monocytes into the wound. Monocytes are essential to wound healing and become wound macrophages. They are important sources of growth factors. Monocytes may coalesce and form multinucleated giant cells, which also have phagocytic functions. Monocytes may also evolve into epithelial cells and histiocytes. Once acute inflammation subsides, local vascular permeability is restored and blood cells cease to pass into the extravascular space. If foreign material or bacteria remain in the wound, the monocytes undergo proliferation. Proliferation of monocytes is characteristic of chronic inflammation.

The macrophage produces many mediators that modulate wound healing, including fibroblast growth factor (FGF), epidermal growth factor (EGF), platelet-derived growth factor (PDGF), transforming growth factor (TGF)-α and -β, tumor necrosis factor (TNF), interleukins, and the matrix metalloproteinases (MMPs) and their tissue inhibitors (TIMPs). Macrophages present early in healing are important in debridement of the wound through their phagocytic activity. Macrophages present later in the wound, along with neutrophils, are important in modification of the provisional ECM. The provisional ECM that fills the wound, consisting of fibrin, fibronectin, and other products released by platelets and inflammatory cells, is modulated to become granulation tissue.

Repair

Several proliferative processes occur during the repair stage, including angiogenesis, fibroplasia, and epithelialization [1–7]. Wound contraction also occurs during this stage. The transition from the inflammatory to repair stage is marked by the invasion of fibroblasts and an increased accumulation of collagen in the wound. In addition, there is migration and formation of new endothelial structures within the wound. The combination of new capillaries, fibroblasts, and fibrous connective tissue forms the characteristic red fleshy granulation tissue that fills the wound beneath the scab or under the bandage. Granulation tissue protects the wound, provides a barrier to infection, and provides a surface for epithelialization. Granulation tissue also contains special wound fibroblasts called myofibroblasts that are important in wound contraction.

The transition from provisional ECM to granulation tissue is active by 3 to 5 days after injury; hence, the first 3 to 5 days are sometimes referred to as the lag phase of healing. This reflects a lag in gain in wound strength and not a lag in wound healing. It is clear that wound elements are considerably active during these early days.

Angiogenesis
Angiogenesis is the growth of new capillaries from preexisting vessels at the wound edges into areas previously unoccupied by vascular tissue. Angiogenesis is a complex event, relying on interaction of the ECM with mediators that stimulate the migration and proliferation of endothelial cells (Fig. 3) [8]. The earliest phase of angiogenesis involves cell migration rather than cell division; intact or recently broken capillary blood vessels are stimulated by angiogenic factors to allow migration of columns of capillary endothelial cells toward

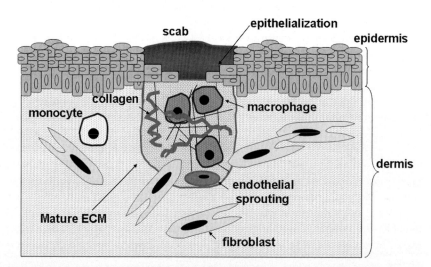

Fig. 3. During repair, angiogenesis (endothelial sprouting) and fibroplasia (fibroblasts and collagen) contribute to formation of the mature ECM. Epithelialization also occurs. The macrophage, derived from the wound monocyte, is integral to the process.

the site of injury. While capillary cell invasion into the wound is occurring, endothelial proliferation also begins. The most likely stimuli for angiogenesis are mitogenic and chemotactic factors for the endothelial cells produced by the macrophage, including FGF, vascular endothelial growth factor (VEGF), TGFβ, angiogenin, angiotropin, angiopectin 1, and thrombospondin [8–10]. Low oxygen tension and increased lactic acid may also be stimuli for angiogenesis through their effects on mediator production [11].

Early granulation tissue has a rich capillary bed with a characteristic deep red color. As wound healing progresses, the new blood vessels disintegrate because of apoptosis and the wound color becomes paler. Many ECM molecules regulate this cell death, including thrombospondin 1 and 2 and antiangiogenic factors, such as angiostatin, endostatin, and angiopoietin 2 [12–14].

Fibroplasia

One or more populations of mesenchymal cells also move into the wound with the endothelial cells. Mediators produced by macrophages, including PDGF, TFGβ, and FGF, in concert with ECM molecules, stimulate fibroblasts in the surrounding tissue to proliferate, express appropriate integrin receptors, and migrate into the wound [15,16]. Integrin receptors are a family of protein molecule pairs that are embedded in the cell surface and link specific molecules in the ECM to intracellular structures and signal pathways. Integrin receptors are essential for cell migration in the wound (Fig. 4) [17].

The wound fibroblast is unique and differs from the normal fibroblast of healthy mesenchymal tissue [18]. The pericyte, a microvascular accessory cell that corresponds to the vascular smooth muscle cell of larger vessels,

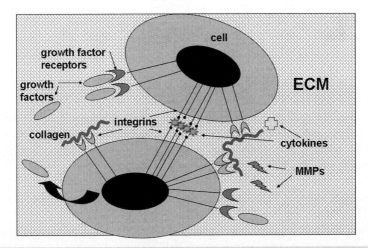

Fig. 4. Integrins facilitate interaction between cells and the ECM that is mediated by growth factors, cytokines, and MMPs. Cell-to-ECM and cell-to-cell interactions are important in ECM maturation and remodeling.

may be a source of these cells. The wound fibroblasts have a characteristic my-ofibroblastic appearance, with phenotypic features of abundant contractile fila-ments, intercellular tight junctions, and a distorted nuclear envelope. The wound fibroblasts contain varying amounts of actin, a smooth muscle protein, as well as intermediate filament proteins, desmin, and vimentin [18].

Fibrin, fibronectin, and hyaluronan within the provisional ECM provide a conduit for cell migration. The appearance of fibronectin and the appropriate integrin receptors that bind the fibroblasts is the rate-limiting step in the forma-tion of granulation tissue [16,19]. Fibroblast movement into the tightly woven provisional ECM requires active proteolytic enzymes, including plasminogen activator, collagenases, gelatinase A, and stromelysin, which cleave a path for cell migration [20,21].

The wound fibroblasts synthesize the true ECM of the wound. The provi-sional ECM is gradually replaced by a collagenous ECM. Type III collagen, which is relatively abundant in blood vessels and associated with the capillary content of the granulation tissue, is replaced by type I collagen produced by the wound fibroblast. There is a marked increase in the ratio of type I to type III collagen as the wound matures. The wound fibroblast also secretes proteogly-cans and ECM glycoproteins that fill the ECM.

The elaboration, orientation, and contraction of the ECM components by the wound fibroblast organize the fibrin-filled wound into a durable connective tissue. The greatest rate of accumulation of connective tissue occurs at the wound site between 7 and 14 days after injury, after which the collagen content stabilizes. The wound fibroblasts then stop producing collagen, and there is re-gression of the capillary content of the granulation tissue. The once fibroblast-rich granulation tissue becomes a relatively acellular scar as cells in the wound undergo apoptosis [22].

Epithelialization

The predominant early activity in epithelialization is one of mobilization and migration of epithelial cells at the margin of the wound, followed by prolifera-tion of epithelial cells behind these leading cells [23]. In partial-thickness skin wounds, epidermal migration over the wound surface begins almost immedi-ately from the wound margins and adnexal appendages, such as hair follicles and sweat glands. In full-thickness skin wounds, the wound can only be resur-faced from the wound margins after adequate granulation tissue has formed. Generally, new epithelium is not visible at the wound edges until 4 to 5 days after injury. In an incised wound that is sutured with the skin edges apposed, epithelialization may be complete as early as 24 to 48 hours after injury.

Soon after injury, the epidermal cells at the margin of the wound undergo phenotypic alteration, which includes retraction of intracellular monofilaments [24], dissolution of most desmosomes that provide physical connections be-tween the cells, and formation of peripheral cytoplasmic actin filaments that al-low cell movement [25,26]. Lateral movement of the epidermal cells is facilitated by the lack of adherence between epidermal and dermal cells to one another because of the dissolution of hemidesmosomal links between the epidermis and the basement membrane induced by collagenases and MMPs produced by the epidermal cells [20,27]. Integrin receptors on the epidermal cells allow them to interact with a variety of ECM proteins, including fibronectin and vitronectin, which are interspersed in the type I collagen at the margin of the wound and in the provisional ECM in the wound space [28]. The path of migration of the epidermal cells is determined by integrins expressed on the membranes of migrating epidermal cells. In the presence of a scab, the epidermal cells move onto the wound under the scab and separate it from the wound surface.

Epidermal cells behind the migrating cells begin to proliferate 1 to 2 days after injury. There are multiple stimuli for the migration and proliferation of epidermal cells, including EGF, TGFα, and keratinocyte growth factor (KGF) produced by epithelial cells, wound fibroblasts, and wound macrophages. As re-epithelialization occurs, there is progressive accumulation of new basement membrane material (laminin) under the migrating cells, starting at the margin of the wound and continuing inward. The epidermal cells revert to their normal phenotype and become firmly attached to the basement membrane and the underlying dermis. Over time, the epidermal layer stratifies. In large open wounds, this may take weeks to months. Re-epithelialization may not be complete, leaving exposed granulation tissue in the center of the wound. The epidermis toward the center of the wound may be thin and easily traumatized. In full-thickness wounds, adnexal structures do not regenerate. Pigmentation of the epidermis is variable and inconsistent across subjects. In general, melanocytes in the skin adjacent to the wound undergo mitosis and migrate into the regenerating epidermis [29]. Integrin receptors on the melanocytes seem to be important in modulating the migration of melanocytes along the basement membrane of the newly formed epithelium and in the intercellular recognition of epithelial cells [30]. Repigmentation is noted progressively from the periphery of the wound to the center, and there is a lag of 1 to 2 weeks before pigmentation is noted [31]. Maximal melanocyte proliferation may not be seen for several months [32].

Contraction

Contraction refers to the reduction in the wound size that corresponds to changes in the tension of the wound and surrounding tissue. Visible wound contraction is evident by 5 to 9 days after injury. Significant fibroblastic invasion into the wound is necessary for contraction to begin. Wound contraction involves a complex interaction of cells, ECM, and mediators, including TGF-β1, TGF-β2, and PDGF [33]. During the second week of healing, the appearance of wound fibroblasts with a myofibroblast phenotype corresponds to contraction of the wound. As healing progresses, the number of wound fibroblasts with myofibroblastic phenotypes decreases in the wound, corresponding to a decrease in wound contraction. Collagen in the granulation tissue does not have contractile properties.

During wound contraction, the surrounding skin stretches (intussusceptive growth) and the wound takes on a stellate appearance. Wound contraction continues until the wound edges meet and negative feedback from touching cells halts the process. Contraction also ceases if the tension of the surrounding skin equals or exceeds the force of contraction. If contraction ceases and the wound has remaining exposed granulation tissue, epithelialization may continue to occur and cover the wound. In some wounds, low myofibroblast content in the granulation tissue may result in failure of a wound to contract despite laxity in the surrounding skin.

Maturation

The transition from ECM to scar requires remodeling of the connective tissue content of the wound. The random and haphazard appearance of the cellular and collagen fiber content of the granulation tissue is altered (Fig. 5) [1–7]. The cellularity of the granulation tissue is reduced as cells die. The collagen fiber bundles become thicker, show increased cross-linking, and take on a specific orientation along the lines of tension. The reorganization of the connective tissue and rearrangement of collagen bundles may take months or even years to occur. The increase in mechanical strength is extremely slow.

Remodeling is also characterized by a reduction in the collagen content of the ECM [33]. Collagen already deposited within the ECM provides negative feedback, first reducing the rate of collagen deposition and then decreasing the overall collagen content. Collagen is degraded by proteolytic enzymes (MMPs) secreted by macrophages, epithelial cells, endothelial cells, and fibroblasts

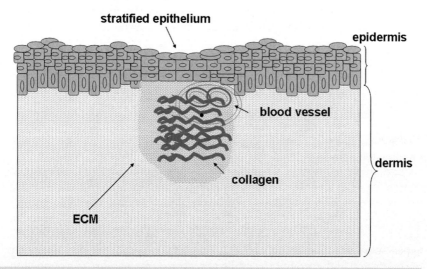

Fig. 5. Maturation and remodeling of the ECM results in a reduction in the cellular, collagen, and vascular content of the ECM, with reorientation and cross-linking of the collagen to increase wound strength. The epidermis thickens as the epithelium stratifies.

within the ECM [34]. Remodeling is a balance between MMP and TIMP expression, in which the ECM has a key role [35].

Although there is no dramatic gain in wound strength in the first 3 to 5 days after injury, some strength is provided by the fibrin in the blood clot (Fig. 6) [36]. In addition, early ingrowth of capillaries and any epithelialization across an apposed wound provide some strength. There is no evidence that the other elements of the provisional ECM contribute to wound strength at this time. The most rapid gain in wound strength occurs between 7 and 14 days after injury, corresponding to the rapid accumulation of collagen in the wound. Wounds gain only approximately 20% of their final strength in the first 3 weeks after injury. Thereafter, the gain in wound strength is slow, reflecting a relatively slower rate of collagen accumulation and the process of remodeling. Wounds never attain the same tensile strength of normal tissue; at maximum strength, a scar is only 70% to 80% as strong as normal tissue [37].

CLINICAL RELEVANCE
Recognition of Wound Stages
Recognition of the stages of wound healing based on macroscopic features allows the clinician to make an association between the microscopic and biochemical events [38]. Knowledge of these events directs appropriate management of the wound.

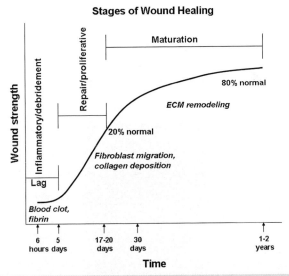

Fig. 6. Changes in wound strength during wound healing. Axes are not drawn to scale. (*Modified from* Hosgood G, Basset DJ. Wound healing, wound management and bandaging. In: McCurnin DM, Basset JM, editors. Clinical textbook for veterinary technicians. 6th edition. Philadelphia: WB Saunders; 2005. p. 136.)

Inflammatory and debridement phase

The macroscopic features of the inflammatory and debridement stage for an open wound include a fresh blood clot, serosanguineous to purulent exudates, denuded surface without granulation tissue, and no visible contraction (Fig. 7). An apposed wound may begin to epithelialize during this stage.

Repair phase

The overwhelming macroscopic feature of this stage is the presence of granulation tissue (Fig. 8). This can vary from red, fleshy, and finely granular to pale pink to white and nodular depending on the vascular and collagen content. A wound must be 3 to 5 days old to show visible granulation tissue. Tissue with low vascularity, such as intact periosteum, fascia, tendon, and nerve sheaths, produces granulation tissue more slowly; thus, aging a wound based on this criterion alone may be misleading. The wound should show visible contraction at 5 to 9 days; however, the degree varies depending on the location of the wound and the laxity of neighboring skin. New epithelium should be present at the wound edges but can only cover a smooth granulating surface.

Maturation phase

The mature wound has an intact epithelial surface that is initially bright pink because of the vascularity of the underlying granulation tissue (Fig. 9). As wound maturation progresses, the epithelial surface becomes paler as the vascularity of the underlying granulation tissue is reduced during the remodeling of the ECM. The epithelium becomes thicker as it stratifies. Wound contraction may continue as the underlying ECM matures. There is less epithelium on a wound with considerable contraction.

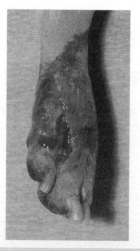

Fig. 7. A fresh wound entering the inflammatory and debridement phase. There are fresh blood clots on the wound surface.

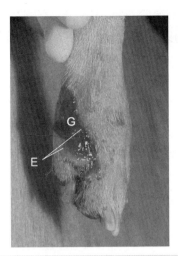

Fig. 8. The wound from Fig. 7 is shown in the repair phase. Note the granulation tissue (G) and epithelialization (E) at the wound edges.

Enhancing Wound Healing

Inflammation and debridement phase

The goal of managing a wound in the inflammatory stage is to reduce wound contamination to favor host defenses and prevent development of wound infection. This necessitates appropriate cleansing and debridement of the wound, protection of the wound from further contamination, and possible application

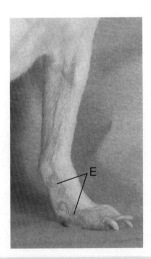

Fig. 9. A different wound in the maturation phase. There is complete epithelialization (E) of the wound surface.

Table 2
Indications for wound dressings and topical agents

Description	Stage of wound healing	Indication and purpose	Products
Wound dressings			
Adherent	Inflammatory	Occasionally used but being replaced by other dressings (see below)	Dry gauze (dry-to-dry) Wet gauze (wet-to-dry)
Hypertonic Saline dressings	Inflammatory	Hypertonic is bactericidal and facilitates natural debridement by drawing fluid and debris from wound	Hypertonic Saline–impregnated gauze dressing
Antimicrobial dressings	Inflammatory	Reduces bacterial colonization; hence, most useful in early wound management; may facilitate management of infected wound in any stage	Gauze impregnated with 0.2% poly-hexamethylene bioguanide (chlorhexidine-related antiseptic); slow-release silver dressings
Hydrophilic dressings	Inflammatory, repair	Wounds with moderate or copious exudates; absorb exudates and keep wound surface moist, enhance natural debridement, and promotes granulation tissue formation	Copolymer starches (maltodexrin), calium alginate
Foam dressing	Inflammatory, repair	Minimal to copious exudates; absorbs exudates and keeps wound moist, promotes granulation tissue formation, and can deliver fluid or medication	Polyurethane foam
Hydrogels	Inflammatory, repair	Wounds with minimal to no exudate, especially partial-thickness wounds (abrasions); keep wound surface moist, promote epithelialization, and rehydrate dry wounds	Hydrogel dressings, amorphous gels, hydrocolloids
Nonadherent, semiocclusive	Maturation	Wound with intact surface; non-adherent layer protects fragile epidermis; not indicated for open wound because it is nonhydrophilic and drying	Petrolatum-impregnated gauze dressings, rayon or Teflon pads

Table 2
(continued)

Description	Stage of wound healing	Indication and purpose	Products
Biologic dressings	Repair	Provide an exogenous source of collagen I, II, and IV, as well as fibronectin, hyaluronic acid, chondroitin sulfate, heparin, heparan, and growth factors; can act as a scaffold for fibroplasia and becomes incorporated into ECM of wound; stem cell attractant with cells differentiating to wounded tissue type	Bovine collagen sheets; porcine small intestinal submucosa sheets, porcine urinary bladder extracellular matrix
Topical agents			
Honey, sugar	Inflammatory, early repair	Antibacterial because of hydrogen peroxide, hypertonicity, low pH, and inhibin content; enhance natural debridement by keeping exudate at surface; reduce edema/inflammation; enhance granulation tissue/epithelialization	Commercial granular sugar, nonpasteurized honey. Medihoney; Medihoney Pty Ltd, Richlands, Australia; raw sterilized Manuka honey (Summerglow Apiaries Ltd, Hamilton, New Zealand)
Copper tripeptide (GHK-Cu)	Repair	Attracts macrophages, mast cells, and monocytes, which release multiple growth factors	Commercial hydrogel
Acetylated mannan	Early inflammatory	Aloe vera extract purported to enhance macrophage production of mediators that stimulate granulation tissue formation and epithelialization	Delivered in a hydrogel or freeze-dried gel
Phenytoin	Inflammatory, early repair	May enhance gene expression of PDGF in macrophages and monocytes, and hence stimulate fibroplasia and angiogenesis; antibacterial; minimal systemic absorption	Topical powder
Topical antimicrobials	Inflammatory	Reduce surface microbial burden	Triple-antibiotic ointment, silver sulfadiazine

(continued on next page)

Table 2
(continued)

Description	Stage of wound healing	Indication and purpose	Products
Topical antiseptics	Inflammatory	Reduce surface microbial burden	Chlorhexidine (0.05%), povidone-iodine (0.019–0.1%)
Growth factors	Content dependent	Content dependent; should be used when target cells or mediators are active; assumption that wound is deficient in or contains excessive target cell or mediator	Equine recombinant growth hormone daily injection; effects equivocal
Topical modulators	Indicated stage dependent on modulator	Content dependent; should be used when target cells or mediators are active; results equivocal; assumption that wound is deficient in or contains excessive target cell or mediator; platelet-rich gel accelerates epithelialization and promotes organization of collagen matrix in horses [50]	Platelet-rich preparations, blood dialysates, and serotonin inhibitors
Enzymatic agents	Inflammatory and debridement, early repair	Enzymatic debridementl; adjunct to surgical debridement or superficial debridement of wound; liquefy coagulum for easier absorption; stimulate granulation tissue	Trypsin-containing preparations
Maggots	Inflammatory and debridement, early repair	Secrete digestive enzymes to dissolve necrotic tissue and promote granulation tissue formation; may be useful when surgical debridement is prohibitive	Medicinal maggots (Monarch Labs, LLP, Irvine, California)

See articles by Krahwinkel and Booth and Campbell elsewhere in this issue.
Abbreviations: ECM, extra cellular matrix; PDGF, plateled derived growth factor.

of topical antimicrobial substances to reduce the bacterial load. Systemic antibiotics are indicated in an infected or heavily traumatized wound. Infection requires bacterial proliferation in the tissue and takes time to develop. Infection delays the wound healing process, however, and it may be difficult to determine the age of an infected wound based on physical appearance. Enhancing natural wound debridement (autolytic debridement) and promoting wound healing by keeping mediator-rich wound exudate at the wound surface are important and are achieved through the application of appropriate wound dressings (Table 2).

Repair phase

The goals of managing a wound in the repair stage are multifocal. The wound must continue to be protected from contamination, because infection inhibits all stages of wound healing. The deposition of vascular granulation tissue and epithelialization are facilitated through the topical application of stimulants and appropriate wound dressings that maintain a moist wound surface (see Table 2; see articles by Krahwinkel and Booth and Campbell elsewhere in this issue). Wound contraction is facilitated by promoting a healthy ECM and can be enhanced by using skin-stretching devices (see article by Hedlund elsewhere in this issue). In locations of excessive motion, which stimulates wound contraction (eg, over flexion surfaces, where contraction can result in contracture), wound contraction can be inhibited through immobilization of the wound or by some form of wound closure. In other areas of excessive motion (eg, over extensor surfaces), flexion can pull wounds apart. Thus, immobilization is indicated.

The presence of wound infection is best confirmed through microbial culture of a piece of tissue from within the wound and is especially important in strategizing treatment for nonhealing wounds (see article by Amalsadvala elsewhere in this issue). Surface contaminants do not reflect wound infection. If wound infection is present, systemic antimicrobial treatment based on antimicrobial sensitivity testing results is indicated. A wound with a healthy granulation tissue bed is unlikely to be infected. The granulation tissue acts as a barrier to surface contaminants invading the deeper tissue in the wound. Topical antimicrobial therapy is not necessary in the presence of a healthy granulation tissue bed and may be detrimental to wound healing, depending on the formulation.

Maturation phase

The goal of managing a maturing wound is to continue to protect the fragile epidermis until it is able to withstand abrasion associated with normal activity (see Table 2).

Decision making in wound management must be based on the integration of knowledge of wound healing with an understanding of the role a clinician can play in facilitating the process. The clinician does not cause wound healing but simply facilitates and modulates the natural process. Other articles in this issue describe techniques and strategies for wound management, the success of which is contingent on implementation in the right wound at the right time.

References

[1] Birch M, Tomlinson A, Ferguson MW. Animal models for adult dermal wound healing. Methods Mol Med 2005;117:223–35.
[2] Cohen IK, Diegelmann RF, Lindblad WJ, editors. Wound healing: biochemical and clinical aspects. 1st edition. Philadelphia: WB Saunders; 1992.
[3] Cohen K, Mast BA. Models of wound healing. J Trauma 1990;30(Suppl):S149–55.

[4] Hackam DJ, Ford HR. Cellular, biochemical, and clinical aspects of wound healing. Surg Infect (Larchmt) 2002;3(Suppl 1):S23–35.

[5] Singer AJ, Clark RAF. Cutaneous wound healing. N Engl J Med 1999;341:738–46.

[6] Yamaguchi Y, Yoshikawa K. Cutaneous wound healing: an update. J Dermatol 2001;28: 521–34.

[7] Yang GP, Lim IJ, Phan TT, et al. From scarless fetal wounds to keloids: molecular studies in wound healing. Wound Repair Regen 2003;11:411–8.

[8] Li J, Zhang Y-P, Kirsner RS. Angiogenesis in wound repair: angiogenic growth factors and the extracellular matrix. Microsc Res Tech 2003;60:107–14.

[9] Liekens S, De Clerq E, Neyts J. Angiogenesis: regulators and clinical applications. Biochem Pharmacol 2001;61:253–70.

[10] Iruela-Arispe ML, Dvorak HF. Angiogenesis: a dynamic balance of stimulators and inhibitors. Thromb Haemost 1997;78:672–7.

[11] Detmar M, Brown LF, Berse B. Hypoxia regulates the expression of vascular permeability factor/vascular endothelial growth factor (VPF/VEGF) and its receptors in human skin. J Invest Dermatol 1997;108:263–8.

[12] Armstrong LC, Bornstein P. Thrombospondins 1 and 2 function as inhibitors of angiogenesis. Matrix Biol 2003;22:63–71.

[13] Banerjee DK. Angiogenesis: characterization of a cellular model. PR Health Sci J 1998;17: 327–33.

[14] Ilan N, Mahooti S, Madri JA. Distinct signal transduction pathways are utilized during the tube formation and survival phases of in vitro angiogenesis. J Cell Sci 1998;111:3621–31.

[15] Gray AJ, Bishop JE, Reeves JT, et al. Aa and Bb chains of fibrinogen stimulate proliferation of human fibroblasts. J Cell Sci 1993;104:409–13.

[16] Xu J, Clark RAF. Extracellular matrix alters PDGF regulation of fibroblast integrins. J Cell Biol 1996;132:239–49.

[17] Stupack DG. Integrins as a distinctive subtype of dependence receptors. Cell Death Differ 2005;12:1021–30.

[18] Eyden B. The myofibroblast: a study of normal, reactive and neoplastic tissues with an emphasis on ultrastrucutre. Part 1—normal and reactive cells. J Submicrosc Cytol Pathol 2005;37:109–204.

[19] McClain SA, Simon M, Jones E, et al. Mesenchymal cell activation is the rate-limiting step in granulation tissue induction. Am J Pathol 1996;149:1257–70.

[20] Mignati P, Ritkin DB, Welgus HG, et al. Proteinases and tissue remodelling. In: Clark RAF, editor. The molecular and cellular biology of wound repair. 2nd edition. New York: Plenum Press; 1996. p. 171–94.

[21] Vaalamo M, Mattila L, Johansson N. Distinct populations of stromal cells express collagenase-3 (MMP-13) and collagenase-1 (MMP-1) in chronic ulcers but not in normally healing wounds. J Invest Dermatol 1997;109:96–101.

[22] Desmouliere A, Redard M, Darby I, et al. Apoptosis mediates the decrease in cellularity during transition between granulation tissue and scar. Am J Pathol 1995;146:56–66.

[23] Shirakata Y, Kimura R, Nanba D, et al. Heparin-binding EGF-like growth factor accelerates keratinocyte migration and skin wound healing. J Cell Sci 2005;111(Pt 11):2363–70.

[24] Paladini RD, Takahashi K, Bravo NS, et al. Onset of re-epithelialization after skin injury correlates with a reorganization of keratin filaments in wound edge keratinocytes: defining a potential role for keratin 16. J Cell Biol 1996;132:381–97.

[25] Gabbiani G, Chaponnier C, Huttner I. Cytoplasmic filaments and gap junctions in epithelial cells and myofibroblasts during wound healing. J Cell Biol 1978;76:561–8.

[26] Goliger JA, Paul DL. Wounding alters epidermal connexin expression and gap junction-mediated intercellular communication. Mol Biol Cell 1995;6:1491–501.

[27] Pilcher BK, Dumin JA, Sudbeck BD, et al. The activity of collagenase-1 is required for keratinocyte migration on a type I collagen matrix. J Cell Biol 1997;137:1445–57.

[28] Clark RAF, Ashcroft GS, Spencer M-J, et al. Re-epithelialization of normal human excisional wounds is associated with a switch from α vβ5 to α vβ6 integrins. Br J Dermatol 1996;135: 46–51.

[29] Hirobe T. Proliferation of epidermal melanocytes during healing of skin wounds in newborn mice. J Exp Zool 1983;227:423–31.

[30] Zambruno G, Marchisio PC, Melchiori A, et al. Expression of integrin receptors and their role in adhesion, spreading and migration of normal human melanocytes. J Cell Sci 1993;105:179–90.

[31] Sowemimo GO, Naim J, Harrison HN, et al. Repigmentation after burn injury in the guinea-pig. Burns Incl Therm Inj 1982;8:345–57.

[32] Cox PM, Dhillon AP, Howe S, et al. Repopulation of guinea-pig skin by melanocytes during wound healing: a morphometric study. Br J Exp Pathol 1989;70:679–89.

[33] Midwood KS, Williams LV, Schwarzbauer JE. Tissue repair and the dynamics of the extra-cellular matrix. Int J Biochem Cell Biol 2004;36:1031–7.

[34] Mott JD, Werb Z. Regulation of matrix biology by matrix metalloproteinases. Curr Opin Cell Biol 2004;16:558–64.

[35] Chakraborti S, Mandal M, Das S, et al. Regulation of matrix metalloproteinases: an over-view. Mol Cell Biochem 2003;253:269–85.

[36] Hosgood G, Burba DJ. Wound healing, wound management and bandaging. In: McCurnin DM, Basset JM, editors. Clinical textbook for veterinary technicians. 6th edition. Philadelphia: WB Saunders; 2005. p. 135–64.

[37] Levenson SM, Geever EF, Crowley LV, et al. The healing of rat skin wounds. Ann Surg 1965;161:293–308.

[38] Baum CL, Arpey CJ. Normal cutaneous wound healing: clinical correlation with cellular and molecular events. Dermatolog Surg 2005;31:674–86.

[39] Roberts AWG. CSF: a key regulator of neutrophil production, but that's not all!. In: Growth Factors 2005;23:33–41.

[40] Grotendorst GR. Connective tissue growth factor: a mediator of TGF-β action on fibroblasts. Cytokine Growth Factor Rev 1997;8:171–9.

[41] Nimni ME. Polypeptide growth factors: targeted delivery systems. Biomaterials 1997;18: 1201–25.

[42] Wieldlocha A, Sorensen V. Signaling, internalization, and intracellular activity of fibroblast growth factor. Curr Top Microbiol Immunol 2004;286:45–79.

[43] Kahari VM, Saarialho-Kere U. Matrix metalloproteinases in skin. Exp Dermatol 1997;6: 199–213.

[44] Graiani G, Emanueli C, Desortes E, et al. Nerve growth factor promotes reparative angio-genesis and inhibits endothelial apoptosis in cutaneous wounds of Type I diabetic mice. Di-abetologia 2004;47:1047–54.

[45] Westermark B. The molecular and cellular biology of platelet derived growth factor. Acta Endocrinol (Copenh) 1990;123:131–42.

[46] Lambert E, Dasse E, Haye B, et al. TIMPs are multifacial proteins. Crit Rev Oncol Hematol 2004;49:187–98.

[47] Guo YH, Gao W, Li Q, et al. Tissue inhibitor of metalloproteinases-4 suppresses vascular smooth muscle cell migration and induces cell apoptosis. Life Sci 2004;75:2483–93.

[48] Massague J. The transforming growth factor-β family. Annu Rev Cell Biol 1990;6:597–641.

[49] Byrne AM, Bouchier-Hayes DJ, Harmey JH. Angiogenic and cell survival functions of vascu-lar endothelial growth factor (VEGF). J Cell Mol Med 2005;9:777–94.

[50] Carter CA, Jolly DG, Worden CES, et al. Platelet-rich plasma gel promotes differentiation and regeneration during equine wound healing. Exp Mol Pathol 2003;74:244–55.

Vet Clin Small Anim 36 (2006) 687–692

VETERINARY CLINICS
SMALL ANIMAL PRACTICE

Differences in Cutaneous Wound Healing Between Dogs and Cats

Mark W. Bohling, DVM[a],*, Ralph A. Henderson, DVM, MS[b]

[a]Department of Small Animal Clinical Sciences, College of Veterinary Medicine,
C247 Veterinary Teaching Hospital, University of Tennessee,
Knoxville, TN 37996, USA
[b]Department of Clinical Sciences, College of Veterinary Medicine, Hoerlein Hall,
Auburn University, Auburn, AL 36849, USA

F or most of its history, the study of wound healing has focused on the similarities rather than on the differences between species, and the general assumption has developed that wound healing is more or less homogeneous across species lines, at least among mammals [1]. Although the same basic phases of wound healing involving the same cells and cytokines are present in the same chronologic order in all species, clinical experience argues that there are significant differences between mammalian species. For example, chronic wounds of the distal limbs with production of exuberant granulation tissue seem to be an almost exclusively equine phenomenon compared with other animals [2–6]. This observation has stimulated several landmark investigations into the nature of problem wounds in horses. One surprising result of these studies was the discovery that although horses and ponies are closely related (actually just different breeds within the same species, *Equus caballus*), ponies heal differently than horses. Ponies have a more intense early inflammatory response to wounding than do horses, which typically leads to more complete wound contraction and uncomplicated healing [6]. Horses, conversely, have a weak inflammatory response that persists and frequently leads to the formation of large amounts of poorly vascularized exuberant granulation tissue, with the ultimate result being a more chronic and indolent course of wound healing [4–6]. It is well known that rodent skin heals primarily via contraction, whereas human skin heals primarily by epithelialization, indicating that rodent models may not be adequate for the study of human wounds and their treatment [7]. Recent studies by the authors have revealed significant differences between the cat and the dog in cutaneous healing [8]. These differences may similarly cause us to reconsider wound care dogma as applied to the feline species.

*Corresponding author. E-mail address: mbohling@utk.edu (M.W. Bohling).

0195-5616/06/$ – see front matter
doi:10.1016/j.cvsm.2006.02.001

NORMAL CUTANEOUS ANATOMY: THE CAT AS A UNIQUE SPECIES

A number of gross and microscopic differences have been noted in the cutaneous anatomy of the cat compared with the dog [9]. Cats also differ from dogs with respect to the cutaneous vascular supply. Studies were performed on the cutaneous angiosomes of nine species, including the cat and dog, with the purpose of evaluating the validity of certain animal models for human wound healing research. Comparison of the cutaneous angiosomes of the dog and cat revealed that the dog has a much higher density of tertiary and higher order vessels than the cat, particularly on the trunk [10]. This gross anatomic difference seems to translate to a functional difference based on the authors' laser Doppler perfusion studies, which revealed significantly less cutaneous perfusion in noninjured feline skin [8]. A link between tissue perfusion and wound healing has been well established [11,12].

FIRST-INTENTION CUTANEOUS HEALING

As part of the authors' investigation, the breaking strength of linear sutured wounds at 7 days after wounding was measured. Results demonstrated that wound breaking strength in cats is significantly inferior to that in dogs. The mean wound breaking strength for sutured wounds in cats at 7 days after wounding was only half of the wound breaking strength for dogs [8]. It was hypothesized that this difference in early first-intention healing reflects significantly lower collagen production in wounds in cats compared with those in dogs.

SECOND-INTENTION CUTANEOUS HEALING

Significant qualitative and quantitative differences between cats and dogs are also seen in second-intention healing. These differences begin in the early inflammatory phase of wound healing. Within 2 days after wounding, wounds in dogs can be grossly seen to produce more wound fluid and to be more edematous and erythematous than identically created wounds in cats. Interestingly, laser Doppler perfusion studies performed in open wounds at weekly intervals after wounding failed to show differences in wound perfusion between cats and dogs. This finding is surprising, because laser Doppler perfusion imaging has been well documented to be correlated with the degree of wound inflammation [13–15]. One possible explanation for this apparent contradiction is that the comparative laser Doppler studies missed the period of time for maximum differences between cats and dogs because of a sampling interval that was too long. Daily imaging for the first 5 to 7 days after wounding would have been more appropriate.

Although the results of the perfusion studies were somewhat equivocal, the rate of granulation tissue formation provided unequivocal evidence of differences by postwounding day 7. Granulation tissue production in cats lagged behind that in dogs for the entire 21-day observation period; the mean time for dogs to complete granulation was only 7.5 days, whereas cats took an average of more than 19 days. The visual character of the granulation tissue also differed between cats and dogs, with that in the latter having a deep red color and that in the former being much paler by comparison. Granulation tissue also seemed to originate from different areas of the wound in cats and dogs. In dogs, granulation tissue develops simultaneously from the entire exposed subcutis, whereas in cats, granulation tissue first appears at the wound edges and then slowly advances across the wound surface. The slower and less abundant production of granulation tissue in wounds in cats may be a major factor in the explanation of their overall slower healing rate compared with wounds in dogs. The rates of wound contraction, epithelialization, and total healing (overall reduction in open wound area attributable to contraction and epithelialization combined) are all reduced in cats compared with dogs.

PSEUDOHEALING AND INDOLENT POCKETS: ROLE OF THE SUBCUTIS IN CUTANEOUS HEALING

It has been the authors' clinical experience that routinely managed wounds in cats can have unexpected adverse outcomes. One such outcome is the phenomenon that the authors have termed *pseudohealing*. This event is characterized by a sutured skin incision that, on cursory inspection, seems to have healed normally at the time of skin suture removal. After suture removal, however, when the cat places ordinary physiologic stress on the closure (eg, grooming, jumping), complete dehiscence occurs with little or no bleeding. Examination of these dehisced wounds reveals little if any adhesion of the muscle fascial tissue to the adjacent deep layer of the skin.

The skin may heal sufficiently to remain intact when stressed, but if wound re-entry is required, as with recurrence of a neoplasm, it is often found that the subcutis has formed a chronic pocket lined with mature smooth collagen and containing a thin, serous, modified transudate. This observation is supported by the literature reporting a condition termed *indolent pocket wounds*, in which a granulation tissue–lined pocket forms that fails to contract or fill [16]. It was the authors' hypothesis that this phenomenon occurs when skin has been closed over areas in which the underlying subcutis has been damaged (eg, abscess) or extensively resected (eg, major tumor resection). These observations led to the examination of the role of the subcutis in cutaneous wound healing.

The role of the subcutis in healing was studied by creating open and sutured wounds in dogs and cats in which the subcutis was completely removed from the wound bed. These wounds were compared with control wounds in which the subcutis was left intact [17]. Comparisons of wound healing between treatments and between species resulted in the following observations regarding the role of the subcutis:

1. Removal of the subcutis resulted in no change in the time to first appearance of granulation tissue but did cause a marked reduction in the rate of production of granulation tissue. The observed reduction in wound granulation tissue was much more marked in cats than in dogs.

2. Creation of subcutaneous defects resulted in a decrease in cutaneous perfusion for cats and dogs, with measurable effects until the end of the second week after wounding.
3. Wound contraction was reduced by removal of the subcutis; this effect is also significantly more pronounced in cats than in dogs.
4. Removal of the subcutis also reduced the rate of wound epithelialization, although this seemed to affect cats and dogs more evenly.
5. No significant effect on first-intention healing was noted from removal of the subcutis. This was attributed to a flaw in the experimental design (insufficient size of subcutaneous defect under closed wounds).

It was concluded that the subcutis is a major source of precursors for granulation tissue and an important contributor to wound healing, at least for second-intention healing [17].

CLINICAL APPLICATION

The clinical application of this knowledge is as yet rather limited. One obvious application relates to our finding that the 7-day sutured wound strength in cats was only half of that seen in dogs. Although it may be fairly said that veterinarians have been closing wounds in cats for a long time without any special attention, it might also be possible that incisional dehiscence in cats, particularly in wounds in which a large volume of subcutis has been removed, may be an unrecognized problem that has been blamed on characteristics of the individual patient rather than on any inherent weakness or relative indolence in feline cutaneous healing.

The question remains: "Can we do better?" For uncomplicated wounds, the routine apposition of subcutis and skin seems to be sufficient. In cases in which this is not possible, however, the appropriate use of subcutaneous "tacking" sutures is warranted to help ensure adequate skin-subcutis contact. For wounds that require resection of significant portions of subcutis, the surgeon should take extra measures to ensure a closure that is strong and tension-free and provides an extended duration of mechanical support to the wound edges. Specific examples of desirable techniques for these situations may include (but are not limited to) the following: the use of "walking" sutures, various stenting techniques, multiple layer closures, and slight eversion of the skin (to maximize the surface area of dermal-to-dermal contact). An even higher risk exists whenever subcutis is to be removed from a cat and another factor is present that may be detrimental to healing, such as an area of high motion like the axilla or groin. In these situations, the risk of pseudohealing increases. For these situations, postoperative drainage and wound immobilization may be beneficial (see the articles by Amalsadvala and Swaim, and Hedlund elsewhere in this issue).

Once a chronic wound is established in the cat, an adequate blood supply is essential for adequate healing. The authors have had the best success when treating with compound flaps that provide their own subcutis or, better yet, with myocutaneous transfers. It is possible that microvascular free tissue transfer may provide an answer to enhancing blood supply to wounds in cats to stimulate healing. Occasionally, nonhealing wounds in cats lead to eventual euthanasia. There is an adage in surgical oncology: "The first surgeon who has the opportunity to treat a neoplasm is the one who is most likely to cure it." A modification of this could be: "The surgeon who prevents wound dehiscence in a cat is the one most likely to be responsible for preventing euthanasia of the cat."

Any further clinical application of this work remains to be seen. In light of the newness of this knowledge, it would be premature to extend clinical application far. As has often been observed, more is missed because of not looking than because of not seeing, and until now, veterinarians have not been looking at the cat as a unique species in regard to wound healing. It is the authors' hope that when problematic wound healing occurs in feline patients in the future, veterinarians are willing to consider the possibility of feline-specific factors and try to identify them so that cats may be more effectively managed. This may well be the greatest value of this preliminary work.

SUMMARY

Cutaneous wound healing in the cat proceeds more slowly than in the dog, with significantly lower strength of closed wounds and lower rates of contraction and epithelialization of open wounds. The subcutaneous tissues play an important supportive role in second-intention wound healing, and removal of large amounts of subcutis seems to retard wound healing in the cat to a greater degree than in the dog. Based on this knowledge, certain recommendations have been made to improve outcomes with potentially problematic wound closures in cats.

References

[1] Fretz PB. Traumatic and incisional wounds: how they heal. In: Proceedings of the 18th Annual Surgical Forum of the American College of Veterinary Surgeons. Washington, DC: American College of Veterinary Surgeons; 1990. p. 25–7.

[2] Chvapil M, Pfister T, Escalada S, et al. Dynamics of the healing of skin wounds in the horse as compared to the rat. Exp Mol Pathol 1979;30(3):349–59.

[3] Dinev D, Dzhurov A. Histogenesis of the granular tissue in wounds of second intention healing in horses and cattle. Vet Med Nauki 1987;24:72–9.

[4] Bertone AL. Principles of wound healing. Vet Clin North Am Equine Pract 1985;48(5):449–63.

[5] Bertone AL. Management of exuberant granulation tissue. Vet Clin North Am Equine Pract 1985;48(5):551–62.

[6] Wilmink JM, Stolk PWT, van Weeren PR, et al. Differences in second-intention wound healing between horses and ponies: macroscopical aspects. Equine Vet J 1999;31:53–60.

[7] Gottrup F, Ågren MS, Karlsmark T. Models for use in wound healing research: a survey focusing on in vitro and in vivo adult soft tissue. Wound Repair Regen 2000;8:83–96.

[8] Bohling MW, Henderson RA, Swaim SF, et al. Cutaneous wound healing in the cat: a macroscopic description and comparison with cutaneous wound healing in the dog. Vet Surg 2004;33(6):579–87.

[9] Affolter VK, Moore PF. Histologic features of normal canine and feline skin. Clin Dermatol 1994;12:491–7.

[10] Taylor GI, Minabe T. The angiosomes of the mammals and other vertebrates. Plast Reconst Surg 1992;89:181–215.

[11] Jonsson K, Jensen JA, Goodson WH III, et al. Tissue oxygenation, anemia, and perfusion in relation to wound healing in surgical patients. Ann Surg 1991;214(5):605–13.

[12] Hartmann M, Jonsson K, Zederfeldt B. Effect of tissue perfusion and oxygenation on accumulation of collagen in healing wounds. Eur J Surg 1992;158:521–6.

[13] Scardino MS, Swaim SF, Morse BS, et al. Evaluation of fibrin sealants in cutaneous wound closure. J Biomed Mater Res 1999;48:315–21.

[14] Tyler MPH, Watts AMI, Perry ME, et al. Dermal cellular inflammation in burns. An insight into the function of dermal microvascular anatomy. Burns 2001;27:433–8.

[15] Nanney LB, Wamil BD, Whitsitt J, et al. CM101 stimulates cutaneous wound healing through an anti-angiogenic mechanism. Angiogenesis 2001;4:61–70.

[16] Lascelles BDX, Davison L, Dunning M, et al. Use of omental pedicle grafts in the management of nonhealing axillary wounds in 10 cats. J Small Anim Pract 1998;39(10):475–80.

[17] Bohling MW, Henderson RA, Swaim SF, et al. Comparison of the role of the subcutaneous tissues in cutaneous wound healing in the dog and cat. Vet Surg 2006;35(1):1–12.

Vet Clin Small Anim 36 (2006) 693–711

VETERINARY CLINICS
SMALL ANIMAL PRACTICE

Management of Hard-to-Heal Wounds

Tannaz Amalsadvala, DVM, MS[a],
Steven F. Swaim, DVM, MS[a,b,*]

[a]Department of Clinical Sciences, College of Veterinary Medicine, Auburn University,
Auburn, AL 36849, USA
[b]Scott-Ritchey Research Center, College of Veterinary Medicine, Auburn University,
Auburn, AL 36849, USA

A wound is an interruption of anatomic, physiologic, and functional integrity of the body's tissue [1]. The healing process begins immediately after infliction by means of a complex and finely orchestrated continuum of stages (ie, inflammatory, debridement, repair, maturation) [2]. The process involves sophisticated synchronization of molecular and biochemical events at the cellular level, resulting in a healed wound (see article by Hosgood elsewhere in this issue) [3]. Malfunction of any component of the process or interruption of any stage results in delayed healing and chronic or nonhealing wounds.

TYPES OF PROBLEM WOUNDS
Disrupted Wounds
Wound disruption can result from tension, infection, underlying hematoma, suturing nonviable tissue, and wound molestation by the animal. Attention to preventing these factors helps to prevent the extra time and expense of attending to the wound a second time.

Wound tension
When planning a surgical incision or excision in an area in which skin is sparse or where a large defect may result, tension on the resulting closure can be reduced if the suture line can be oriented to run parallel to the tension lines in the skin. Skin tension lines result from the predominant pull of skin fibrous tissue. They have been mapped for dogs but vary with breed, confirmation, gender, and age. Suture lines parallel to tension lines gape less, have less tension when closed, heal faster, and do not tend to widen over time. With traumatic wounds, manipulation of wound edges should be used to plan a closure with the least amount of tension [2,4].

*Corresponding author. Scott-Ritchey Research Center, College of Veterinary Medicine, Auburn University, Auburn, AL 36849. E-mail address: swaimsf@auburn.edu (S.F. Swaim).

0195-5616/06/$ – see front matter
doi:10.1016/j.cvsm.2006.02.002

When large wounds are present, techniques and materials should be considered that reduce the tension of closure. These include the use of undermining and skin stretching techniques (see article by Hedlund elsewhere in this issue). Relaxing incisions (Z-plasty, V-to-Y plasty, and multiple punctate incisions) can also be considered (see article by Fowler elsewhere in this issue). Tension-relieving suture patterns can be used to help relieve skin tension. These can be suture patterns that concentrate tension at the wound edges, such as alternating narrow- and wide-bite simple interrupted sutures, interrupted horizontal or vertical mattress sutures (with or without stents), combination apposition and tension sutures (far-near-near-far or far-far-near-near), and an adjustable horizontal mattress suture. It should be remembered that interrupted horizontal mattress sutures tend to obstruct capillary blood flow to the wound edge because of their box-like configuration. The other suture patterns all lie in the same plane and do not have this disadvantage. When these suture patterns are used in combination with a subdermal or subcuticular pattern, they provide added security to the suture line [2,4,5]. A tension suture pattern that advances the skin edges together and also distributes tension away from the wound edges is the "walking" suture pattern (see article by Hedlund elsewhere in this issue) [2,4–6].

When a wound is near a joint, movement of the joint may place tension on suture lines. Use of some of the previously mentioned tension suture patterns along with bandaging and splinting the joint to prevent movement can help to avoid wound disruption (see article by Campbell elsewhere in this issue).

When selecting suture material, it should be remembered that small-gauge material has lower tensile strength, larger gauge material may tend to lacerate tissue, and multifilament material could cause more tissue trauma. All these factors could cause wound disruption. Therefore, clinical judgment should be used to select a monofilament material of sufficient size to close the wound without causing tissue trauma.

Infection

Infection delays wound healing. Bacterial, granulocyte, and macrophage collagenases degrade collagen, thereby decreasing wound strength [1]. Decreased pH and oxygen tension, interruption of blood supply, and mechanical interference by exudate are also factors that contribute to nonhealing [7]. In addition, decreased fibroblast activity of infection has a negative effect on healing [1]. The end result is a tendency for wound disruption. Thus, use of proper initial wound management along with systemic and topical medication is important to prevent disruption (see articles by Dernell, and Krahwinkel and Booth elsewhere in this issue).

Underlying hematoma or seroma

A hematoma or seroma can result from incomplete hemostasis and the presence of dead space. These can cause pressure on suture lines and provide a rich environment for infection, thus leading to disruption [8]. Adequate hemostasis and drainage of wounds are indicated (see article by Dernell elsewhere in this issue).

Suturing nonviable tissue

The unclosed wound is the unmet challenge. Unfortunately, veterinarians may tend to close a traumatic wound too quickly. Adequate debridement is necessary (see article by Dernell elsewhere in this issue) [8]. If staged debridement is used until all nonviable and questionable tissue has been removed from the wound, disruption does not occur because of sutures pulling out of nonviable tissue.

Wound molestation

A major cause of wound disruption is the animal molesting the suture line. Several methods can be used to prevent this. Often, a comfortable bandage is adequate. To keep a dog away from its hindquarters, side braces made from aluminum splint rods or other rigid material can be used (see article by Campbell elsewhere in this issue). Basket-type muzzles come in varying sizes, are commercially available, and can be used to prevent molestation of sutures at almost any point on the dog's body. Likewise, an Elizabethan collar or bucket with a hole in the bottom can be affixed to an animal's collar. They keep the animal's paws away from the head area and the animal's teeth and tongue away from other body areas [2]. To prevent wound disruption around the lips, the authors use stainless steel simple interrupted sutures with sharp tag ends to discourage licking. In the authors' experience, use of distasteful substances around sutures or on bandages has not been successful in preventing wound molestation.

Pressure Wounds

Decubital ulcers

Decubital ulcers are a problem in dogs at locations of bony prominences, such as the ischial tuberosity, greater trochanter, tuber coxae, acromion of the scapula, lateral humeral epicondyle, lateral tibial condyle, lateral malleolus, sides of the fifth digits, olecranon, calcaneal tuberosity, and sternum. They result from tissue compression between the bony prominence and the surface on which the animal is lying. Capillary compression results in ischemia and avascular necrosis. Further vasoconstriction by tissue thromboxane A_2 elevation and reperfusion injury contributes to tissue damage [2,4,9,10]. Ulcers are classified from grade I through grade IV, with increasing severity as grades increase [2].

There are numerous predisposing factors for decubital ulcers. These include thin and sparsely haired skin as seen in Greyhounds, shearing forces, friction between skin and bedding or skin and a bandage [10,11], improper bedding material [9,10], and skin maceration from urine and feces [9–11].

Prevention and treatment of decubital ulcers is centered around reducing pressure and maintaining skin hygiene. A vinyl-coated thick foam rubber pad with an artificial sheep skin (Dubicrest Padding 4700; Alpha Protech, Tulsa, OK) covering helps to prevent pressure and wicks urine away from the skin of the incontinent dog, respectively (Fig. 1). Changing the animal's position every 1 to 5 hours is helpful. When an animal is placed in sternal recumbency, the pelvic limbs should be extended caudally to prevent joint contracture. Tetraplegic dogs should be placed in a sling for 2 to 4 hours daily to relieve pressure on the acromion of the scapulae, tuber coxae, and trochanter major [2,4,10].

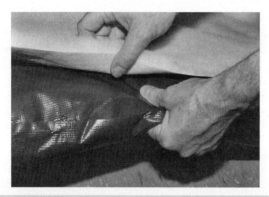

Fig. 1. Vinyl-covered thick foam rubber pad for pressure relief. The artificial sheep skin covering wicks urine away from the skin of the incontinent dog.

Skin over bony prominences should be frequently observed for signs of impending ulcers, such as hyperemia, moisture, and easily epilated hair. Clipping, gentle washing, drying, and padding such an area are important. Whirlpool or warm-water baths two to three times daily help to keep skin clean and promote circulation [2,4,10]. If skin over the ischial tuberosities develops a decubital ulcer, a piece of rubber sheeting (eg, back of a surgeon's glove) can be sutured across the perineal area to reduce fecal contamination in the incontinent dog (Fig. 2) [2].

A high-protein and high-carbohydrate diet with vitamin supplements is indicated for animals with decubital ulcers. Such diets promote healing [2,10].

Bandage-, splint-, and cast-induced wounds
Similar to decubital ulcers, casts, splints, and bandages over bony prominences can compress tissues, causing wounds and preventing their healing. Contrary to the thinking that additional padding is needed over these areas, less padding

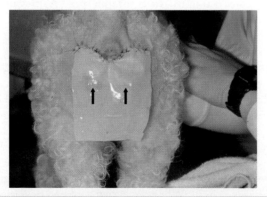

Fig. 2. A piece of rubber sheeting (back of a surgical glove) is sutured over the perineal area under the anus using 3-0 nylon or polypropylene suture to help prevent fecal contamination of underlying pressure wounds (*arrows*).

is actually needed. Additional padding increases pressure when outer bandage layers are applied, especially with elastic materials. The pressure counteracts the action of fibroblasts and myofibroblasts that are trying to contract the wound. Thus, it is better to keep pressure off of the wound by distributing it around the wound (see article by Campbell elsewhere in this issue) [2,12].

Rigid cast or splint immobilization of open wounds over areas of potential mobility (ie, tarsal flexion surface) inhibits wound contraction. This retarded contraction has been attributed to the passive pressure of the cast or splint on the wound [13]. Thus, immobilization should be attained such that it does not place pressure on the wound (eg, rigid fixation on the side of the limb opposite the wound) (see article by Campbell elsewhere in this issue) [12].

Early application of a fully encasing cast after trauma to a lower limb can result in avascular necrosis. As the limb swells within the cast, circulatory embarrassment can occur. Application of a bivalved cast with periodic changing of the cast and padding can help to prevent this.

Acute and Chronic Wounds
Orthopedic conditions
Osteomyelitis and sequestra. Chronic osteomyelitis may present as a draining sinus, recurrent cellulitis, or an abscess. Progressive destruction and proliferation of bone or sequestra may be present [14]. These may be present beneath a non-healing wound (Fig. 3). Infections may be monomicrobial, with *Streptococcus intermedius* or *Staphylococcus aureus*, or polymicrobial, with *Streptococcus* spp or *Proteus* spp. Anaerobes, such as *Actinomyces* spp, *Clostridium* spp, *Peptostreptococcus* spp, *Bacteroides* spp, or *Fusobacterium* spp, can also cause infections as well as mycotic organisms like *Blastomyces* dermatitidis and *Coccidioides* immitis [14].

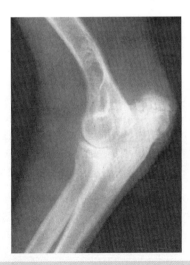

Fig. 3. Radiograph of the olecranon area of a dog with osteomyelitis underlying a nonhealing wound over the point of the olecranon.

Sources of infection are hematologic or posttraumatic. A common source of infection is surgical site contamination during open-fracture reduction [14]. Chronic osteomyelitis is a problem wound that can appear radiographically as lysis of the medullary cavity or sequestra formation, with sclerosis and lysis being interspersed throughout the bone [14,15].

A biopsy of affected bone should be obtained for culture and sensitivity testing for aerobes and anaerobes. If the animal has been on antibiotics, these should be discontinued for at least 24 hours before taking biopsies [15]. Biopsies should be obtained from the bone at the time of surgical intervention or via a fine-needle biopsy from tissue immediately adjacent to the infection site [14]. With an open wound, bone can be taken with a small trephine introduced via aseptically prepared intact skin adjacent to the wound. This helps to ensure getting the causative organism and avoiding surface contaminants.

In the presence of sequestra, exudate pockets, and necrotic tissue, debridement of necrotic tissue and drainage are necessary. If osteomyelitis is present in conjunction with a fracture, the degree of fracture stability should be determined by palpation and radiographs. If the fracture and implants are stable, the implants should be left; however, with loose implants and an unhealed fracture, implants are removed, sequestra are removed, and the fracture is rigidly stabilized [14].

Direct antibiotic therapy can be applied, with the advantage of higher local drug concentration for prolonged periods [15]. Antibiotic-impregnated polymethyl methacrylate beads may be used in chronic infections [14]. In one case, one author (SFS) has packed the infected bone with the appropriate antibiotic mixed with a bioactive glass (Consil; Nutramax, Edgewood, MD) that is used in dental reconstruction, with good results.

After obtaining a biopsy for culture and sensitivity testing, the animal may be placed on a bacteriocidal broad-spectrum antibiotic, such as a cephalosporin, intravenously for 3 to 5 days until culture results are available [15]. Once these results are available, the appropriate systemic antibiotic is started. This should be given for 4 to 6 weeks (see article by Krahwinkel and Booth elsewhere in this issue) [14].

Exposed bone. Exposed bone is often encountered in distal limb degloving wounds and inhibits wound contraction and epithelialization [16,17]. When allowed to heal by second intention, a bed of granulation tissue is required for second-intention healing to progress [2,17]. Such a bed is also necessary for skin grafting [2].

In the healing process, granulation tissue is produced by the vascular soft tissue at the wound periphery and gradually advances over the bone. A freeze-dried acemannan-containing medication (Carrasorb-M; Carrington Laboratories, Irving, Texas) has been shown to stimulate granulation tissue formation over exposed bone (see article by Krahwinkel and Booth elsewhere in this issue) [12,18]. The drilling of small holes in the bone (forage) into the marrow cavity stimulates granulation tissue. A clot forms over the bone and serves as a matrix for fibroblast ingrowth and neovascularization of granulation tissue [2,4,12,19,20].

Movement and pressure
Wounds over joints. Wounds over joints present a challenge to healing in that they are subject to tension, compression, or shearing forces. The desired result of wound healing is for the two sides of a wound to heal together. If they are exposed to these forces, however, healing is impaired. Wounds over extension surfaces of joints (eg, carpus, stifle) are subject to tension when joint flexion pulls wound edges apart. Thus, meticulous closure is necessary. Casting or splinting the joint is necessary to prevent joint flexion for proper healing (see article by Campbell elsewhere in this issue) [2,12].

Paw pad wounds. Paw pads are shock absorbing and spread as weight is applied. Thus, in the presence of an open wound, edges are pushed apart, impeding healing [21,22]. If sutures are present in the pad, such pad spreading results in sutures tearing through the tissues [22]. It is therefore necessary to relieve pressure on paw pads to attain adequate healing, especially in large dogs. Various bandaging and splinting techniques have been evaluated as to their efficacy in reducing pressure on digital and metacarpal or metatarsal pads using various forms of foam rubber pads, metal splints, and combinations of these [22]. Aside from the complete absence of weight bearing using a Velpeau bandage (forelimb) or Robinson sling (pelvic limb), a localized crutch in the form of a "clam shell" bandage or splint has been found to give the best pressure relief on pads (see article by Campbell elsewhere in this issue) [22,23].

Axillary and inguinal wounds. Wounds in the axillary and inguinal areas may result from forelimb entrapment in a collar, vehicular trauma, burns, neoplasias, and infections [24,25]. A primary factor in the impaired healing of such wounds is the shearing movement between the two wound surfaces as the animal ambulates [2]. If such wounds have been present for a long period, it is possible that there may be infection with an atypical organism. Thus, a biopsy for culture and sensitivity testing is indicated. Techniques for closing such wounds have included meticulous closure and the use of skin fold flaps, omental pedicle flaps, axial pattern skin flaps, or combinations of these (see article by Hedlund elsewhere in this issue).

Immobilization of the surgically repaired site is an important aspect of attaining healing. This is more of a challenge in cats than in dogs. For immobilization of the axillary and inguinal areas of a cat, the authors have found an empty cardboard box to be effective. A box large enough to accommodate the cat has an access hole cut in it, and it is placed upside down in the cat's cage. The cat gets in the box and takes a sternal recumbent position with the limbs flexed under it, thus immobilizing the axillary and inguinal areas to enhance healing.

Sinus tracts
Sinus tracts can be considered to be tubular ulcers that are lined with a poor quality of granulation tissue that is thick and fibrotic. The opening is surrounded by thick, fibrotic, inelastic skin that has hyperplastic epidermal edges. It is not uncommon to have bacterial or fungal infections with pain, swelling,

and a serous to purulent drainage. A malodorous serous discharge and crepitants may be present in the presence of a foreign body and anaerobic infection [2,9,26]. Sinus tracts are associated with foreign bodies, including suture remnants, cotton gauze strands, wood chips, plant awns, pieces of straw, insect mouth parts, or even broken teeth from an attacker [2,9,26,27]. Chronic, draining, nonhealing tracts may also be associated with surgical implants [26] and bone sequestra (Fig. 4). Sinus tracts occur at various body locations depending on their point of entry and their migratory path. Common points of entry of a foreign body include the interdigital spaces, ear canal, conjunctiva, oral mucosa, nares, and other cutaneous areas. The foreign bodies may migrate, causing abscesses in the middle or inner ear, retrobulbar area, perianal area, interdigital spaces, or on the neck and trunk [2,9]. With a foreign body, the phenomenon of "tissue intelligence" takes place. In an attempt to rid the tissues of the foreign material, host defense mechanisms do not allow healing to progress to completion [2]. Thus, the wound does not heal, or if it does, it opens and drains at a later time [26].

Diagnostic procedures for sinus tracts include impression smears, culture and sensitivity tests for aerobic and anaerobic organisms, and fungal cultures. Biopsies are indicated for histopathologic examination and microbiologic evaluation [2,9,26,28]. Radiographs and ultrasonography may help to locate radiopaque and radiolucent foreign bodies, respectively. Careful probing of a tract may reveal a foreign body or may give an idea of the lesion's extent. Scintigraphy and MRI scans have been described for locating organic debris [27].

The extent of a sinus tract may be determined by positive-contrast sinography [2,26]. Because most contrast media have an iodine base, which may be microbiocidal, samples for culture should be gathered before sinography is performed [2,9]. For large-diameter tracts, a Foley catheter is used for catheterization, with bulb inflation preventing backflow of medium. With small-diameter tracts, backflow of medium can be prevented by a purse-string suture or digital pressure around the catheter entrance point. These procedures are important, because retrograde flow of contrast medium onto the skin cannot be differentiated from that in the tract. Prefilling the catheter with contrast medium

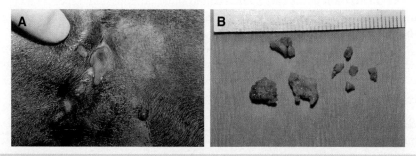

Fig. 4. Sinus tract. (A) Sinus tract opening with purulent exudate. (B) Bone sequestra removed from the end of the sinus tract.

prevents air bubble injection, which could result in misrepresentation of tracts on radiographs [2,9].

Surgical intervention is indicated to remove any foreign body, along with appropriate antimicrobial medication. Surgery may be by incisional dissection, excisional dissection, or nidus removal. For incisional dissection, the tract is catheterized as previously described for sinography [2]. A purse-string suture around the catheterization site is tied as the catheter is removed to prevent backflow of the injected sterile 1% methylene blue. Massaging the area during injection may help to distribute the methylene blue into the depths of the tracts. Twenty-four hours after injection, the stained tracts are traced to their origin using careful incisional dissection following the blue stain (Fig. 5A). Major factors for good dissection are (1) caution when undermining in areas of vital structures, (2) hemostasis, (3) sharp tissue division, (4) tissue traction with countertraction, and (5) adequate exposure [2]. This technique should not be used in cats, because methylene blue causes methemoglobinemia.

For excisional dissection, the tract is catheterized with a flexible fine catheter, which is advanced progressively as dissection proceeds around the tract [2]. An elliptic excision is made around the sinus opening, followed by sharp and blunt dissection to isolate the tract. A low-blended cutting or coagulation electrosurgical current helps to attain hemostasis for better structure identification during dissection (Fig. 5B).

The third technique for surgical removal of a foreign body involves removal of a known nidus, such as a bone sequestrum or surgical implant. The sinus tract is not removed. It heals spontaneously after removing the foreign body (Fig. 5C) [2,26].

An emerging technology for removing foreign bodies from sinus tracts is "woundoscopy" [29]. A small-gauge flexible endoscope is inserted in the opening of the sinus tract. If a foreign body is visualized during examination, endoscopic rat-toothed forceps are used for removal. Deep tissue biopsies may be collected using endoscopic biopsy forceps. With the growing use of endoscopy in veterinary practice, woundoscopy may become a useful technique in veterinary wound management.

Neoplasia

Various skin and subcutaneous neoplasms may appear as nonhealing wounds (eg, squamous cell carcinoma). In some cases, the wound is the result of a tumor outgrowing its vascular supply, followed by ulceration and necrosis. A wound biopsy is necessary for diagnosing such neoplastic lesions. After diagnosis, appropriate medical, radiologic, or surgical therapy is provided as indicated for the type of neoplasia [9].

Infection

The pathologic changes in a chronic wound differ from those in an acute wound. In an acute wound, the host defense mechanism is primed by an inflammatory response. This facilitates phagocytosis, which is advantageous to the host as the wound progresses into the repair stage of healing. In a chronic

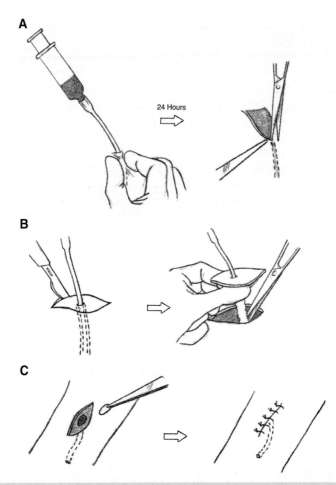

Fig. 5. Three techniques for treating a sinus tract. (A) Incisional dissection: methylene blue is injected into the sinus tract 24 hours before surgery, after which the sinus tract is incised and dissected. (B) Excisional dissection: catheter is inserted into the tract, an elliptic incision is made around the tract opening, and blunt excisional dissection is performed around the tract. (C) Nidus removal: known nidus (eg, bone sequestrum) is removed without removing the tract.

wound, however, persistent infection sustains the inflammatory response, which results in further trauma to wound tissue. The immune mechanism is dulled, and there is a decrease in the microbial clearance rate. These changes result in delayed healing. Chronically infected wounds have unhealthy, pale, weak, frangible granulation tissue, which results in impaired contraction and epithelialization [30]. A practitioner should strongly suspect an infectious cause of a chronic wound when there are smaller wounds adjacent to a large wound.

Organisms causing chronic wounds may be bacterial or fungal. There may be a mix of gram-positive and gram-negative bacteria. Aerobe and anaerobe mixtures are also possible [30]. Examples of infectious organisms are *Pseudomonas* spp, *Streptococcus* spp, and *Staphylococcus* spp, to include methicillin-resistant *S aureus*. Other infections include atypical mycobacterial granulomas, actinomycosis, actinobacillosis, and nocardiosis. Subcutaneous fungal infections include mycetomas, phaeohyphomycosis, pythiosis, zygomycosis, and sporotrichosis. Chronic wounds can also be associated with histoplasmosis and blastomycosis [2,9,28,30].

A biopsy is indicated to provide an accurate qualitative microbial assessment of the wound. Before obtaining a biopsy, the practitioner should consult with the microbiologist, who should be informed that atypical organisms are suspected so that special culture media, stains, and other identification techniques can be used [2]. It should also be ascertained whether any special transport media are needed to submit the sample.

Chronic wounds often have surface bacterial contamination and possible colonization. These microorganisms do not interfere with healing, however [30]. It is necessary to differentiate surface microorganisms from those causing the infection and nonhealing [30,31]. The wound surface should be thoroughly cleansed using a presurgical scrub technique to remove contaminants and biopsies taken from the center and edge of the wound. Cultures should be performed for aerobes, anaerobes, and fungi [9,28].

Once the causative organism and appropriate therapy have been identified, treatment can be instituted. The animal owner should be informed that some organisms may require prolonged therapy. Thickened indurated skin around the wound usually contains the organism; thus, removal or debridement of such skin can be advantageous in that a large amount of the causative organism can be removed and therapy is not solely dependent on medication. In the authors' experience, however, wound closure should not be attempted until the organism is completely controlled. Premature closure, even if it is easily accomplished, is futile, and the wound is likely to disrupt.

Corticosteroids and chemotherapy

Corticosteroids are potent anti-inflammatory agents. It should be remembered that inflammation is an important stage in the wound healing process. Thus, reducing it with the use of corticosteroids during early wound healing can decelerate the healing process. Steroids have their greatest effect early in the healing process [1] but can also be detrimental to the later stages of healing. Cyclooxygenase and 5-lipoxygenase are inhibited by corticosteroids. The arachidonic acid inflammatory cascade is thus blocked.

Steroids retard angiogenesis, reduce vascular permeability, decrease phagocytosis, and stabilize lysosomal membranes. Glucocorticoids suppress fibroblasts to inhibit collagen synthesis and have antimitotic effects on keratinocytes, thus decreasing the rate of epithelialization. Impaired healing is the result [1,32].

When treating slow-healing wounds, any exogenous steroid therapy, including any topical steroids, should be discontinued while continuing other therapy for the wound. Continuation of steroids increases the risk of or susceptibility to new infection and potentiation of existing infection. In the presence of starvation and protein depletion, the effects of cortisone are enhanced such that a low dose markedly inhibits fibroplasia. Single doses have no effect on healing [1].

Cytotoxic agents used in chemotherapy can influence the rate of wound repair [1,32,33]. Such drugs affect dividing cells and thus could influence such cells in wound healing. The mechanism of action, dose, and timing of administration all affect wound repair. This has made interpretation of clinical and experimental studies difficult; therefore, no general conclusion can be made regarding the effects of these drugs on wound healing. No set recommendations can be made regarding the use of these agents in animals after surgery. It seems that they have their greatest effect on healing in high doses given before or soon after injury [1].

Perivascular injections

Perivascular injection of some intravenous drugs (eg, thiobarbiturates, arsenicals, doxorubicin, large volumes of parenteral fluid) may cause necrosis and tissue slough as well as a chronic open wound [2,9]. The size and severity of the wound are dependent on the type of medication, its volume and pH, and whether an attempt was made to prevent an impending lesion. With some medications other than doxorubicin, corticosteroids diluted in physiologic saline or lactated Ringer's solution or mixed with lidocaine may be locally infiltrated to dilute caustic effects of the drug and to speed absorption. Additionally, dimethyl sulfoxide applied topically every 12 hours, together with soaks in a warm-water solution of magnesium sulfate two or three times daily, may help to reduce the pain and edema of the perivascular injection. If tissue does slough, staged debridement, lavage, and open-wound management are in order, followed by some form of reconstructive surgery [2,9].

With large volumes of parenteral fluid, physiologic saline and steroids are not indicated; however, reduction of edema is necessary. Use of dimethyl sulfoxide and magnesium sulfate soaks as well as diuretics may be helpful [2].

Doxorubicin in the tissue nearly always causes a large wound. The duration and extent of tissue damage are prolonged by release of the drug from dying cells with subsequent binding to adjacent viable cells, thus setting up a vicious cycle that results in radially progressing slough. A radical therapeutic approach is indicated. After gentle aseptic preparation of the involved area to prevent drug spreading, a bold incision with wide excision of the subcutis and infusion vein (after its ligation) is indicated. Skin should be spared at this time in hopes of its survival for use in reconstruction later. After several days of open-wound therapy with use of topical hydrophilic agents to draw body fluids and doxorubicin out of tissues, closure may be considered [2].

Envenomization: Loxosceles recluses *(brown recluse spider)*

The brown recluse spider's bite can result in severe nonhealing wounds (dermonecrotic arachnidism). The venom contains a number of enzymes, with sphingomyelinase-D being a major component. It is usually difficult to state definitively that the wound is of this origin because of the elusive nature of the spider. The "red, white, and blue" lesion with its centripetal progression of vasodilation, ischemia, and thrombosis, which are characteristic of the lesion, is not observed because the animal's hair coat obscures the skin. The veterinarian should suspect a brown recluse spider bite when a circular patch of necrotic skin sloughs from an animal for no known reason and the animal has been in an area in which such spiders are present. The lesion is an indolent nonhealing ulcer. Usually, the veterinarian sees the lesion in the later stage of the condition when it has an eschar of dead skin. At this point, therapy is surgical debridement of the eschar [34,35]. The authors have found the use of wound healing stimulant drugs to be helpful in enhancing the healing of such wounds (see article by Krahwinkel and Booth elsewhere in this issue).

Malnutrition
A catabolic state with a negative nitrogen balance attributable to malnutrition is a major contributing factor to nonhealing wounds. In such a state, the body does not have the necessary protein and energy sources (fats and carbohydrates); therefore, existing stores of protein are broken down to maintain basal functions. Thus, the increased caloric and protein demands for healing are not available, and the wound becomes quiescent [36].

Glucose and protein are important for normal progression of normal healing. Glucose is the primary source of energy for leukocytes and fibroblasts. It is the integral molecule within the ground substance that is laid down by the fibroblasts. Deposition of this is necessary before collagen formation [2]. Thus, glucose deficiency can affect collagen formation and wound strength.

Depletion of protein stores can result in attenuated fibroplasia and prolonged healing time [8]. The normal plasma protein levels range from 7.0 to 7.5 g/dL. A level of 6.0 g/dL slows healing, and below 5.5 g/dL, there is a 70% chance of wound disruption. Thus, adequate protein levels are necessary for animals undergoing healing. Sufficient protein levels help to prevent edema and promote increased fibroplasia with increased wound strength [37]. Feeding DL-methionine or cysteine to a protein-depleted animal prevents delayed repair [1,8].

Vitamins affect wound healing. Excess vitamin A labilizes lysosomes to enhance inflammation. Because steroids stabilize lysosomes and inhibit wound repair, vitamin A can counteract this negative effect [1,8]. Likewise, vitamin E stabilizes lysosomes similar to steroids and thus can inhibit healing in large doses [1,8]. Again, vitamin A can reverse the effects of vitamin E. Vitamin C deficiency can impair healing in that it is necessary for the hydroxylation of proline and lysine in collagen synthesis [1,8]. Although dogs and cats do not require exogenous sources of vitamin C, there is the possibility that the vital levels of ascorbic acid may decrease after trauma (ie, wounding). This could be an indication for vitamin C supplementation in these animals [8].

Zinc deficiency can result in lack of replication of epithelial cells and fibroblasts, causing a weak wound and lack of epithelialization. At the other extreme, an elevated zinc concentration can inhibit macrophages, decrease phagocytosis, and interfere with collagen cross-linking to have a negative effect on healing [1,8].

Radiation
An undesirable side effect of radiation therapy for neoplasia is the radiation injury it induces [2,38]. Radiation can have similar effects on neoplastic and adjacent normal tissue [32], thus being simultaneously beneficial and detrimental to the patient.

Radiation is deleterious to cells needed for the progression of normal wound healing (rapidly dividing cells, such as epithelial cells, endothelial cells, fibroblasts, and myofibroblasts) [32,39]. Tissues that have a rapid cell turnover, such as the skin, oral mucosa, bone marrow, urinary bladder, and intestine, are the most susceptible to early and/or acute radiation injury. In the skin, the early clinical changes are seen as edema, desquamation, and erythema. Early changes are observed within 2 to 4 weeks after radiation therapy [2,38]. Four degrees of radiation injury have been described, with increasing pathologic changes as the degrees increase [2,4]. The most significant late change is a progressive decrease in circulation with chronic progressive endarteritis [4,38]. The late changes may be seen months to years after conclusion of treatment [38].

Techniques for dealing with radiation injury include prevention of wound healing problems and treating dermal lesions. When radiation therapy is to be used after surgery, the surgical wound can be safely irradiated 7 to 14 days after surgery [2,39]. If radiation therapy is to be used before surgery, it should be done 2 to 8 weeks before surgery [2,39]. Because of a potentially compromised blood supply, aseptic technique should be strictly adhered to and any manipulation that would further insult the blood supply should be avoided [2,4].

To help diminish radiation injury, an acemannan-containing hydrogel (CarraVet Wound Gel; Veterinary Products Laboratories, Phoenix, Arizona) can be applied to the skin daily, beginning on the day radiation therapy starts and continued for at least 2 weeks [2,40].

Treatment of dermal lesions includes keeping the area clean and preventing self-mutilation, especially when the sign is moist desquamation [2,39]. Topical application of an acemannan-containing hydrogel or silver sulfadiazine cream can be used [2].

Staged debridement over a longer period than for other wounds should be used on ulcers caused by progression of necrosis [39]. Debridement should only remove visible necrotic tissue and not be taken back to bleeding edges [39]. Enzymatic and adherent bandage debridement can be considered for use in conjunction with surgery. Any debrided tissue should be submitted for histopathologic examination for tumor recurrence [2,4,39].

Prophylactic antibacterial therapy should be considered, because irradiated tissue has lowered resistance to infection. Antibacterial agents that sensitize to radiation should be avoided (ie, metronidazole), however [39]. Because of impaired circulation in the irradiated tissue, topical antibacterial agents may have an advantage over systemic antibiotics (see article by Krahwinkel and Booth elsewhere in this issue) [2].

If a skin graft is considered for reconstruction of an irradiated area, the area must be completely debrided to healthy vascular tissue. Skin, muscle, myocutaneous, and omental flaps should be considered for reconstruction because they carry their own inherent circulation. In addition, a graft can be applied or skin is provided with a muscle or myocutaneous flap. Small local flaps may be considered for small local lesions; however, it should be remembered that regional skin may have been negatively affected by radiation. Axial pattern skin flaps from an area distant to the irradiated area are well suited for reconstruction [2,4,39]. There exists the possibility that one of the wound healing stimulant drugs (see article by Krahwinkel and Booth elsewhere in this issue) can enhance vascularization of an irradiated area and result in a good graft bed.

Problem wounds in cats

In clinical practice, chronic wounds are not encountered as often in cats as in dogs [24]. Nonhealing wounds in cats have been associated with underlying causes, such as foreign bodies, neoplasms, immunosuppressive therapy, immunodeficiency, and hyperadrenocorticism, however [24]. Other causes associated with chronic wounds in cats include mycobacterial infections, bacterial L-forms, and viral feline cow pox [24,28]. Immunocompromised cats with feline immunodeficiency virus (FIV) or feline leukemia virus (FeLV) may have chronic open wounds [41]. Treatment of such chronic wounds centers around determining the underlying cause of the wound and correcting it if possible. The use of a wound healing stimulant medication could also be considered in treating such wounds (see article by Krahwinkel and Booth elsewhere in this issue). One author (SFS) has noticed, empirically, that some nonhealing wounds in cats that have not responded to other therapies have responded positively to topical application of a tripeptide-copper complex medication (see article by Krahwinkel and Booth elsewhere in this issue).

Underlying metabolic disease

Three underlying diseases of which a practitioner should be aware that can affect wound healing are Cushing's syndrome, diabetes mellitus, and hypothyroidism. Cushing's syndrome, hyperadrenocorticism, may be a spontaneous pituitary-related disorder manifested by a collection of clinical and biochemical abnormalities, or it may be iatrogenic. There is an overproduction of cortisol by the adrenal cortices or prolonged administration of corticosteroids, respectively [42]. The effect on wound healing would be similar to what is seen with the effects of corticosteroids on healing (see section on corticosteroids and chemotherapy in this article).

Diabetes in human beings has a marked effect on wound healing related to a combination of peripheral neuropathy and angiopathy. There are also abnormalities in leukocyte function, cell adherence, chemotaxis, and collagen synthesis. Although diabetes has not been reported to cause complications in surgery or delayed wound repair in animals, the possibility should be considered. A diabetic animal may be more susceptible to wound infections because of compromised leukocyte function [1].

Hypothyroidism may also have a negative effect on wound healing. A thyroid function test should be included in the evaluation of chronic wounds. One author (SFS) has found hypothyroidism to be associated with the chronic infection or wounds associated with chronic fibrosing interdigital pyoderma [43].

PSEUDOHEALING

"Pseudohealing" is a phenomenon that is usually associated with animal bite wounds [2,8]. As teeth puncture the skin, subcutaneous tissue is inoculated with bacteria from the attacker's mouth and the skin and hair coat of the victim. The puncture wound may be small; however, the "iceberg" effect may be present (ie, what is seen on the surface is minor compared with what is below the surface). Underlying tissue is badly damaged as the attacker shakes its head. The puncture wound heals quickly (pseudohealing); however, the extensive damage to underlying tissue combined with its inoculum provides an environment conducive to abscessation. The authors' experience has been that the condition is more prevalent in cats than in dogs and that cat-fight abscesses are common in practice. The abscess spreads beneath the skin, going unnoticed until a large segment of skin sloughs, leaving a sizable open wound (Fig. 6). A similar situation can occur with premature closure of a contaminated wound after insufficient debridement [2,8]. It is best to debride bite wounds thoroughly and to manage them as open wounds for a few days before delayed closure (see article by Trout and Pavletic elsewhere in this issue).

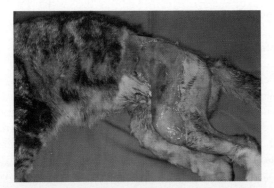

Fig. 6. Extensive wound on a cat's hindquarters resulting from skin slough subsequent to pseudohealing and large subcutaneous abscess development.

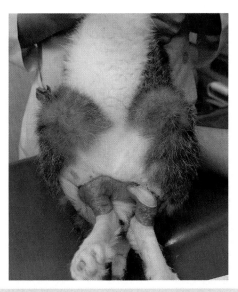

Fig. 7. Severe wound contracture deformity on a cat resulting from open-wound healing of a large wound that covered the flexion surfaces of the stifle joints, medial femoral areas, and ventral pelvic area.

ABNORMAL HEALING (WOUND CONTRACTURE)

With open-wound healing, fibroblasts, myofibroblasts, and collagen of granulation tissue represent the seat of the contraction that occurs during the repair stage [2,12]. When the contraction of second-intention healing of a large wound takes place over the flexion surface of a joint, folding or bunching and bonding of collagen fibers may occur with flexion. The result is contracture such that joint extension is severely limited, which can lead to disuse atrophy of muscles (Fig. 7). Physical therapy, including passive range-of-motion exercises, during the healing stages can help to prevent this contracture. The principles of closing a large wound over a flexion surface and correcting a wound contracture scar are the same; however, with the latter, the scar tissue is removed first. Depending on the size and location of the wound, moving local tissue, a skin flap, or a skin graft can be used to close the wound [2,12]. If the contracture is in the form of a narrow band (ie, bow-string scar), multiple Z-plasties along the scar can lengthen the area to relieve contracture [2].

SUMMARY

There are numerous reasons why some wounds do not heal in a normal manner as described in the article by Hosgood elsewhere in this issue. When the practitioner encounters such a wound, it is not uncommon to follow the natural instinct to place various medications and dressings on the wound to control microorganisms or to enhance healing. When a wound does not heal properly, however, it is important to consider the history, animal, wound, and environment to ascertain the reason why the wound is not healing or has not healed properly. In other words, underlying causes need to be assessed, and appropriate corrective measures need to be taken for treatment.

Acknowledgments

The authors thank Barbara Glass for her assistance in preparing the manuscript of this article.

References

[1] Hosgood G. Wound repair and specific tissue response to injury. In: Slatter DH, editor. Textbook of small animal surgery. 3rd edition. Philadelphia: WB Saunders; 2003. p. 66–86.

[2] Swaim SF, Henderson RA. Small animal wound management. 2nd edition. Baltimore: Williams & Wilkins; 1997. p. 1–12,143–90, 87–141, 295–370.

[3] Gregory CR. Wound healing and influencing factors. In: Fowler D, Williams JM, editors. Manual of canine and feline wound management and reconstruction. Shurdington, Cheltenham (UK): British Small Animal Veterinary Association; 1999. p. 13–23.

[4] Pavletic MM. Atlas of small animal reconstructive surgery. 2nd edition. Philadelphia: WB Saunders; 1999. p. 41–63, 65–106, 131–71.

[5] Trout NJ. Principles of plastic and reconstructive surgery. In: Slatter DH, editor. Textbook of small animal surgery. 3rd edition. Philadelphia: WB Saunders; 2003. p. 274–92.

[6] Hedlund C. Surgery of the integumentary system. In: Fossum TW, editor. Small animal surgery. 2nd edition. St. Louis (MO): Mosby; 2002. p. 134–228.

[7] Mason LK. Treatment of contaminated wounds, including wounds of the abdomen and thorax. In: Harari J, editor. Surgical complications in wound healing in the small animal practice. Philadelphia: WB Saunders; 1993. p. 33–62.

[8] Swaim SF. Surgery of traumatized skin management and reconstruction in the dog and cat. Philadelphia: WB Saunders; 1980. p.119–213.

[9] Swaim SF, Angarano DW. Chronic problem wounds of dog limbs. Clin Dermatol 1990;8(3/4):175–86.

[10] Swaim SF, Hanson RR, Coates JR. Pressure wounds in animals. Compend Contin Educ Pract Vet 1996;18(3):203–19.

[11] Nwomeh B, Yager DR, Kelman CI. Physiology of the chronic wound. Clin Plast Surg 1998;25(3):341–56.

[12] Swaim SF, Hinkle SH, Bradley DM. Wound contraction: basic and clinical factors. Compend Contin Educ Pract Vet 2001;23(1):20–34.

[13] Swaim SF, Lee AH, Henderson RA. Mobility vs. immobility in the healing of open wounds. J Am Anim Hosp Assoc 1989;25:91–6.

[14] Johnson AL, Hulse DA. Other diseases of bones and joints. In: Fossum TW, editor. Small animal surgery. 2nd edition. St. Louis (MO): Mosby; 2002. p. 1168–91.

[15] Bubenik CJ, Smith MM. Orthopaedic infections. In: Slatter DH, editor. Textbook of small animal surgery. 3rd edition. Philadelphia: WB Saunders; 2003. p. 1862–75.

[16] Hurwitz DJ. Osseous interference of soft tissue healing. Surg Clin North Am 1984;64: 699–704.

[17] Bradley DM, Swaim SF, Stuart SW. An animal model for research on wound healing over exposed bone. Vet Comp Orthop Traumatol 1998;11:131–5.

[18] Bradley DM. The effects of topically applied acemannan on the healing of wounds with exposed bones [doctoral dissertation]. Auburn (AL): Auburn University; 1998.

[19] Lee AH, Swaim SF, Newton JC, et al. Wound healing over denuded bone. J Am Anim Hosp Assoc 1987;23(1):75–84.

[20] Clark GN. Bone perforation to enhance wound healing over exposed bone with shearing injuries. J Am Anim Hosp Assoc 2001;37(3):215–7.

[21] Swaim SF, Riddell KP, McGuire JA. Effects of topical medications on healing of open pad wounds in dogs. J Am Anim Hosp Assoc 1992;28(6):499–502.

[22] Swaim SF, Marghitu DB, Rumph PF, et al. Effects of bandage configuration on paw pad pressure in dogs: a preliminary study. J Am Anim Hosp Assoc 2003;39(2):209–16.

[23] Swaim SF. Bandaging and splinting techniques. In: Bistner SI, Ford RB, Raffe MR, editors. Handbook of veterinary procedures and emergency treatment. 7th edition. Philadelphia: WB Saunders; 2000. p. 549–71.

[24] Brockman DJ, Pardo AD, Conzemius MG, et al. Omentum-enhanced reconstruction of chronic nonhealing wounds in cats: techniques and clinical use. Vet Surg 1996;25(2): 99–104.

[25] Hunt GB. Skin fold advancement flaps for closing large sternal and inguinal wounds in cats and dogs. Vet Surg 1995;24(2):172–5.

[26] Wykes PM. Cutaneous sinus tracts of the dog. Compend Contin Educ Pract Vet 1982;4(4): 293–6.

[27] White RAS. Surgical treatment of specific skin disorders. In: Slatter DH, editor. Textbook of small animal surgery. 3rd edition. Philadelphia: WB Saunders; 2003. p. 339–55.

[28] Beale KM. Nodules and draining tracts. Vet Clin North Am Small Anim Pract 1995;25(4): 887–97.

[29] Kehoe A, Elmore M. Woundoscopy: a new technique for examining deep nonhealing wounds. Ostomy Wound Manage 2002;48(4):30–3.

[30] Dowe G, Browne AMB, Sibbald RG. Infection in chronic wounds: controversies in diagnosis and treatment. Ostomy Wound Manage 1999;45(8):23–40.

[31] Browne AMB, Dowe G. Infected wounds: definitions and controversies. In: Falanga V, editor. Cutaneous wound healing. London (UK): Martin Dunitz; 2001. p. 203–19.

[32] Laing EJ. The effects of chemotherapy and radiation on wound healing. In: Harari J, editor. Surgical complications and wound healing in the small animal practice. Philadelphia: WB Saunders; 1993. p. 125–41.

[33] Cornell K, Water DJ. Impaired wound healing in the cancer patient: effects of cytotoxic therapy and pharmacologic modulation by growth factors. Vet Clin North Am Small Anim Pract 1995;25(1):111–31.

[34] Forks TP. Brown recluse spider bites. J Am Board Fam Pract 2000;13(6):415–23.

[35] Sams HH, Dunnick CA, Smith ML, et al. Necrotic arachnidism. J Am Acad Dermatol 2001;44(4):561–73.

[36] Crane SW. Nutritional aspects of wound healing. Semin Vet Med Surg (Small Anim) 1989;4(4):263–7.

[37] Noffsinger GR, McMurray BL, Jones TJ. Proteins in wound healing. J Am Vet Med Assoc 1957;131(10):481–5.

[38] Dernell WS, Wheaton LG. Surgical management of radiation injury: part I. Compend Contin Educ Pract Vet 1995;17(2):181–93.

[39] Dernell WS, Wheaton LG. Surgical management of radiation injury: part II. Compend Contin Educ Pract Vet 1995;17(4):499–510.

[40] Roberts DB, Travis EL. Acemannan-containing wound dressing gel reduces radiation induced skin reaction in C3H mice. Int J Radiat Oncol Biol Phys 1995;32(4):1047–52.

[41] Norsworthy GD. Fight wound infections. In: Norsworthy GD, Crystal MA, Tilley LP, editors. The feline patient: essentials of diagnosis and treatment. Baltimore: Williams & Wilkins; 1998. p. 215–8.

[42] Kintzer PP, Peterson ME, Mullen HS. Diseases of the adrenal gland. In: Birchard SJ, Sherding RG, editors. Saunders manual of small animal practice. 2nd edition. Philadelphia: WB Saunders; 2000. p. 259–73.

[43] Swaim SF, Lee AH, MacDonald JM, et al. Fusion podoplasty for treatment of chronic fibrosing interdigital pyoderma in the dog. J Am Amin Hosp Assoc 1991;27(3):264–74.

Vet Clin Small Anim 36 (2006) 713–738

VETERINARY CLINICS
SMALL ANIMAL PRACTICE

Initial Wound Management

William S. Dernell, DVM, MS

Animal Cancer Center, Colorado State University, Veterinary Teaching Hospital,
300 West Drake, Fort Collins, CO 80523, USA

INITIAL PATIENT ASSESSMENT

The steps involved in initial patient assessment are dependent on the cause of the wound. The algorithm in Fig. 1 is an example of potential decision making in the initial management of a wound. All wound management needs to be done as part of the overall patient assessment. Classic traumatic wounds, such as vehicle or animal fight trauma, require careful and detailed patient assessment before any intensive wound care is initiated. At the same time, the wound needs to be protected so that further injury or contamination is limited. Some form of protective bandage, with or without rigid stabilization, is indicated. For truncal wounds, this may be more complicated but may be as simple as a topical wound dressing. In more serious wounds, an adhesive drape material can be placed over the wound, with or without topical medications. If microbial assessment of the wound is planned, culture samples should be taken before topical or systemic antimicrobial treatment is initiated. Body wraps can also be used, but care must be taken when manipulating the patient before a detailed assessment is performed.

Posttrauma Patient Assessment

Immediate assessment of the "ABC's" (airway, breathing, and circulation) is warranted in any severely traumatized patient and should be assessed before addressing wound coverage or further assessment. Hemorrhagic wounds should have pressure bandages applied immediately to prevent hypotensive shock, however. Once the patient is stabilized, a thorough physical examination should be performed to assess critical systems first and then to assess the wound(s). Analgesics should be administered to patients that are in pain, especially before manipulation; however, the adverse effects of such drugs in light of the patient's overall condition need to be considered. For example, the potential for respiratory depression from narcotics in patients with respiratory compromise should be considered. It is essential that a thorough neurologic examination be completed before the administration of analgesics. Table 1 lists analgesic and sedative agents commonly used for trauma patients

E-mail address: wdernell@colostate.edu

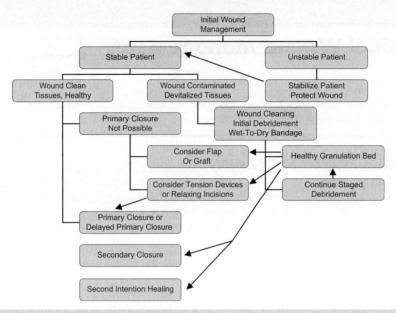

Fig. 1. Flow chart of representative decision points and options for initial would management.

[1,2]. If fractures or joint instability are encountered, some form of temporary stabilization should be applied. This might be in the form of a splint or rigid bandage (see the article by Campbell elsewhere in this issue). If the wound area is also involved in this area of stabilization, a temporary dressing may be needed. Until the patient is sufficiently stabilized that the wound can undergo initial treatment, the wound can be covered with sterile water-soluble jelly or a water-soluble antibacterial ointment (see the article by Krahwinkel and Boothe elsewhere in this issue) [3–13] and then with a light cotton wrap, followed by an outer wrap [3,14]. Again, microbial sampling should take place before antimicrobial therapy. The topical treatment keeps bandage material from adhering to the tissues and decreases further contamination. A water-soluble topical dressing also facilitates wound cleaning later.

Initial Wound Assessment

Once any life-threatening injuries are assessed and the patient is stabilized, a thorough examination of the wounded area should proceed. The cause of the wound, if not known, should be determined if possible. Wounds caused by different types of insults can have disparate levels of tissue damage, contamination, treatment approaches, and prognoses (Table 2,3) [3,14]. In some cases, such as postoperative incisional dehiscence, the degree of damage can more easily be assessed and visual inspection alone can provide sufficient information to allow the formulation of an initial treatment plan. Assessment of the degree of damage can be more difficult in some wounds. For example, crushing injuries can be associated with little external tissue damage noted early; however, because of deeper tissue damage and vascular compromise, the result can be progression of the wound over 12 to 24 hours to extensive tissue loss. Bite wounds can also appear minor superficially yet be associated with extensive deep tissue damage, and they can be associated with vascular damage because of tearing of the dermis from the subcutaneous plexus (ie, the "iceberg effect"), with most of the significant damage being below the surface. The article by Pavletic and Trout elsewhere in this issue discusses specific factors and treatment involved in burn, bullet, and bite wounds. If such injuries are known or suspected, initial wound cleaning, minor debridement, and temporary wound dressing may be preferred over any aggressive wound treatment so as to allow time for better establishment of tissue damage (ie, the use of staged debridement). Aggressive immediate intervention in these cases can result in removal of tissue that may actually be viable but was in a state of vascular stasis. Placing the patient under sedation or anesthesia for a procedure that might need to be repeated later might end up in a much more aggressive procedure (eg, amputation because of extensive tissue damage), or might be putting that patient at unnecessary risk.

The level of tissue damage and risk can usually be assessed adequately within 24 hours [14]. It is rare that the risk of delaying aggressive wound management immediately after trauma exceeds the risk of acting too quickly, resulting in inadequate or excessive treatment. During this waiting period, analgesic (see Table 1), systemic (Table 4), and topical anti-infective agents and physical support are warranted [2,3]. Systemic antibiotics should be considered if muscle and fascia are disturbed, if the animal is severely immunocompromised, or if signs of local or systemic infection exist. The most common bacterial organisms involved in external (surface) wounds are coagulase-positive staphylococci and *Escherichia coli* [2,3].

Clipping of the hair around the wound is part of the preoperative preparation, and it facilitates wound inspection. Before clipping, the placement of sterile water-soluble gel within the wound or packing the wound with sterile saline-soaked gauze keeps hair from further contaminating the wound. The hair on the wound edges can be removed using scissors with sterile gel on the blades to trap the hair [3]. Initial wound cleaning may facilitate wound inspection, especially that of the deeper tissues. This can sometimes be done without chemical restraint, but for the severely traumatized or painful patient, sedation can facilitate adequate cleaning (see Table 1). In cases of severe contamination, simple initial cleansing can be performed with warm tap water. This is best done using a gentle spray device. The advantage to this method is that large volumes can be used, facilitating removal of debris. In addition, the spray action facilitates debris removal. Tap water has been shown to be cytotoxic to fibroblasts, but in cases in which removal of debris and initial contamination outweigh the risk of tissue damage, this is appropriate [2]. If there is minimal to moderate contamination, initial wound cleaning should be facilitated with

Table 1
Analgesic, sedative, and induction agents commonly used for trauma patients

Analgesic agent	Dose[a]	Advantages	Disadvantages	Comments
Local blocks	Lidocaine[b,c] 2%, 2.0 mg/kg Bupivicaine[c] 0.5%, 1.5 mg/kg	Inexpensive Low toxicity Minimal systemic effects	No systemic sedation	Lidocaine can be sprayed onto sterile gauze packed within the wound
Analgesic tranquilizer[d]	Ketamine: Dog: 10–21 mg/kg IM, 2.2–4.4 mg/kg IV Cat: 6–10 mg/kg IM Diazapam: 0.25–0.75 mg/kg IV	Immobilization Sedation	Mild to moderate analgesia	Can be used as induction agent
Bupenorphine	0.006–0.02 mg/kg IV, IM, SQ	Good for moderate pain	Mild respiratory depression	Has dose plateau
Medetomidine	0.0025–0.01 mg/kg IV, IM, SQ	Profound immobilization Good analgesia	Respiratory depression (especially with opioid)	Often combined with local analgesia
Butorphanol	Dog: 0.2–0.5 mg/kg IM, SQ, IV Cat: 0.2–0.8 mg/kg	Can be partially reversed	Limited analgesic efficacy and duration	Good for restraint with tranquilizer
Morphine	Dog: 0.2–1 mg/kg Cat: 0.1–0.4 mg/kg IM, SQ	Rapid onset Potent Inexpensive	Controlled substance Respiratory depression Vocalization and dysphoria Vomiting Histamine release if given IV	Can follow-up with oral (sustained release) tablets
Oxymorphone	Dog: 0.05–0.2 mg/kg IM, SQ, IV Cat: 0.02–0.1 mg/kg IM, SQ, IV	Rapid onset Potent Less vocalization or dysphoria	Controlled substance Respiratory depression	More consistent response than morphine

	Dose			
Hydromorphone	Dog: 0.05–0.2 mg/kg IM, SQ, IV Cat: 0.02–0.1 mg/kg IM, SQ, IV	Rapid onset Potent Inexpensive	Respiratory and cardiovascular depression Vomiting	More readily available than oxymorphone
Fentanyl	2–10 ug/kg[e]	Potent analgesic Rapid onset Rapid clearance	Short acting Potential apnea	Best used as a constant rate infusion
NSAIDs	Variable	Low toxicity Anti-inflammatory	Inadequate for higher level pain	Often used in combination Contraindicated with steroids
Thiobarbiturates[f]	10–15 mg/kg IV	Ultrashort-acting induction agent	No residual analgesia Rough recovery if not premedicated	Usually used for induction of general anesthesia
Propofol	Dog: 4–6 mg/kg IV Cat: 6–8 mg/kg IV	Induction agent Moderate anesthesia length High safety index	No residual analgesia Respiratory depression Induction apnea	Usually used for induction of general anesthesia

Abbreviations: IV, intravenous; IM, intramuscular; NSAID, nonsteroidal anti-inflammatory drug; SQ, subcutaneous.

[a] Unless specified, dose is the same for the dog and the cat.
[b] Adding sodium bicarbonate (0.1) per milliliter of lidocaine decrease's the initial discomfort.
[c] Lidocaine/bupivicaine doses are maximum tolerated systemic doses (MTDs). Local anesthetics are generally dosed to effect, remaining below the MTD.
[d] Ketamine: valium as an example. One may combine a narcotic with a sedative agent. In such cases, the narcotic can be reversed if needed.
[e] Also available in transdermal patches (Duragesic; Janssen Pharmaceutical, Titusville, NJ); dosing is not well established and absorption/blood levels are variable and delayed.
[f] Thiopental as an example.
Data from Bellah JR, Williams JM. Wound closure options and decision making. In: Fowler D, Williams JM, editors. Manual of canine and feline wound management and reconstruction. Chellenham (UK): British Small Animal Veterinary Association; 1999. p. 25–36; and Williams JM. Open wound management. In: Fowler D, Williams JM, editors. Manual of canine and feline wound management and reconstruction. Chellenham (UK): British Small Animal Veterinary Association; 1999. p . 37–46.

Table 2
Unique features of common wound classifications

Classification	Causes	Unique features	Treatment approaches
Incisional	Surgical scalpel Knife blade Needles Arrows Nails Glass	Depth may vary Deep tissue damage possible Relatively clean injuries Increased blood loss Minimal tissue trauma	May be closed primarily if early from wounding Usually minimal debridement needed Inspection of deeper tissue important
Puncture	Fight injury Knife blade Needles Arrows Nails Glass Plant parts	Can be extensive deep injury Vascular compromise possible Contamination via puncture wounds Body cavity penetration possible Retained foreign body	Delayed closure beneficial Deep exploration beneficial Systemic anti-infective agents beneficial Thorough patient assessment essential
Abrasions	Automobile trauma Pad trauma	Heavy contamination common Deep penetration of debris and organisms Potential skin loss	Extensive cleaning and debridement needed Delayed closure beneficial If epidermis intact, should heal without surgery
Traumatic degloving or shearing injury	Automobile trauma Fight injury	Vascular damage possible May be associated with orthopedic injury Minimal to moderate contamination	Stabilization/treatment of orthopedic injury Delayed or secondary closure beneficial May require flaps/grafts
Physiologic degloving	Vascular injury	Minimal contamination Slow progressive course of tissue damage/loss	Delayed treatment, repeated debridement essential

Etiology	Cause	Characteristics	Management
Avulsion	Fight injury	Can be extensive deep injury; Vascular compromise possible; Contamination via puncture wounds of bites	Delayed closure beneficial; Deep exploration beneficial; Systemic anti-microbial agents beneficial
Cast/bandage	Inappropriate bandage application or care	Vascular compromise possible pressure; Joint injury possible; Gangrenous changes possible	If epidermis intact, should heal without surgery; Surgical repair of full-thickness wound; Amputation of avascular tissues if severe
Projectiles (see the article by Pavletic and Trout in this issue)	Low-velocity firearms	Deep tissue damage possible; Entry contamination possible	May not require surgical management (without body cavity penetration, surgical exploration with body cavity penetration); Systemic anti-microbial agents beneficial
Projectiles (see the article by Drs. Pavletic and Trout in this issue)	High-velocity firearms	Deep tissue damage likely; Large exit wounds likely; Orthopedic injury likely	Wound exploration/tissue debridement (with body cavity penetration)
Venomous bites	Snakes Spiders Scorpions	Vascular damage possible; Slow progressive course of tissue damage/loss	Second-intention or delayed closure beneficial; Systemic therapy may be essential
Burns (see the article by Drs. Pavletic and Trout in this issue)	Thermal Chemical Electrical	Systemic effects possible; Secondary infection common; Deep tissue damage possible; Wound contraction complications possible for deep burns	Assess patient for systemic effects; Early and repeated debridement beneficial; Reconstructive surgery for deep burns

Data from White RAS. The aetiology and classification of wounds and skin deficits. In: Fowler D, Williams JM, editors. Manual of canine and feline wound management and reconstruction. Cheltenham (UK): British Small Animal Veterinary Association; 1999. p. 5–12.

Table 3
Unique features of wounds classified by level and duration (class) of contamination (3)

Classification[a]	Degree of contamination	Duration of contamination	Comments
Clean class I	Minimal	0–6 hours	Surgically created under asepsis. No invasion of contaminated organ systems
Clean-contaminated class I	Minimal	0–6 hours	Operative wounds of contaminated organ systems (respiratory, alimentary, urogenital)
Contaminated class II or class III	Significant or gross	6–12 hours (class II) >12 hours (class III)	Open traumatic wounds ± debris Operative wounds without asepsis Incisions into inflammation/ contamination
Dirty/infected class III	Gross	>12 hours	Old traumatic wounds Infected wounds Perforated viscera

[a]Class of the wound relates to its duration.
   Data from Swaim SF, Henderson RA. Wound management. In: Swaim SF, Henderson RA, editors. Small animal wound management. 2nd edition. Baltimore (MD): Williams & Wilkins; 1997. p. 13–51.

normal saline or dilute antiseptic solution, such as 0.05% chlorhexidine or 1% povidone-iodine solution. The former can be safely used in any situation, and the latter aids in decreasing bacterial contamination without resulting in substantial damage to exposed tissues. Because it is the physical aspect of wound cleansing (flushing) that is beneficial, antiseptic solutions may not be necessary, depending on the level of contamination. Physical flushing with saline or other sterile liquids can be facilitated by connecting a syringe to a three-way stopcock, which, in turn, is connected to a fluid bag. This allows rapid filling of the syringe without the potential for contamination by filling by pouring or placing the syringe tip into a bowl. Appropriate pressure (4–15 psi) can be accomplished using a 20-mL syringe fitted with an 18-gauge needle. Higher pressures can result in driving debris and bacteria deeper into tissues rather than facilitating their removal [2].

Diagnostic wound evaluations
Once the wound is assessable, a careful examination needs to be performed. Analgesia or sedation may be needed, because the wound needs to be aggressively explored (probed) to assess the level of injury and the tissue involved. This exploration must be conducted carefully, especially for wounds over body cavities, to safeguard against inadvertent contamination of deep tissues or exposure of the pleural or peritoneal cavities [15]. Wound communication with body cavities and the degree of deep tissue involvement must be determined, however. Sterile instruments and aseptic technique should be practiced

Table 4
Systemic antimicrobial agents commonly used for trauma patients

Agent	Dose[a]	Advantages	Disadvantages	Comments
Clavulanic acid-potentiated amoxicillin	13.75 mg/kg BID	Broad spectrum Inexpensive	Pseudomonas spp show resistance	Potential gastrointestinal upset
Second-generation cephalosporins	20 mg/kg TID	Broad spectrum Inexpensive	Pseudomonas spp show resistance	Not effective for anaerobes
Potentiated sulphonamides	Variable	Broad spectrum Inexpensive	Poor tissue penetration into abscesses or necrotic tissue	Resistance common
Fluoroquinolones	5–11 mg/kg SID to BID	Broad spectrum	Anaerobes show resistance Expensive	Cartilage damage risk in young dogs
Aminoglycosides	Variable	High gram-negative affinity	Potential renal toxicity	Not for continuous use

Abbreviations: BID, twice daily; SID, once daily; TID, three times daily.
[a]Dosages apply for dogs and cats unless specified. Dosages are for oral or intravenous (when applicable) administration.
Data from Bellah JR, Williams JM. Wound closure options and decision making. In: Fowler D, Williams JM, editors. Manual of canine and feline wound management and reconstruction. Cheltenham (UK): British Small Animal Veterinary Association; 1999. p. 25–36.

during the initial wound exploration, regardless of the level of wound contamination.

Orthopedic injuries are to be noted, and an assessment of the importance of addressing them above and beyond the wound itself needs to be determined [3]. Radiographs or other imaging can then be planned based on the level of suspicion of orthopedic injury. If a fracture is found, temporary stabilization is essential before approaching any wound care. If the fracture is open, it is important not to push the penetrating fracture ends back beneath the skin; rather, the limb should be splinted in its present position. Reduction of this open fracture needs to be delayed until sterile operative conditions can be met so as to minimize deep tissue contamination from the skin penetration.

If tendons, supportive ligaments, or major nerves are found to be severed, an attempt at aggressive surgical debridement of the wound and these structures as well as primary suturing should be planned as soon as the patient is stabilized. Any delay in attempts at primary reanastomosis of tendons, ligaments, or nerves results in tissue contraction and an inability to appose the ends later without undue tension. If severe trauma to the surrounding tissues exists, primary anastomosis of tendons, ligaments, and nerves can be performed to combat contraction while the surrounding tissues undergo staged debridement. Delayed secondary anastomosis can then be performed once the surrounding tissues are healthy. Suturing techniques have been described for posttraumatized tendons, ligaments, and nerves [16–20].

In most cases, severed vessels need not be repaired, because collateral circulation maintains viability. Repair of large vessels is feasible and can be attempted [21]. Evidence of an open joint (usually after shearing injury) also mandates immediate care [22]. After cleaning and copious lavage, an attempt should be made to suture any remaining joint capsule and ligament structures to help stabilize the joint. After wound debridement and joint closure, external stabilization should be used (as part of the bandage support) to decrease continued damage to capsular and intra-articular tissues.

If significant contamination is suspected or there is evidence of established infection, initial antimicrobial therapy (see Table 4) can be guided by a Gram stain of the wound to establish the predominant bacterial population [3]. Culture samples can be obtained from the wound during the initial wound exploration or during initial debridement. The advantage of obtaining culture samples during initial debridement is that sampling can occur from deeper tissues after removal of superficial (highly contaminated) tissues, resulting in a sample more representative of the level of infection and the organisms involved. In addition, it is easier to obtain a small sample of tissue for submission during initial debridement. This is usually more effective in obtaining representative cultures than surface swabs, which are often the only viable culturing method if the patient is not sedated or anesthetized. If antimicrobial flush solutions are employed during initial debridement, however, samples need to be obtained before these solutions are used. Tissue samples are best submitted using a culture transport device (medium). Surface swabs are often not representative of deeper and more pathogenic organisms that may be present. Systemic antimicrobial therapy is initiated or changed (if previously initiated) based on culture results or clinical changes.

If vascular compromise to area larger than the immediate wound is suspected, ultrasound and scintigraphy techniques may be beneficial, if available [23]. These diagnostics may help in the decision regarding the timing of attempted closure. Any indication of vascular compromise warrants a delay in closure and reassessment. It is certainly possible that collateral circulation may compensate and regions initially compromised may remain viable. More definitive tests of tissue vascularity and viability are presently lacking beyond clinical reassessment over time.

For chronic draining wounds or tracts, preoperative diagnostic steps can include plain radiographs or ultrasound to look for the presence of a foreign body, CT or MRI to evaluate for levels and degrees of tissue disruption, and contrast studies (sinography) to evaluate invasion of drainage tracts [24,25]. Before surgical exploration and debridement, (sterile) methylene blue or scarlet red can be injected into a draining sinus to aid in location of dissecting tracts (see the article by Amalsadvala and Swaim elsewhere in this issue).

DECISION OF CLOSURE

There are various factors that influence the timing of wound closure (see Fig. 1). Once the wound has been thoroughly assessed, the first decision to be made is if and when to close the wound. If there is any question as to the level of contamination, potential for deep tissue injury, tissue viability, or vascular compromise, a delay in closure with repeated wound assessment should be considered. Patients with a high level of wound contamination or extensive tissue damage are at high risk for wound dehiscence unless appropriate initial wound care is undertaken. If there is a high likelihood of wound dehiscence, putting a patient through sedation or anesthesia to obtain primary closure may be placing that patient under undue risk for little potential gain. Clean wounds treated within 24 hours of initial wounding (especially incisional injuries) can be managed by wound cleaning and primary closure. Beyond immediate primary closure, wound closure options include delayed primary closure, secondary closure, and second-intention healing (Table 5) [1]. If tissue loss exists but the wound is fresh and clean, partial primary closure can be attempted

Table 5
Wound closure options based on time from wounding and wound factors

Technique	Time from wounding	Factors
Primary closure	Within 24 hours	Minimal tissue damage Minimal contamination Closure at the time of initial wound cleaning and debridement Local tissue available for closure
Delayed primary closure	Within 3–5 days (before granulation tissue)	Minimal to moderate tissue damage Minimal to moderate contamination Closure after temporary dressing and several debridement attempts Closure timing based on healthy mobile wound tissues Local or distant tissue available for closure
Secondary closure	Longer than 5 days (after granulation tissue)	Extensive tissue damage or contamination Wounds requiring repeated debridement Closure timing based on healthy granulation bed Local or distant tissue available for closure
Second-intention healing	Variable	Variable wound factors Local or distant tissues may not be available Closure based on wound contraction and epithelialization

Data from Bellah JR, Williams JM. Wound closure options and decision making. In: Fowler D, Williams JM, editors. Manual of canine and feline wound management and reconstruction. Cheltenham (UK): British Small Animal Veterinary Association; 1999. p. 25–36; and Swaim SF, Henderson RA. Wound management. In: Swaim SF, Henderson RA, editors. Small animal wound management. 2nd edition. Baltimore (MD): Williams & Wilkins; 1997. p. 13–51.

with a plan to treat the unclosed portion as an open wound or closed using skin grafts or flaps.

The second decision involves that of in-house care versus referral to another facility. If referral is elected, initial wound care should involve basic wound cleaning and application of a bandage. Rigid limb support through the use of a splint or brace may be beneficial, especially if motion of the tissues could further compromise healing. The bandage may or may not include a topical treatment or specific wound dressing (see the articles by Hosgood, Krahwinkel and Boothe, and Campbell elsewhere in this issue). Systemic antimicrobial therapy and analgesics may be indicated (see Tables 1 and 4). The decision for referral can also be deferred to a later time point, depending on the response to initial care combined with the comfort level of the clinician concerning the prospective level of care needed or difficulty of final closure.

If in-house care is elected and immediate primary closure is not possible, the third decision involves multiple factors:

1. Need for further systemic patient support or stabilization
2. Need for further wound cleansing and debridement (Table 6)
3. Need for further diagnostic procedures
4. Prognosis for wound healing and return to function
5. Use of topical and systemic agents (see Table 4 and the article by Krahwinkel and Booth elsewhere in this issue)
6. Need for wound coverage and the type of bandage needed (see the articles by Hosgood and Campbell elsewhere in this issue)
7. Time frame of wound care expected
8. Outpatient versus inpatient care [26–30]

Debridement

Debridement is indicated any time that necrotic tissue or debris exists within a wound that was not removed by basic initial wound cleansing. Small amounts of debridement may be feasible without sedation or anesthesia, but it is more likely that some form of analgesia and chemical restraint are necessary, especially if aggressive surgical debridement is indicated (see Table 1). Minor wound debridement may be accomplished by spraying a topical anesthetic on the wound or by placing a gauze sponge soaked in local anesthetic. There are several techniques for accomplishing wound debridement (see Table 6 and the article by Krahwinkel and Booth in this issue).

Surgical debridement is most commonly used, especially in the earlier stages of wound care. It allows efficient and rapid removal of necrotic tissue and debris as well as thorough wound exploration. For large wounds and those with deep tissue injury, initial surgical debridement is imperative. The goal of surgical debridement is to remove all "obvious" necrotic tissue and debris. The most common method of surgical debridement uses a "layered" approach, removing the more superficial devitalized tissues first, followed by debridement of deeper tissues [3]. The assessment of tissue viability is subjective. The most reliable indicators of viability are color and attachment. If tissues are

Table 6
Common methods of wound debridement

Method	Agent(s)	Advantages	Disadvantages	Application
Surgical		Aggressive Rapid Effective Can apply to large areas	Viable tissues may be sacrificed Hemorrhage can be an issue	Extensive necrosis or debris Deep tissue damage
Enzymatic	Proteolytic enzymes	May not require anesthesia/surgery Used to supplement surgical debridement	Minimally effective	Minimal necrotic tissue and debris Liquefy tenacious exudate Outpatient treatment
Mechanical/bandage	Wet-to-dry or dry-to-dry dressings	Incorporated as part of bandage Exudate absorption occurs Used to supplement surgical debridement	Painful removal Can require multiple anesthesias	Minimal to moderate necrosis or debris
Interactive dressings	Hydrogels Hydrocolloids Alginates	Autolytic wound debridement Provides an environment to enhance healing	Expensive Can require frequent bandage changes	Moderate necrosis or debris Exudative wounds
Larval	Maggots (Lucillia sericata)	Specific to necrotic tissue only	Technicalities of application are involved Availability Limited to smaller wounds	Small wounds in locations in which minimal normal tissue can be sacrificed

Data from Williams JM. Open wound management. In: Fowler D, Williams JM, editors. Manual of canine and feline wound management and reconstruction. Cheltenham (UK): British Small Animal Veterinary Association; 1999. p. 37–46; and Swaim SF, Henderson RA. Wound management. In: Swaim SF, Henderson RA, editors. Small animal wound management. 2nd edition. Baltimore (MD): Williams & Wilkins; 1997. p. 13–51.

extremely light or dark and are not attached, they should be removed. Questionable tissue should be left in place and re-evaluated at a later time. Active bleeding from the cut surface can be one factor used to assess tissue viability. In nonvital tissue areas, aggressive sequential (layer by layer) debridement is often performed to the level where active bleeding is present from all remaining tissues in the wound. The surgeon must be aware that certain factors can affect the degree and volume of bleeding from tissues, such as systemic or local hypotension (decreases), tissue temperature (cold decreases and heat increases), vasodilation (increases), vasoconstriction (decreases), and coagulation defects (increases). The surgeon should be aware that vessels within a wound may initially be constricted as part of the response to trauma and the body's attempt to attain hemostasis. Thus, using active bleeding as a criterion for debridement could result in removing viable tissue. Multiple factors must be considered when assessing tissue viability by tissue blood loss.

Debridement of wounds while attempting to spare tissue requires a more conservative approach. A clear line of demarcation between dark tissues (dark blue or black) and normal color is a good indicator that the dark tissues are not viable. Blue or gray tissues are suspect, and pink or red tissues are usually viable. Numerous factors can also affect color, such as hypotension, vasodilation, edema, and tissue type. For example, tendinous and ligamentous tissues are more likely to be gray in color, despite being viable, whereas these colors in muscle are not favorable. Conservative debridement usually involves removal of obviously necrotic tissue only, with the plan to repeat this debridement later, thus allowing time to differentiate true tissue viability (ie, staged debridement).

Copious lavage should be done during debridement. For a description of the technique, the reader is referred to the section in this article on initial wound lavage for wound assessment. This can aid in the removal of debris, and rehydration of tissues can assist in the assessment of true tissue viability based on color changes. Surgical debridement is generally followed by mechanical debridement (ie, wet-to-dry bandages, interactive dressings). Interactive dressings interact with the wound tissues to enhance the healing process. These dressings include the hydrogels, hydrocolloids, alginates, and polyurethane foams. They retain varying amounts of moisture over a wound. The hydrogels, hydrocolloids, and alginates enhance autolytic debridement of wounds, and the moist environment associated with these dressings stimulates the healing process. A disadvantage of dressings that retain moisture is the danger of tissue maceration if tissue becomes too wet and excoriation (tissue damage from excessive proteolytic enzymes in chronic wounds) (see the articles by Hosgood and Campbell in this issue).

Another method of surgical debridement is en bloc debridement (Fig. 2). This method involves complete excision of all affected tissue, with a border of normal tissue. The primary wound can be packed with gauze and is temporarily closed. The excision is performed in normal tissue surrounding the wound, and the wound is not entered. This technique would be similar to

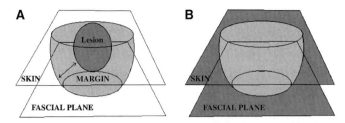

Fig. 2. Principle of en bloc debridement of a wound (lesion) within the skin and subcutaneous tissue. (A) Debridement is planned for complete removal of the lesion, with a cuff of normal tissue (margin) surrounding it. (B) Newly created wound (light area) is within normal healthy tissue. (*Modified from* Dernell WS, Withrow SJ. Preoperative patient assessment and margin evaluation. Clin Tech Small Anim Pract 1998;13(1):20; with permission.)

surgical removal of a malignancy [31]. En bloc resection is generally reserved for wounds that are obviously infected or where layered debridement would not likely result in a healthy wound. This method is best applied when there is adequate surrounding normal tissue to allow closure. Alternatively, the newly created wound can be treated as an open wound.

For fresh wounds with minimal to moderate contamination and without progressive damage, where surgical debridement and lavage are successful in removal of all necrosis and debris, delayed primary closure can be attempted at the time of initial surgical debridement. Alternatively, follow-up mechanical debridement may be enough to result in a wound bed (in a matter of days) that allows secondary closure. The veterinarian has wound closure options based on time from wounding and specific wound factors (see Table 5).

In many instances, a single debridement procedure is not adequate to result in a sufficiently healthy wound for primary or delayed primary closure. This is especially true for injuries that might involve progressive tissue changes attributable to vascular compromise or deep tissue injury. When multiple debridement attempts are anticipated or reassessment over time is important, covering the wound with an appropriate bandage or dressing after the initial debridement is essential (see the article by Campbell in this issue) [26–29]. This affords the opportunity to apply mechanical and/or bandage debridement or the interactive dressings [1,3].

Although there are numerous newer bandage materials that interact with wound tissues, a commonly used technique in early wound management is wet-to-dry dressings. Wet-to-dry dressings provide wound protection and coverage, initially maintain a moist environment, provide mechanical debridement, and absorb moderate amounts of exudates. These dressings are specifically applicable to wounds with viscous exudates and necrotic debris. Many early wounds, irrespective of the wound injury, fit into this category; therefore, wet-to-dry dressings have widespread application. After surgical debridement and wound cleaning, a moistened gauze square is unfolded and carefully layered within the wound, making an attempt to maximize contact with all surfaces of the wound. Several layers of wet gauze, followed by several layers of dry gauze, are sequentially added. The gauze is covered with an absorptive layer and, finally, an external layer. Modern wound care is finding that wet-to-dry dressings have limited indications, however. A controlled objective study comparing wet-to-dry dressings with interactive dressings in veterinary medicine is in order.

In truncal areas or areas in which it is difficult to apply a standard bandage, tie-over bandages can be used to maintain wet-to-dry dressings. A tie-over bandage can also be combined with wound tensioning devices to facilitate stretching of the skin during the initial wound care period, thus facilitating delayed closure. The standard technique of a tie-over bandage involves the placement of suture loops in the skin at the periphery of the wound. The saline-soaked gauze is placed over the wound, and a lap sponge, cotton roll, or some other absorptive material is then placed over this primary dressing (Fig. 3A, B). A nonpervious layer, such as paper drape material, is then placed (over the

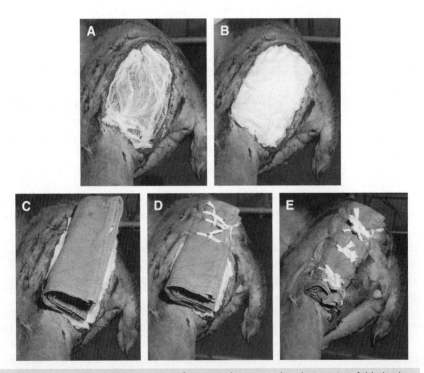

Fig. 3. Steps involved in the creation of a wet-to-dry tie-over bandage. (A) Unfolded saline-moistened gauze is placed over all surfaces of the wound in layers. (B) Laparotomy pad is placed over the gauze for absorption. (C) Folded surgical towel is placed over the laparotomy pad. (D) Tying umbilical tape segments over the towel between peripheral suture loops holds the dressing in place. (E) Connecting the umbilical tape cross-ties with bands of latex cut from latex gloves places constant inward tension on wound edges to facilitate wound contraction.

absorptive layer) to hold the moisture within the deeper layers as well as to protect the wound from ascending contamination. The bandage materials are then held on the wound by lacing umbilical tape between the suture loops with moderate tension (see Fig. 3C, D). Tension devices, such as segments of latex rubber, may be incorporated in the tie-over bandage to apply inward pressure on the wound edges (see Fig. 3E). It is recommended that two or three rows of suture loops be placed to permit the bandage lacing to progress outward from the wound as the skin stretches, allowing maintenance of wound edge tension. It is possible that interactive dressings could be applied in a similar way. An advantage to this type of wet-to-dry dressing compared with the use of some of the newer commercially available interactive dressings is its relative affordability.

Wet-to-dry bandages are typically changed daily. Ideally, the bandage should be changed before fluid strike-through is noted. Longer delays between changing any "wet" bandage often result in loss of the bandage's ability to absorb exudates. This causes prolonged contact between the exudate and the wound, which can cause a delay in wound healing and increase the chances of wound infection [27]. The ideal scenario is to have the wetness of the bandage dilute exudates so that they are absorbed in the secondary bandage layer. With evaporation of fluid from the bandage, it becomes partially dry. Debris and necrotic tissue adhere to the bandage in its dry state and are removed with the bandage (ie, mechanical debridement). If strike-through occurs, there is insufficient absorptive layering or the bandage was left on too long. Prolonged periods between bandage changes usually result in a profound odor to the bandage because of the biodegrading of exudates. Wet-to-dry bandages are usually combined with surgical debridement until the wound progresses to the point that debridement is no longer needed. At an early stage, this might be when wound tissues appear healthy and there is minimal exudate present. At this point, delayed primary closure can occur (see Table 5). At a later stage, this may be when a healthy granulation bed is forming within the wound and secondary closure can be considered. Once a healthy granulation bed has formed, wet-to-dry dressings are no longer needed. At this point, a semiocclusive nonadherent pad or polyurethane foam can be used. Occlusive hydrogel or hydrocolloid dressings are also appropriate (see the articles by Hosgood and Campbell in this issue). Throughout the initial wound management and healing process, topical treatments may be used (see the article by Krahwinkel and Boothe in this issue). In general, these do not add significantly to the progression of wound healing but may be applicable in specific circumstances.

Other less traditional wound debridement techniques can also be used as well, alone or in combination with surgical, mechanical, and autolytic debridement (see Table 6). Enzymatic debridement through the use of proteolytic enzymes or derivatives of bacteria (*Bacillus subtillus*) can be used in wounds with minimal necrotic tissue or debris (see the article by Krahwinkel and Boothe in this issue). These products offer little advantage over surgical, mechanical, or autolytic debridement, with the exception that they may be better adapted to outpatient treatment than repeated wet-to-dry bandaging [3].

Although more commonly employed in human medicine than in veterinary medicine, medical maggots (*Lucillia sericata*) can also be used for debridement. The advantage to these is that they debride necrotic tissue and spare healthy tissue. This may be advantageous for wounds in areas in which vital structures exist and aggressive surgical or mechanical debridement could result in loss of essential tissues [7,32,33].

For wounds with moderate to marked exudates in which the exudates may contact the skin, protection of the skin with petroleum-based ointments can help to avoid the dermatitis that can occur associated with contact from the exudates. Care must be taken to avoid placement of the petroleum ointments within the healing wound tissues, because this can delay healing [5].

Continued Therapy and Wound Reassessment

Depending on the type of wound care and the interval of any treatments, patients can be treated on an inpatient or outpatient basis. This also depends on financial constraints and the comfort level of owners. If any procedures are to be performed by an untrained owner, it is best to observe the owner doing the procedure to ensure that it is being done properly. For wounds that require prolonged and repeated treatments, a compromise can usually be achieved once the intensive initial therapy is replaced by less aggressive and more routine treatments.

Throughout the initial wound management phase, regardless of the plan for closure, continuous wound reassessment is essential. The response to surgical, mechanical, autolytic, or enzymatic debridement, as reflected in the appearance of the tissues, should guide the clinician as to the next logical step in the process as well as allowing more accurate assessment of the time involved to each point of wound progression. The response to initial management can also alert the clinician to problems in the healing process and related management so that adjustments can be made. An example might be that the lack of formation of healthy granulation tissue in a portion of a wound through the use of repeated mechanical debridement may prompt the intervention of surgical debridement to that area of tissue.

Alternative Therapies

Alternative therapies, such as acupuncture, electrical stimulation, laser light, stimulants, and growth factors, may have application in open wounds to accelerate healing and can be incorporated in the early management of wounds (see the article by Krahwinkel and Boothe in this issue) [11,12,34–37]. The factors that can influence wound healing are discussed (see the article by Hosgood in this issue).

There have been a considerable number of publications in the human literature as well as some recent work in veterinary medicine regarding the potential benefit of vacuum-assisted wound care [38]. This technique involves the placement of porous foam over the open wound. An egress tube is placed above the foam and covered by nonporous tape or another covering to seal the wound. The egress tube is then connected to a suction apparatus, and suction is applied to the wound. In one human study, vacuum-assisted treatment was shown to decrease the time to healing compared with wet-to-dry dressings from 42 to 22 days [39]. Proposed mechanisms include the continuous evacuation of exudates, bacteria, and proteolytic enzymes; mechanical stimulation of the tissue to accelerate granulation tissue formation; neovascularization; and a skin-stretching response at the periphery. Commercial vacuum units are available; however, units can be constructed. Caution must be used, because there may be a narrow range of effective pressures and there is some evidence that intermittent pressure or cycling may be of greater benefit than continuous cycling [40]. Different pressures may be needed for different types of wounds. Complications that have been reported include patient discomfort, sepsis, and anemia [40]. This method is not recommended in wounds with marked exudates or in those in which hemostasis is not adequate. More evaluation is needed in veterinary patients before this method can be routinely recommended.

DELAYED PRIMARY AND SECONDARY CLOSURE AND SECOND-INTENTION HEALING

Delayed primary closure involves initial wound cleaning and debridement, followed by one or two additional debridement attempts with or without bandage debridement (see Table 5). If this results in healthy tissues with minimal exudate in a relatively short time, closure can then be attempted using local tissues. Delayed primary closure is usually performed within 3 to 5 days after initial wounding, before the formation of granulation tissue and wound contraction. If mild to moderate tension is present, it can be overcome by undermining the wound edges and the use of various tension suture patterns with or without tension-relieving devices (eg, buttons, rubber tubing) and relaxing incisions [41–43]. The use of temporary tie-over pressure bandages can assist in management of wound tension immediately after surgery. If the wound is under excessive tension, further delay in closure (secondary closure) may be warranted and can be assisted through the use of skin-stretching devices or tissue expanders [43,44]. Alternatively, flaps or grafts can be used at the time of delayed primary closure (see the articles by Amalsadvala and Swaim, Fowler, and Hedlund elsewhere in this issue).

Secondary closure can occur at varying times after wounding but usually involves initial and follow-up wound cleaning after a healthy granulation bed has formed (see Table 5). Healthy granulation tissue signals the point at which necrotic tissue and debris have been adequately removed and the wound has sufficient blood supply. Areas within a wound that lack granulation tissue, or where the tissue is of questionable health, usually indicate the presence of damaged tissue or inadequate blood supply. In these instances, additional debridement or wound exploration is indicated. Granulation tissue formation over exposed bone may be facilitated by the technique of forrage, where small holes are drilled through the cortex into the medullary canal or the bone cortex is debrided, allowing neovascularization to occur from the inside of the bone

[45,46]. The use of swine intestinal submucosa (an acellular matrix dressing) has also been evaluated for enhancing wound healing over exposed bone [13].

Once secondary closure is elected, options include removal of the epithelium from the wound edge, with separation of the edge from the granulation tissue. This is followed by advancing the skin over the granulation bed for wound closure. Alternatively, the granulation tissue can be removed, followed by wound closure. This decision depends on the thickness of granulation tissue, the mobility of the skin edges, and the overall health of the granulation bed. Although removal of the granulation tissue sounds counterintuitive, granulation tissue can delay wound healing for flaps and local tissue plasties [3].

Granulation tissue is also an essential stage in wound healing by second intention (see the article by Hosgood in this issue). Granulation tissue contains fibroblasts and myofibroblasts that cause wound contraction. Granulation tissue also supplies nutrition and chemotaxis for epithelial cell migration from the wound edges to the center. In cases in which second-intention healing is elected, wound protection through bandaging, restraint devices, and exercise restriction is essential to protect the fragile healing tissues, specifically the newly forming epithelium [47]. If second-intention healing is selected and the wound reaches a point of stagnation (interrupted healing), secondary closure can again be considered.

WOUND DRAINAGE

The veterinarian has several options for wound drainage (Table 7) [48]. Surgical drains facilitate obliteration of dead space and provide a means for wound lavage. With primary, delayed primary, or secondary closure, the obliteration

Table 7
Common wound drainage methods

Drain method	Advantages	Disadvantages
Passive	Simple Inexpensive Can be used on outpatient basis	Can introduce organisms Messy Needs to be covered Must exit distant to primary wound Slower elimination of dead space
Active (suction)	More rapid elimination of dead space Less messy Can exit primary wound Does not require bandaging	Patient should be maintained in the hospital More expensive (commercial drains)
Combination (sump)	Used for wounds requiring lavage	Should be kept covered Risk of ascending contamination

Data from Swaim SF, Henderson RA. Wound management. In: Swaim SF, Henderson RA, editors. Small animal wound management. 2nd edition. Baltimore (MD): Williams & Wilkins; 1997. p . 13–51; and Baines SJ. Surgical drains. In: Fowler D, Williams JM, editors. Manual of canine and feline wound management and reconstruction. Cheltenham (UK): British Small Animal Veterinary Association; 1999. p. 47–55.

of dead space is an important consideration to facilitate wound healing. This is especially true for primary closure of contaminated wounds and closure of wounds with moderate exudates or transudates. Drains may also be beneficial in cases in which deep tacking sutures need to be avoided in closure because of the potential for compromising blood supply to a skin flap.

Passive drains are most commonly used. Penrose drains are placed within the dead space of a wound. They are tacked dorsally using a suture placed through the skin into the drain and back out of the skin. The ventral exit point is beyond the wound edge and in a location that uses gravity to help pull fluid along the drain and out of the wound. The use of double-exit (dorsal and ventral) passive drains is usually not necessary and can lead to an increased chance of ascending contamination. Multiple drains can be used in deep wounds closed in multiple layers. Passive drains should be covered with extra absorptive material within the bandage to collect drainage fluid. The frequency of bandage change needed is dependent on the amount of drainage that occurs. Drains should be left in place until the amount of drainage steadily decreases or the quality of the drainage changes from an exudate to a transudate. Drainage is not likely to stop completely, because the drain itself causes enough irritation to result in some drainage. A guideline for removing a drain is to remove it when drainage becomes minimal or is of approximately the same amount on consecutive days.

Active drains have the advantage of a more rapid effect on tissue attachment and drainage cessation. A negative suction drain tube is placed within the wound dead space and tacked using a suture if needed. It can exit from a small puncture wound adjacent to the closed wound or, alternatively, distant from the wound. These drains do not have to exit in a dependent location because they do not rely on gravity. Negative suction drains can be purchased from commercial suppliers (eg, Jorgensen Labs, Loveland, Colorado) or can be made from a syringe and intravenous tubing (Fig. 4A, B). For the latter, intravenous extension tubing is fenestrated after removal of the male end. The female end is connected to a large syringe, and holes are drilled into the syringe plunger. Once the tubing is placed into the wound and the drain exit site is sealed around the tube with a purse-string suture, negative pressure is applied to the syringe and a pin or large-gauge hypodermic needle is placed across the plunger to hold it in position for negative pressure in the syringe barrel. As the syringe fills and the negative pressure abates, the plunger is further withdrawn and a new pin or needle is placed. Once the syringe fills, it is disconnected and emptied. For smaller dogs and cats or for small wounds, a similar apparatus can be made using a butterfly catheter and red-topped Vacutainer tubes (see Fig. 4C). The female end is removed from the butterfly catheter, and the distal tube is fenestrated. The tube is buried in the wound through a small stab incision, with the needle end exiting. The needle is then placed into a Vacutainer tube, and the negative pressure draws fluid from the wound. Once the tube fills, it is replaced.

Combination drains can be placed to allow ingress and egress. This would be applied to a draining wound with dead space in which continuous or

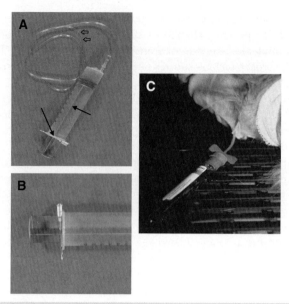

Fig. 4. Two forms of negative suction drainage. (A) Syringe system. Holes (*open arrows*) are made in intravenous extension tubing after removal of the male end. The female end is connected to a 60-mL syringe, and holes are drilled into the syringe plunger (*area between closed arrows*) so that a large hypodermic needle can be placed through them. (B) Close-up view of the hypodermic needle through the syringe plunger. (C) Vacutainer system. A fenestrated butterfly catheter with the female end removed has been placed in a closed wound. The male (needled) catheter end is inserted into a Vacutainer tube.

periodic wound lavage was needed. Continued wound lavage might be indicated for primary closure or delayed primary closure if there is concern that the wound may be highly contaminated or truly infected but closure is still elected. Wounds closed by secondary closure do not generally need lavage, because granulation tissue signals that contamination and/or infection is minimal. Combination drains can be purchased or can be made by inserting a stiff, fenestrated, red-rubber feeding tube or silastic tube through a Penrose or other passive drain tube. Both are secured within the wound. The stiff inner tube is used for ingress of lavage solution, and the passive tube is used for egress. In larger wounds, the ingress and egress drains can be placed separately (not one within the other). The egress drain in this case can be a negative suction drain. Ingress drains need to be well protected to minimize contamination when fluids are passed through them into the wound.

Regardless of the drain type, it is helpful to premeasure the drain length before implantation so that if problems arise on removal, it can be documented that the entire drain has been removed. Most drains are radiopaque; thus, broken segments can be located in a wound using radiography or in the gastrointestinal tract if the drain has been ingested.

FOLLOW-UP CARE AND WOUND REASSESSMENT

Once the wound has been closed, appropriate protection from self-trauma and environmental insult is needed. For most extremity and some truncal lesions, the placement of a short-term bandage is appropriate. This not only protects the wound from self-trauma and contact with the environment but helps to absorb any exudates. In addition, mild pressure to a wound surface can result in some local analgesia to the wound. If a drain is in place, bandaging is essential. For some truncal wounds, circumferential bandaging may not be feasible. In these cases, a tie-over bandage or another covering, such as a child's T-shirt, stockinet, or commercial Lycra body suit, can be used (see the article by Campbell in this issue). Elizabethan collars or restrictive neck collars or braces should be used in any case in which self-trauma is possible. Owners are often unaware of the deleterious effects of animals licking their wounds or of the short time frame within which an animal can completely destroy any closure attempt. If an open wound must be left uncovered, a water-soluble topical ointment can sometimes help to keep the wound surface moist and trap debris on the surface that might otherwise penetrate the wound. For a sutured wound, such ointment can help to keep the wound edges moist. If the wound is in an area in which there is a potential for urine or fecal soiling, a petroleum-based ointment affords better protection. If a passive drain is in place, the use of a petroleum-based ointment over the skin at the drain exit site can help to avoid the dermatitis that can result from contact with exudates.

Repeated follow-up is also essential to ensure rapid wound healing and to minimize complications. Evaluation of the closed wound would ideally be performed within 2 to 3 days to check the bandage or covering and to observe the condition of the wound. At this point, if there are questionable areas of the wound (ie, color changes), it is usually best to be conservative in management and allow the wound to define itself. Frequent rechecks until days 5 through 7 after closure are indicated. By day 7, most wound closures show evidence of healing, stasis, or dehiscence. If a wound is stagnant, continued observation may be best unless there are other clinical parameters that dictate otherwise. If dehiscence occurs, immediate resuturing is only indicated if the wound breakdown is thought to be a result of trauma or excessive tension if tension-relieving steps can be used to overcome the tension. Wound breakdown attributable to loss of tissue viability or infection is best treated as an open wound, returning to the steps initially described in the section of this article on initial management. Even if wound breakdown occurs, it is rare that no progress has been made toward healing. Even in the worst case scenario of wound dehiscence, some skin stretching has likely occurred, some granulation tissue has formed, and tissue viability is now better defined. Wound treatment and closure options at this point are the same as those after the initial wounding. Trimming granulation tissue from the edges of such wounds may result in a more cosmetic closure. Leaving a small amount of granulation tissue may result in an earlier gain in wound strength, however. As the maturation stage of wound healing occurs, scar cosmesis improves.

SUMMARY

No matter what the cause, initial wound management often follows similar pathways. A successful wound closure and healing outcome is often dependent on adherence to basic principles of wound assessment, appropriate care, and reassessment. Initial patient assessment is followed by wound assessment and the decision as to the first course of wound management action. Wound management often involves cleaning and determination of the feasibility of primary closure or delayed closure after open wound management. Open wound management generally involves wound debridement and lavage, together with bandaging and frequent reassessment with further debridement. Delayed closure options include delayed primary closure, secondary closure, or second-intention healing. The latter two occur after the establishment of healthy granulation tissue within the wound. If delayed closure is attempted, the use of surgical drains often facilitates healing and can decrease the incidence of wound dehiscence. Strict adherence to appropriate wound management principles and careful reassessment and adaptation of planning should result in consistent and successful wound closure in all but the most difficult wounding scenarios.

References

[1] Bellah JR, Williams JM. Wound closure options and decision making. In: Fowler D, Williams JM, editors. Manual of canine and feline wound management and reconstruction. Cheltenham (UK): British Small Animal Veterinary Association; 1999. p. 25–36.

[2] Williams JM. Open wound management. In: Fowler D, Williams JM, editors. Manual of canine and feline wound management and reconstruction. Cheltenham (UK): British Small Animal Veterinary Association; 1999. p. 37–46.

[3] Swaim SF, Henderson RA. Wound management. In: Swaim SF, Henderson RA, editors. Small animal wound management. 2nd edition. Baltimore (MD): Williams & Wilkins; 1997. p. 13–51.

[4] Lee AH, Swaim SF, McGuire JA, et al. Effects if nonadherent dressing materials on the healing of open wounds in dogs. J Am Vet Med Assoc 1987;190:416–22.

[5] Swaim SF, Wilhalf D. The physics, physiology and chemistry of bandaging open wounds. Compend Contin Educ Pract Vet 1997;7:146–56.

[6] Swaim SF, Riddell KP, McGuire JA. Effects of topical medications on the healing of open pad wounds in dogs. J Am Anim Hosp Assoc 1992;28:499–502.

[7] Hendrix CM. Facultative myiasis in dogs and cats. Compend Contin Educ Pract Vet 1991;13:86–94.

[8] Canapp SO, Farese JP, Schultz GS, et al. The effect of topical tripeptide-copper complex on healing of ischemic open wounds. Vet Surg 2003;32:515–23.

[9] Mathews KA, Binnington AG. Wound management using honey. Compend Contin Educ Pract Vet 2002;24:53–60.

[10] Mathews KA, Binnington AG. Wound management using sugar. Compend Contin Educ Pract Vet 2002;24:41–50.

[11] Hosgood G. Wound healing: the role of platelet-derived growth factor and transforming growth factor beta. Vet Surg 1993;22:490–5.

[12] Swaim SF, Vaughn DM, Kincaid SA, et al. Effects of locally injected medications on healing of pad wounds in dogs. Am J Vet Res 1996;57:394–9.

[13] Winkler JT, Swaim SF, Sartin EA, et al. The effect of a porcine-derived small intestinal submucosa product on wounds with exposed bone in dogs. Vet Surg 2002;31:541–51.

[14] White RAS. The aetiology and classification of wounds and skin deficits. In: Fowler D, Williams JM, editors. Manual of canine and feline wound management and reconstruction. Cheltenham (UK): British Small Animal Veterinary Association; 1999. p. 5–12.

[15] Shahar R, Shamir M, Johnston DE. A technique for management of bite wounds of the thoracic wall in small dogs. Vet Surg 1997;26:45–50.

[16] Swiontkowski MF, Mackenzie EJ, Bosse MJ, et al. Factors influencing the decision to amputate or reconstruct after high-energy lower extremity trauma. J Trauma 2002;52: 641–9.

[17] Slutsky DJ, editor. Nerve repair and reconstruction: a practical guide. Atlas Hand Clin 2005;10.

[18] Berg RJ, Egger EL. In vitro comparison of three loop pulley and locking loop suture patterns for repair of canine weightbearing tendon and collateral ligaments. Vet Surg 1986;15: 107–10.

[19] Krackow KA, Thomas SC, Jones LC. A new stitch for ligament-tendon fixation. J Bone Joint Surg Am 1986;68:764–6.

[20] Tomlinson J, Moore R. Locking loop tendon suture use in five calcaneal tendons. Vet Surg 1982;11:105–9.

[21] Kerstetter KK, Sackman JE. Principles of vascular surgery. In: Bojrab MJ, editor. Current techniques in small animal surgery. 4th edition. Baltimore (MD): Williams & Wilkins; 1998. p. 643–50.

[22] Beardsley SL, Schrader SC. Treatment of dogs with wounds of the limbs caused by shearing forces: 98 cases (1975–1993). J Am Vet Med Assoc 1995;207:1071–5.

[23] Wisner ER, Pollard RE. Trends in veterinary cancer imaging. Vet Comp Oncol 2004;2: 49–74.

[24] Lamb CR, White RN, McEvoy FJ. Sinography in the investigation of draining tracts in small animals: retrospective review of 25 cases. Vet Surg 1994;23:129–34.

[25] Fredlin J, Funkquist B, Hansson K, et al. Diagnostic imaging of foreign body reactions in dogs with diffuse back pain. J Small Anim Pract 1999;40:278–85.

[26] Swaim SF. Management and bandaging of soft tissue injuries of dog and cat feet. J Am Anim Hosp Assoc 1985;21:329–40.

[27] Morgan PW, Binnington AG, Miller CW, et al. The effect of occlusive and semi-occlusive dressings on the healing of acute full-thickness skin wounds on the forelimbs of dogs. Vet Surg 1994;23:494–502.

[28] Swaim SF, Lee AH, Henderson RA. Mobility versus immobility in the healing of open wounds. J Am Anim Hosp Assoc 1989;25:91–6.

[29] Lee AH, Swaim SF, Yang ST, et al. The effects of petrolatum, polyethylene glycol, nitrofurazone and a hydroactive dressing on open wound healing. J Am Anim Hosp Assoc 1985;22: 443–51.

[30] Bauer MS, Aiken S. The healing of open wounds. Semin Vet Med Surg 1989;4:268–73.

[31] Dernell WS, Withrow SJ. Preoperative patient assessment and margin evaluation. Semin Vet Med Surg 1998;13(1):17–21.

[32] Sherman RA. Maggot versus conservative debridement therapy for the treatment of pressure ulcers. Wound Repair Regen 2002;10:208–14.

[33] Sherman RA, Hall MJR, Thomas S. Medicinal maggots: an ancient remedy for some contemporary afflictions. Annu Rev Entomol 2000;45:55–81.

[34] Lucroy MD, Edwards BF, Madewell BR. Low-intensity laser light-induced closure of a chronic wound in a dog. Vet Surg 1999;28:292–5.

[35] Hawkins D, Houreld N, Abrahamse H. Low level laser therapy (LLLT) as an effective therapeutic modality for delayed wound healing. Ann NY Acad Sci 2005;1056:486–93.

[36] Sumano H, Mateos G. The use of acupuncture-like electrical stimulation for wound healing of lesions unresponsive to conventional treatment. Am J Acupunct 1999;27:5–14.

[37] Ojingwa JC, Isseroff RR. Electrical stimulation of wound healing. Invest Dermatol 2003;121:1–12.

[38] Lantz OI. Vacuum assisted closure: a review and current veterinary applications. In: Proceedings of the 2005 American College of Veterinary Surgeons Symposium, San Diego, CA. Madison (WI): Omnipress; 2005. p. 532–6.

[39] McCallon SK, Knight CA, Valiulus JP, et al. Vacuum-assisted versus saline-moistened gauze in the healing if postoperative diabetic foot wounds. Ostomy Wound Manage 2000;46: 28–32.

[40] Argenta LC, Morykwas MJ. Vacuum-assisted closure: a new method for wound control and treatment: clinical experience. Ann Plast Surg 1997;38:563–76.

[41] Dernell WS, Harari J. Surgical devices and wound healing. In: Harari J, editor. Surgical complications and wound healing. 1st edition. Philadelphia: WB Saunders; 1993. p. 349–79.

[42] Austin BR, Henderson RA. Buried tension sutures: force-tension comparisons of pulley, double butterfly, mattress and simple interrupted suture patterns. Vet Surg 2006;35:43–8.

[43] Scardino MS, Swaim SF, Henderson RA, et al. Enhancing wound closure on the limbs. Compend Contin Educ Pract Vet 1996;18:919–51.

[44] Pavletic MM. Use of an external skin-stretching device for wound closure in dogs and cats. J Am Vet Med Assoc 2000;217:350–4.

[45] Lee AH, Swaim SF, Newton JC, et al. Wound healing over denuded bone. J Am Anim Hosp Assoc 1987;23:75–84.

[46] Clark GN. Bone perforation to enhance wound healing over exposed bones in dogs with shearing injuries. J Am Anim Hosp Assoc 2001;37:215–7.

[47] Fitch RB, Swaim SF. The role of epithelialization in wound healing. Compend Contin Educ Pract Vet 1995;17:167–93.

[48] Baines SJ. Surgical drains. In: Fowler D, Williams JM, editors. Manual of canine and feline wound management and reconstruction. Cheltenham (UK): British Small Animal Veterinary Association; 1999. p. 47–55.

Vet Clin Small Anim 36 (2006) 739–757

VETERINARY CLINICS
SMALL ANIMAL PRACTICE

ELSEVIER
SAUNDERS

Topical and Systemic Medications for Wounds

D.J. Krahwinkel, DVM, MS[a],*,
Harry W. Boothe, Jr, DVM, MS[b]

[a]Department of Small Animal Clinical Sciences, The University of Tennessee College of Veterinary Medicine, C247 Veterinary Teaching Hospital, Knoxville, TN 37996–4544, USA
[b]Department of Clinical Sciences, College of Veterinary Medicine, Auburn University, 417 Hoerlein Hall, Auburn, AL 36849–5540, USA

Much of clinical practice is spent in caring for surgical and accidental wounds. Understanding the complexity of wound healing and the biologic chemicals that play essential roles is important in making decisions regarding wound care. The veterinarian's task is to aid in the healing of the wound to reduce the patient's discomfort and the client's expense, and, in so doing, to help the wound to heal as quickly as possible. Wound healing occurs in an environment of various biochemicals, which, in proper balance, provide for optimum wound healing. These biochemical products include a mixture of chemotactic factors, eicosanoids, free radicals, cytokines, growth factors, inflammatory cells, and enzymes. These agents act in concert to break down the undesirable components in a wound (debridement) and to provide the chemical instruction and biologic components necessary for the wound to heal.

Wound healing is a complex sequence of biochemical and physiologic events. Most wounds heal without intervention by the veterinarian; however, the use of proper topical and systemic medications can enhance the healing process, resulting in faster healing with fewer complications and undesirable side effects. Modern wound care medications all play an active role in some phase of wound healing. A proper knowledge of these medications and their actions can help the veterinary practitioner to choose the correct product for each wound. No one medication is essential or best for every wound. Each product has its own individual indications, including the type, condition, and age of the wound. "Type" would be a burn or gunshot, for example. "Condition" would be infected or clean. "Age" would indicate acute or chronic.

Medications used to enhance wound healing function in a variety of different ways. These include maintaining a moist environment (ie, hydrogels, hydrocolloids, alginates), providing a local energy source (ie, maltodextrin, honey,

*Corresponding author. E-mail address: djk@utk.edu (D.J. Krahwinkel).

0195-5616/06/$ – see front matter
doi:10.1016/j.cvsm.2006.04.001

sugar), reducing wound edema by hydrophilic action (ie, alginates, freeze-dried form of acemannan, honey, sugar), increasing the level of growth factors (ie, acemannan, tripeptide-copper complex), providing a source of healing substance (ie, collagen, biologic membrane/extracellular matrix bioscaffolds), increasing the inflammatory response (ie, maltodextrin), controlling infection (ie, topical and systemic antimicrobials), aiding debridement (ie, topical enzymes), increasing the oxygen content (ie, hyperbaric oxygen), and increasing the blood flow (ie, laser, ultraviolet radiation, electrical stimulation). Some medications work in only one of these ways, whereas others have multiple functions.

There is available today on the health care market an abundance of products for use in modern wound care. These products are all aimed at enhancing some phase of wound healing. This article is an overview of some of the numerous products that represent various approaches to wound care. The discussion of these products is not an endorsement of any particular product, and the omission of a product is not meant to infer that it is not of value. Current medical literature contains hundreds of articles evaluating various compounds and their effects on wound healing. It would be impossible to discuss them all in the allotted space. Most modern wound care products speed wound healing compared with a saline or medication vehicle control; however, the improvement may only be a few days. One must consider the enhancement in healing versus the cost of the product. More details on many of these products are available in the article by Campbell elsewhere in this issue. A summary of the products described in this article is available in Tables 1 and 2.

ENHANCEMENT OF HEALING
Hydrocolloids
Hydrocolloids are generally compounds of pectin, gelatin, and carboxymethylcellulose with some form of film or adhesive backing, thus serving as a bandage (see the article by Campbell in this issue) (see Table 1) [1]. In addition to the standard hydrocolloid sheets, pastes and powders are also available to use for filling tracts and sinuses. These products have considerable absorption abilities varying between 75% and 650% of their weight in fluid [2]. They absorb wound fluid and exudate by swelling into a gel-like mass, maintaining a moist environment conducive to healing. The hydrocolloid is held in place by an adhesive border or a securing bandage. Hydrocolloids are indicated for partial- and full-thickness wounds and can safely be used on granulating and necrotic wounds [2]. Wounds covered with hydrocolloids have lower infection rates in people than those covered with gauze, film, hydrogels, or foams [2]. They also help to protect the wound from contamination and aid in autolytic debridement.

These products are designed to remain on the wound for up to 7 days but should be changed whenever strike-through occurs. People who are unfamiliar with hydrocolloids may be concerned by the appearance and odor of the dissolving residue. The purulent appearance and odor may give the false impression of infection; however, when the residue is removed by gentle lavage, the wound appears healthy. Exuberant granulation can occur if the hydrocolloids are used too long. In a study comparing hydrocolloids, hydrogels, and a polyethylene oxide dressing for open wounds on the legs of dogs, the polyethylene dressing and the hydrogels showed better healing than the hydrocolloid [3]. Wounds under the hydrocolloid or hydrogel tended to develop exuberant granulation tissue. The study indicated that wounds must be observed regularly to ensure that any phase of healing does not become excessive.

Hydrogels

Hydrogels are 80% to 90% water- or glycerin-based wound dressings that are available in sheets to serve as bandages (see the article by Campbell in this issue). They are also available in the form of amorphous gels or impregnated gauzes (see Table 1). Hydrogels are able to absorb a minimal amount of fluid but are capable of donating large amounts of moisture to the wound [2]. Hydrogels provide a moist environment that rehydrates a dry wound bed. This facilitates autolytic debridement and the removal of dried eschar and reduces pain at the wound site. The product must be applied only to the wound site and covered with an outer bandage. If applied to the surrounding skin, maceration can occur. Hydrogels may be applied to the wound as often as twice daily; however, sheets can be effective on the wound for up to 5 days [1]. They are indicated for minimal to moderately draining wounds, such as abrasions, blisters, burns, ulcers, and partial-thickness donor sites. Hydrogels are also used in the late stage of healing on wounds that have healthy granulation tissue, decreased drainage, and evidence of epithelialization.

Alginates

Alginates are polysaccharide dressings produced from kelp (seaweed). They are available as twisted fibers or mats and are applied to wounds as a primary dressing (see Table 1). Sodium from the wound exudate and calcium from the alginate undergo ion exchange, resulting in a soluble alginate gel [4]. A secondary dressing is used to secure the alginate. The gel produces a nonadherent moist wound environment that promotes autolytic debridement and wound healing. Alginate products are best used to treat moderately heavy exudating wounds in the early stages of healing [5]. If used on a dry wound, the alginate is moistened with saline to avoid desiccating the wound and to avoid a wet-to-dry bandage. These dressings are particularly useful for wounds in which hemostasis is also desired.

If desiccation does not occur, the dressing can be left in place for up to 7 days or changed when there is strike-through of the secondary dressing [4]. The alginate gel can be gently lavaged away without damage to the underlying tissue. The gel that forms on the wound may emit a putrid odor and have a purulent appearance that can be mistaken for wound infection (see the article by Campbell in this issue).

Table 1
Some commercial products used to enhance wound healing

Classification	Brand name	Action	Ingredient(s)	Manufacturer (location)
Hydrocolloids	Procol	Hydrophilic	Hydrocolloid	DeRoyal (Powell, TN)
	DuoDerm	Hydrophilic	Hydrocolloid	Convatec (Indianapolis, IN)
	Tegasorb	Hydrophilic	Hydrocolloid	3-M (St. Paul, MN)
	Nu-Derm	Hydrophilic	Hydrocolloid	Johnson & Johnson (Arlington, TX)
Hydrogels	Iamin	Increase growth factors	Tripeptide-copper complex	Procyte Corporation (Redmond, WA)
	Nu-Gel	Hydrophilic	Hydrogel with collagen	Johnson & Johnson (Arlington, TX)
	BioDres	Hydrophilic	Polyethylene oxide	DVM Pharmaceuticals (Miami, FL)
	Aquacel	Hydrophilic	Methylcellulose	Convatec (Indianapolis, IN)
	Aquacel Ag	Hydrophilic Antibacterial	Methylcellulose with silver	Convatec Indianapolis, IN)
	Aquasorb	Hydrophilic	Glycerin	DeRoyal (Powell, TN)
	Curafil	Hydrophilic	Curafil	Tyco Health Care Kendall (Mansfield, MA)
Collagens	HyCURE	Epithelialization Hemostasis Collagen deposition Granulation	Hydrolyzed bovine collagen	The HyMed Group (Bethlehem, PA)
	Collasate	Epithelialization Hemostasis Collagen deposition Granulation	Bovine collagen	PRN Pharmacal (Pensacola, FL)
Alginates	Curasorb	Hydrophilic	Kelp (seaweed)	Tyco Health Care Kendall (Mansfield, MA)
	Kalginate	Hydrophilic	Kelp (seaweed)	DeRoyal (Powell, TN)
	Tegagen	Hydrophilic	Kelp (seaweed)	3-M (St. Paul, MN)

Classification	Product	Composition	Effects	Manufacturer
Extracellular matrix scaffolds	VetBioSiST	Porcine intestinal submucosa	Increase growth factors, Fibronectin, Hyaluronic acid	Global Veterinary Products (New Buffalo, MI)
	ACellVet	Porcine vesicular basement membrane	Increase growth factors, Fibronectin, Hyaluronic acid	ACell (Jessup, MD)
Growth factor enhancers	Iamin	Tripeptide-copper complex	Collagen deposition, Wound contraction, Neovascularization, Epithelialization	Procyte Corporation (Redmond, WA)
	Regranex	Platelet-derived growth factor	Epithelialization, Wound contraction, Neovascularization	Johnson & Johnson (Arlington, TX)
	Intracell	Maltodextrin (D-glucose polysaccharide)	Hydrophilic, Granulation, Cell energy, Epithelialization	MacLeod Pharmaceuticals (Fort Collins, CO), DeRoyal (Powell, TN)
	Multidex			
	CarraVet, Carra Sorb M	Acemannan	Increased fibroblasts, Neovascularization, Epithelialization, Collagen deposition	Veterinary Products Labs (Phoenix, AZ)
	Ultrasan	Chitan	Increased growth factors, Increased fibroblasts	BioSyntech (Laval, Quebec)

Some products function in more than one classification.
These are examples of products. There may be other manufacturers of similar products that have different brand names. The reader is referred to various drug/medication references or the Internet for information on other products.

Table 2
Topical wound products used for infection and debridement

Classification	Product	Brand name	Ingredients	Manufacturer (location)
Topical antimicrobial	Gentamicin sulfate	Gentamicin sulfate	0.1% gentamicin sulfate	Fougera (Melville, NY)
	Nitrofurazone	Fura-Septin	0.2% nitrofurazine	Bimeda (Oakbrook, IL)
	Silver sulfadiazine	Silvadene	1% silver sulfadiazine	Marion Laboratories (Kansas City, MO)
	Triple-antibiotic ointment	Neosporin ointment	Bacitracin zinc, neomycin, and polymyxin B sulfate	Burroughs Wellcome Company (Durham, NC)
Topical antiseptics	Povidone-iodine solution	Betadine solution	2% povidone-iodine solution	The Purdue Frederick Company (Norwalk, CT)
	Chlorhexidine solution	Nolvasan	Chlorhexidine diacetate	Fort Dodge Laboratories (Fort Dodge, IA)
	Dakin's solution	Dakin's solution	0.25% solution of sodium hypochlorite	The Clorox Company (Oakland, CA)
	Tris-EDTA	TrizEDTA	Tromethanine edentate disodium dehydrate	Derma Pet (Potomac, MD)
Topical debridement	Granulex-V	Granulex-V	Trypsin, balsam of Peru, and castrol oil	Bertek Pharmaceuticals (Morgantown, WV)
	Elase	Elase	Desoxyribonuclease and fibrinolysin	Fujisawa Healthcare (Deerfield, Il)
	Collagenase	Santyl	Collagenase	Advance Biofactures Corporation (Lynbrook, NY)
	Papain/urea	Accuzyme	Papain and urea	Healthpoint, Ltd (Fort Worth, TX)

These are examples of products. There may be other manufacturers of similar products that have different brand names. The reader is referred to various drug/medication references or the Internet for information on other products.
Abbreviation: EDTA, ethlyenediaminetetraacetic acid.

Extracellular Matrix–Derived Dressings

Collagen

Processed collagen provides a matrix for cellular colonization and subsequent connective tissue formation essential for wound healing. Dressings in the form of sheets, powders, gels, or sponges enhance inflammation and hemostasis and provide a scaffold to accelerate fibroplasia and epithelialization (see Table 1) [6]. The collagen product is placed within the boundary of the wound, covered with a nonadherent bandage, and held in place with a secondary bandage (see the article by Campbell in this issue).

In one study of hydrolyzed collagen on open wounds of dogs, the treated wounds had a significantly greater percentage of epithelialization at 7 days than did control wounds [7]. Topical bovine collagen gel and collagen membranes yielded equivocal results in equine wounds, however [8]. The positive effect seen in dogs may have been related to the hydrophilic nature of the collagen, resulting in a moist environment that enhanced epithelialization (see the article by Campbell in this issue) [7].

Extracellular matrix bioscaffolds

Biologic membranes in the form of bioscaffolds have been used in an effort to enhance wound healing (see Table 1). One of these is a porcine small intestine submucosa (SIS) membrane. It is composed of collagen types I, III, IV, V, VI, and VIII, along with fibronectin, hyaluronic acid, chondroitin sulfate, and heparin [9]. Another scaffold is made from acellular urinary bladder matrix or submucosa (UBM/UBS) and acts as an inductive scaffold for tissue replacement [10]. Either product can be implanted into tissue defects, including skin, in an effort to provide a three-dimensional extracellular matrix for the ingrowth of cells and vasculature. These biomaterials are reported to contain various growth factors essential for tissue healing [9]. They are available as lypholyzed sheets of tissue that are cut to fit the wound and sutured to the wound margin. They are then left in place to be incorporated into the host tissues [11]. Two or three applications of bioscaffold, without removing the previously applied scaffold material, provide cells and other factors of healing enabling one to proceed with routine bandaging. The wounds are covered with a protective bandage over the bioscaffold until healing occurs. Because of the technology required to harvest and prepare these membranes, they are relatively expensive (see the article by Campbell in this issue).

Clinical studies on these products are limited. In one report where intestinal submucosa was used over exposed bone, there was no enhancement of wound healing seen [9]. Similar results were found in equine wounds [12].

Tripeptide-Copper Complex

Tripeptide-copper complex (TCC) has been shown to stimulate several of the mechanisms essential for wound healing (see Table 1). Initially isolated from human plasma, TCC has properties of a growth factor, chemotactic agent, and wound activator. The actions within the wound include neovascularization, epithelialization, collagen deposition, and wound contraction [13].

TCC is a hydrogel with delivery of copper to the wound site. It is indicated for a variety of partial- and full-thickness wounds. Wounds should be debrided and thoroughly cleansed. The TCC gel can be applied under a nonadherent dressing and changed daily. In nonbandaged wounds, the gel can be applied up to four times daily.

Daily topical applications to diabetic ulcers in people resulted in enhanced wound healing compared with controls [14]. A significant decrease in the healing time of ischemic wounds in rats was seen when TCC was compared with the vehicle placebo of TCC and a no-treatment control [13]. An open wound healing evaluation was done in laboratory dogs comparing TCC with the vehicle placebo [15]. The treated wound granulated faster, contracted quicker, and healed 7 days sooner than the controls.

Acemannan

Acemannan is a topical wound medication derived from the aloe vera plant. It is an acetylated mannan that acts as a growth factor, stimulating macrophages to enhance interleukin (IL)-1 and tumor necrosis factor-α (TNFα) at the wound site (see Table 1) [16]. IL-1 enhances fibroblast proliferation, increases neovascularization, stimulates epidermal growth, and enhances collagen deposition [5]. TNFα has a positive effect on wound angiogenesis [5]. It may also have a stabilizing effect on growth factors to promote their effects on fibroplasia [16].

Treatment with acemannan is indicated for partial- and full-thickness burns, lacerations, dermal ulcers, and abrasions and to stimulate slow-healing wounds. The wound should first be debrided and lavaged before acemannan is applied. The product is available as a hydrogel or a hydrophilic freeze-dried foam. It is placed under a nonadherent bandage that is changed daily. Application can begin in the early inflammatory phase of healing and continues into the proliferative phase.

Foot pad wounds in dogs treated with aloe vera containing acemannan were significantly smaller at 7 days than those treated with a triple-antibiotic ointment or those with no treatment [17]. A study on people with pressure ulcers failed to find a difference between acemannan and saline-treated wounds, however [18]. Studies would suggest that the greatest effects may be seen in the first week after injury [16].

Maltodextrin

Maltodextrin, a common ingredient in processed foods, is a D-glucose polysaccharide with 1% ascorbic acid. When applied to a wound, it forms a hydrophilic film dressing that creates a moist environment to nurture wound healing. It also seems to be a chemoattractant for polymorphonuclear cells, lymphocytes, and macrophages to the wound site, which increases the level of growth factors essential for healing (see Table 1) [5,16]. The hydrolysis of the polysaccharide provides glucose, which may be used for cell energy to promote healing [5]. In an equine model, maltodextrin seemed to reduce pain and stimulate granulation and epithelialization compared with topical antibiotics [16]. Clinical findings include softening of necrotic tissue, quick penetration of wound irregularities, nontoxic, no systemic absorption, and effectiveness in infected and noninfected wounds [19].

Maltodextrin comes as a hydrophilic powder and as a gel. The wound should be debrided and lavaged, and maltodextrin should then be applied. The product seems to have an effect from the early inflammatory through repair stages of healing [5]. The powder is preferred for exuding wounds, and the gel is preferred for drier wounds. A primary dressing and absorbent secondary bandage are placed over the wound and changed daily. The wound should be lavaged between bandage changes.

Platelet Gel

Degranulating platelets release numerous growth factors and other substances associated with wound healing [16]. Platelet-derived products offer considerable advantage in wound care, because a large number of growth factors are available in high concentrations when platelets are activated. Topical application of platelet-derived growth factors encouraged repair of previously nonhealing wounds in people [20]. Treated wounds show increased epithelialization, contraction, and neovascularization. A similar result was seen in the experimental treatment of equine wounds using a homologous gel produced from platelet-rich plasma [21]. There are currently no studies available to determine if the same result would be seen in dogs or cats. A recombinant platelet-derived growth factor is approved by the US Food and Drug Administration (FDA) and is commercially available, but it is quite expensive (see Table 1).

Chitosan

Chitosan is a polysaccharide in which the active ingredient is glucosamine, which functions as a wound healing accelerator [22]. Chitosan is derived from chitan, which is found in the exoskeleton of shellfish such as crabs, lobster, and shrimp as well as in shark cartilage. The application of chitosan to wounds enhances the function of inflammatory cells, various growth factors, and fibroblasts (see Table 1). As a result, granulation is promoted and wound healing is accelerated. This enhanced wound healing was confirmed in a group of dogs with experimentally created wounds [22]; however, toxic effects, including fatal hemorrhagic pneumonia, were seen when doses exceeding 50 mg/kg were administered subcutaneously. This has not been seen in other species.

Omentum

Nonhealing wounds in high-motion areas, such as the axillary and inguinal spaces, are common, especially in cats. Conventional closure often results in failure. Omental pedicle transfer has been used successfully to enhance the healing of these wounds [23]. The known functions of the omentum include lymphatic drainage to aid in reducing wound edema, angiogenesis to increase blood supply to the wound, and provision of a source of monocytes and macrophages to provide growth factors to the wound (see the articles by Swaim and Amalsadvala and Hedlund elsewhere in this issue) [24].

Honey

The use of honey as a wound treatment dates back to 2000 BC. It has been used for cleansing and accelerating the healing of wounds for centuries. The scientific basis for its use was not clear until recently, however. The biologic effects of honey on wounds include a decrease in inflammatory edema, stimulation of macrophage migration, acceleration of sloughing of dead tissue, provision of a cellular energy source, formation of a protective layer of protein on the wound, and development of a healthy granulation bed [25]. There is also an antibacterial effect attributed to honey because of its hydrogen peroxide content, which helps to stimulate angiogenesis within the wound [26].

Honey is reported to be effective against a wide variety of gram-positive and gram-negative organisms, including *Escherichia coli*, *Proteus mirabilis*, *Pseudomonas aeruginosa*, *Salmonella typhimurium*, *Serratia marcescens*, *Staphylococcus aureus*, *Streptococcus pyogenes*, and *Candida albicans*. In a study of human patients with burn wounds, those treated with honey showed more rapid healing than those treated with silver sulfadiazine (SSD) [27].

Honey used for wound care should be unpasteurized and not heated above 37°C [25]. Contaminated or infected wounds should be liberally lavaged after surgical debridement. Surgical gauze is soaked in honey (30 mL on 10-cm × 10-cm gauze pad) and then placed on the wound. Absorbent secondary dressings are used to maintain the honey on the wound. The wound is rebandaged one to three times daily depending on the frequency of strike-through.

Care should be exercised when using honey on large wounds because of its hydrophilic property of drawing fluids from the wound. In an animal that is already losing large amounts of fluids, electrolytes, and protein from the wound, a topical medication drawing more of these from the body could exacerbate metabolic imbalances. Monitoring hydration, electrolytes, and protein levels is essential when using honey on large wounds.

Sugar

Finely powdered sugar has been used to clean wounds for hundreds of years. Granulated sugar is now commonly used to treat wounds worldwide. The scientific basis for using sugar is based on the high osmolality created by sugar within the wound [28]. Sugar reduces edema in the wound, attracts macrophages that aid the healing process, accelerates sloughing of devitalized tissue, provides a cellular energy source, promotes the formation of a protective layer of protein on the wound, and encourages a healthy granulation bed [29]. A sugar paste commonly used for wounds is made from castor sugar (400 g), icing sugar (600 g), glycerin (480 mL), and 3% hydrogen peroxide (7.5 mL) [30].

Wounds are thoroughly lavaged, and granulated sugar is placed on the wound at least 1 cm deep. Absorbent bandages are placed over the wound to absorb the excess wound fluid. The bandage is changed and the sugar replaced at least twice a day to help maintain the osmolality of the wound [30]. The bandage should always be changed when strike-through occurs. The wound should be lavaged between bandage changes. Once healthy granulation tissue has formed and there are no signs of infection, the sugar can be discontinued and the wound closed or permitted to heal by second intention.

Hyperglycemia does not develop in sugar-treated patients, because the sugar molecule is a complex molecule that is not absorbed from the wound [29]. Sugar seems to be effective in treating wounds infected with *Staphylococcus*, *Streptococcus*, *Enterobacter*, *E coli*, *Klebsiella*, *Pseudomonas*, and *Serratia* [30].

As with honey, care should be exercised when using sugar on large wounds to avoid fluid, electrolyte, and protein imbalances, because these are pulled from the wound by the hydrophilic action of sugar. It is important to monitor hydration, electrolyte, and protein levels when using sugar on large wounds.

Oxygen Therapy

Adequate tissue oxygen tension (pO_2) is an essential factor in wound healing and infection control [31,32]. The probability of wound healing is extremely high when the pO_2 is greater than 40 mm Hg, but healing is much less likely to occur when the pO_2 is less than 20 mm Hg [33]. Chronic nonhealing wounds are frequently hypoxic, partially because of poor perfusion. In nonhealing wounds, pO_2 values ranging from 5 to 20 mm Hg have been recorded; infected and traumatized tissue typically has values less than 30 mm Hg. Active cell division requires a pO_2 of approximately 30 mm Hg [33]. Cellular responses to tissue injury are enhanced in the presence of oxygen. For example, oxygen is critical for at least some of the antimicrobial properties of polymorphonuclear cells [33]. Cell death and tissue necrosis caused by tissue hypoxia likely contribute to ideal growth conditions for the wound microflora, including fastidious anaerobes [33].

Oxygen delivery is a critical element for the healing of wounds [34]. The clinical challenge is how to improve the delivery of blood and oxygen to wounds when these are deficient [35]. Options for delivering increased levels of oxygen to wounds include the use of hyperbaric (inhaled) oxygen and topical oxygen therapy. Of these two methods, hyperbaric oxygen therapy has been studied more extensively.

The value of hyperbaric oxygen therapy in wound healing is controversial, and its use as a standard treatment for chronic nonhealing wounds has not been widely accepted [33]. In theory, hyperbaric oxygen therapy stimulates cellular processes involved in wound healing, directly impairs the growth of anaerobic pathogens, and enhances the oxygen-dependent mechanisms in white blood cells [33]. Hyperbaric oxygen restores this defense against infection and increases the rate of phagocytic killing of some common bacteria [36]. Hyperbaric oxygen equipment is expensive and poses safety concerns.

The potential benefits of supplemental perioperative oxygen administration on wound healing in human beings have shown variable results on the incidence of wound infection [37]. Well-perfused wounds that are failing to heal as well as acute and rapidly advancing soft tissue infections (eg, necrotizing fasciitis) are likely to gain the most benefit from hyperbaric oxygen therapy [33].

The effect of topical oxygen on wound healing has been variably described as clinically ineffective or exhibiting no detrimental effects on wounds [38,39]. Exposure of open dermal wounds to topical oxygen treatment increased the tissue pO_2 of superficial tissue [34].

Mechanical Stimulants and Physical Therapeutic Modalities

Wound healing may be altered by such mechanical stimulants as a low energy level laser, photodynamic therapy, electrical stimulation, vacuum-assisted devices, and hyperthermia induced by microwave irradiation. Low-level laser therapy (fluency of 2 J/cm^2) induces proliferation of fibroblasts in vivo and in vitro and has a positive biomodulator effect on wound healing. A synergistic effect of a low energy level laser and photosensitizer drugs on wound healing in rats has been shown [40]. Evaluation of the available data on the effect of low-level laser therapy suggests that the addition of laser therapy does not improve wound healing, however [41]. Electrical stimulation, including pulsed electromagnetic field, activates fibroblasts, stimulates migration of other key cells, and enhances microcirculatory flow [31]. Pulsed electromagnetic field treatment enhanced epithelialization of open wounds in dogs [42].

Vacuum-assisted closure is a relatively new technology that applies controlled negative subatmospheric pressure to the wound bed and has applications in a variety of chronic and infected wounds that are difficult to manage [43,44]. Vacuum-assisted closure effectively converts an open wound into a controlled and temporarily closed environment [43]. Mechanisms of action of vacuum-assisted closure are thought to include tissue edema reduction, increased localized blood flow, enhanced granulation tissue formation, and encouraged migration of keratinocytes across wound defects [43,44]. As of 2004, the body of evidence was judged to be insufficient to support conclusions about the effectiveness of vacuum-assisted closure in the treatment of wounds [41].

Use of microwave irradiation on wounds has been quite limited to date. Hyperthermia induced by microwave irradiation has been shown to improve epithelialization in wounds of rabbits and human beings [45].

CONTROL OF INFECTION

Systemic Antimicrobials

All wounds are at least at some risk of becoming infected. Wound colonization is most frequently polymicrobial, with numerous potentially pathogenic bacteria being present [33]. Infected wounds frequently do not heal properly, although the reason for such delayed healing is unclear. Open wounds frequently provide an environment conducive to the formation of biofilms. Bacteria comprising biofilm are frequently characterized by complex antimicrobial resistance patterns [46]. Clinical indicators that the bacterial burden is compromising wound repair include poor-quality granulation tissue, increased volume of exudates, and increased pain [47]. Microbial density ($>10^5$ colony-forming units per gram of tissue), synergic relations between bacterial species (especially aerobic and anaerobic organisms), and the presence of specific microorganisms (eg, *P aeruginosa*, β-hemolytic streptococci) are thought to play a role in wound infection [33,48].

One factor in primary wound healing of open contaminated wounds is the bacterial numbers (ie, $>10^5$ colony-forming units per gram of tissue) [49]. Wound contaminants are likely to originate from three potential sources: environmental, cutaneous, and endogenous. Environmental sources may predominate in traumatic wounds, with flora being polymicrobial. Endogenous sources, especially oral and gastrointestinal flora, often supply most organisms that colonize wounds. Acute and chronic wounds are susceptible to contamination and colonization by a wide variety of aerobic and anaerobic microorganisms [33].

Chronic wounds do not heal in an orderly and efficient manner. Chronic wounds in people are classified into four groups regarding infection status: contaminated, colonized, critically colonized, and infected [48]. Wound contamination is the presence of nonreplicating microorganisms in the wound. In contrast, wound colonization refers to the presence of replicating microorganisms that adhere to the wound but do not cause injury to the host. Colonization becomes critical when bacteria cause delayed wound healing. Wound infection is the presence of replicating microorganisms within the wound and the presence of injury to the host. Bacteria in the latter two groups adversely affect wound healing. In chronic wounds, the pathogen species may be much more important than the number of organisms [31].

A classification scheme for chronic wounds in veterinary patients is not used; hence, the role of bacteria in wounds of veterinary patients is less well understood. Chronic wounds in veterinary medicine are most commonly associated with trauma, neoplasia, pressure necrosis, radiation injury, burns, and indolent ulcers. Approaches to managing chronic wounds in veterinary patients usually include reducing tissue trauma, ischemia, and bacterial contamination [13].

In general, antimicrobial administration should be considered when muscle fascia is disrupted, questionable tissue remains after debridement, an animal is severely immunocompromised, or systemic signs of infection are present [50]. Opinion-based recommendations for wound management in human beings suggest that antimicrobials play an important role in the treatment of chronic infected wounds; however, scientific support for such use, selection, and duration is lacking [48]. Appropriate systemic antimicrobials are considered essential in the management of nonhealing clinically infected wounds, although their appropriateness in nonhealing noninfected wounds is unsubstantiated. The careful use of broad-spectrum antimicrobial agents is likely to be the most successful treatment in the management of clinically infected chronic wounds in people [33]. Systemic antimicrobial therapy should be used in all chronic wounds in which there is active infection beyond that manageable with local wound therapy [31].

Selection of systemic antimicrobials for use with wounds, although frequently empiric, should ideally be based on culture and susceptibility testing results. A Gram stain may aid in identifying bacteria and predicting microbial load in the wound [33,49]. Principles of antimicrobial selection and use should be followed, including knowledge of expected flora, ability of the antimicrobial to reach the wound at appropriate concentrations, bacterial resistance patterns, and antimicrobial pharmacokinetics [51]. Because of the frequency of encountering staphylococcal species in acute superficial wounds of veterinary patients, cephalosporins or amoxicillin-clavulanate combinations may be efficacious [49]. Duration of administration of antimicrobials is determined, in part, by the stage of wound healing. Antimicrobial therapy usually should be discontinued once a healthy bed of granulation tissue is present, in part, because systemic antimicrobials tend not to reach adequate tissue levels in chronic granulation tissue [49,52].

Topical Antimicrobials

Topical therapy, although only one aspect of effective wound care, often plays an important role by removing known impediments to repair and creating a favorable environment for healing [47]. The basic tenant of medicine, "above all else, do no harm," seems particularly applicable to the topical treatment of wounds. Most topical preparations are more effective in preventing wound infection than in treating it [49]. Historically, wounds have been treated with a multitude of topical agents, including antimicrobial agents and antiseptics.

The objective of using topical antimicrobials, including antiseptics, in the contaminated or infected wound is to reduce the number of microorganisms present in the wound. Topical antimicrobials are most appropriate when used to decrease the bacterial burden in chronic wounds with active but localized infection. Topical antimicrobials should have a low sensitization potential, not be used systemically, and have low tissue toxicity [31]. One potential advantage of topical compared with systemic antimicrobials is their ability to deliver high levels to the wound, irrespective of vascular supply [48]. Water-based topical antibacterial creams penetrate the depths of open wounds and can affect bacterial growth in the wound [53]. Topical antimicrobials are generally restricted to those that are toxic when administered systemically [33].

Topical antimicrobial agents commonly used in wounds of small animals include gentamicin sulfate, nitrofurazone, SSD, and triple-antibiotic ointment (bacitracin zinc, neomycin sulfate, and polymyxin B sulfate) (see Table 2) [47,54]. Gentamicin sulfate has efficacy against gram-negative bacteria and *Staphylococcus* spp and has been shown to promote wound contraction [55]. Nitrofurazone is characterized by a broad gram-positive spectrum, has hydrophilic properties, and may have a negative impact on epithelialization [47,54]. SSD is used frequently in burns, in part, because of its efficacy against *Pseudomonas* spp. It can penetrate necrotic tissue and enhances wound epithelialization [54]. SSD may also have a negative effect on fibroblasts, and thus on wound contraction. It can also cause bone marrow suppression [50]. Triple-antibiotic ointment has efficacy against many bacteria, although not usually against *Pseudomonas* spp, and it may stimulate epithelialization because of its zinc content [49]. The three antibiotics have a synergistic effect against organisms. The ointment is poorly absorbed by tissues. It should be used early in wound management before bacteria have penetrated the tissues and caused infection [50]. Topical antimicrobials are applied sparingly and aseptically to the wound. Their use is usually discontinued once healthy granulation is noted within the wound [49].

Topical Antiseptics

The use of antiseptics remains one of the major controversies in human wound care [47]. The ideal wound antiseptic is bactericidal without harming healing tissues [49]. Wounds most likely to benefit from topical antiseptic treatment are those with or without signs of infection that are of a traumatic or chronic nature, heavily contaminated with a variety of microorganisms, and failing to heal [33]. Use of topical antiseptics in wounds should be discontinued once bacterial balance has been restored (see section on use of topical debridement) [47].

Antiseptics are frequently used to cleanse or lavage animal wounds. The more widespread use of antiseptics in animal wounds reflects, in part, their frequent contaminated status. Also, the presence of necrotic or devitalized tissue reduces the quantity of bacteria required for infection [49]. Thus, the use of antiseptics in wounds with such tissue would be indicated. The goal of wound cleansing is to flush nonviable tissue and bacteria from the wound surface mechanically without damaging viable tissue or driving bacteria into underlying tissue [47].

Topical antiseptic agents used most commonly in animal wounds include bisbiguanide chlorhexidine-diacetate solution (0.05%) and povidone iodine (1%) (see Table 2). Chlorhexidine has sustained residual activity and good activity in the presence of organic matter. At appropriate concentrations, chlorhexidine seems to have minimal deleterious effects on wound healing. Povidone iodine has good antimicrobial activity but lacks residual activity because of inactivation of free iodine by organic matter in the wound [49]. Other wound antiseptic agents of potential interest are Tris–ethylenediaminetetraacetic acid (EDTA) and Dakin's solution (0.25% solution of sodium hypochlorite) (see Table 2). Tris-EDTA has antibacterial properties, particularly against certain gram-negative bacteria (*P aeruginosa*, *Proteus vulgaris*, and *E coli*) [56]. Formulations of other germicidal agents (eg, chlorhexidine, chloroxylenol) may contain EDTA [57,58]. Dakin's solution is not used frequently in veterinary wounds, but it may have short-term value in wounds with large amounts of devitalized tissue [49].

TOPICAL WOUND DEBRIDEMENT

The importance of wound debridement has been known for centuries. Necrotic tissue and foreign substances in the wound bed serve to impede healing. Debridement is a major consideration for wound bed preparation, enhances wound assessment, decreases infection potential, activates cellular activity, and removes physical barriers to healing [59]. The positive clinical outcome of wound debridement is a viable wound base [59]. Wound bed preparation is emerging as an essential element for obtaining maximal benefits from wound care products [60].

Types of wound debridement include selective and nonselective methods. Nonselective methods remove necrotic and viable tissue; hence, selective methods are usually preferred. Nonselective types of debridement include mechanical (wet-to-dry dressings, hydrotherapy, and pulsed lavage) and chemical (antiseptics, such as Dakin's solution, hydrogen peroxide, iodine, and chlorhexidine) methods. Selective types include surgical, autolytic (moisture-retentive topical therapy), enzymatic (trypsin, collagenase, and papain-urea products), and biotherapy (maggots) (see the article by Dernell elsewhere in this issue) (see Table 2) [59].

Algorithms to assist with the choice of debridement method in chronic human wounds are available [59]. Such is not the case for chronic animal wounds, where the predominant types of nonsurgical debridement are mechanical and chemical (see the article by Dernell in this issue). Other methods of debridement, including enzymatic and biotherapy (maggots), are offered to veterinary patients.

Enzymatic methods of debridement use topical application of exogenous enzymes to the wound surface, where they work synergistically with endogenous enzymes [31]. Enzymatic debridement of animal wounds is used with some frequency as an adjunct to mechanical and chemical wound debridement, particularly when the patient represents a poor anesthetic risk or when surgical debridement presents other risks [54]. Enzymatic agents liquefy coagulum and break down necrotic tissue while sparing viable tissue [54]. Contact time with the wound must be sufficient to produce the desired effect.

Enzymatic agents containing trypsin (eg, Granulex-V), desoxyribonuclease, and fibrinolysin (eg, Elase) are products used for wound debridement (see Table 2). Trypsin dissolves blood clots and digests necrotic tissue, pyogenic membranes, and crusts [31,61]. Desoxyribonuclease and fibrinolysin break down fibrin and inactivate fibrinogen and several coagulation factors. Products of fibrinolysin degradation are not resorbed and must be removed from the wound by irrigation [31]. Collagenase-containing (eg, Santyl) and papain-urea (eg, Accuzyme) products are used in human wounds (see Table 2). Collagenase digests collagen but is not active against keratin, fat, or fibrin [31]. When tested in a necrotic wound model in pigs, collagenase gel was significantly better than a desoxyribonuclease/fibrinolysin product [62]. Papain digests necrotic tissue by liquefying fibrinous debris, but it requires the presence of activators, such as urea, to function [31].

Biotherapy has been recognized as an effective method of debridement in human wounds for 70 years. Medicinal maggots secrete digestive enzymes that selectively dissolve necrotic tissue, disinfect the wound, and stimulate wound healing. When compared with conservative debridement therapy in the treatment of pressure ulcers in human patients, maggot therapy was more effective and efficient [63]. Additionally, the risk of postoperative wound infection among human patients treated with maggots before surgical closure is low (see the article by Dernell in this issue) [64].

References

[1] Myer A. Dressings. In: Kloth LC, McCulloch JM, editors. Wound healing: alternatives in management. 3rd edition. Philadelphia: FA Davis; 2002. p. 232–63.

[2] Myers BA. Dressing selection and bandaging. In: Wound management. Upper Saddle River (NJ): Prentice Hall; 2004. p. 116–51.

[3] Morgan PW, Binnington AG, Miller CW, et al. The effect of occlusive and semi-occlusive dressings on the healing of acute full-thickness skin wounds on the forelimbs of dogs. Vet Surg 1994;23(6):494–502.

[4] Cho CY, Lo JS. Dressing the part. Dermatol Clin 1998;16(1):25–47.

[5] Swaim SF, Gillette RL. An update on wound medications and dressings. Compend Contin Educ Pract Vet 1998;20(10):1133–44.

[6] Gomez JH, Hanson RR. Use of dressings and bandages in equine wound management. Vet Clin North Am Equine Pract 2005;21(1):91–104.

[7] Swaim SF, Gillette RL, Sartin EA, et al. Effects of a hydrolyzed collagen dressing on the healing of open wounds in dogs. Am J Vet Res 2000;61(12):1574–8.

[8] Yvorchuk-St. Jean K, Gaughan E, St. Jean G, et al. Evaluation of a porous bovine collagen membrane bandage for management of wounds in horses. Am J Vet Res 1995;56(12): 1663–7.

[9] Winkler JT, Swaim SF, Sartin EA, et al. The effect of a porcine-derived small intestinal submucosa product on wounds with exposed bone in dogs. Vet Surg 2002;31(6):541–51.

[10] Badylak SF. The extracellular matrix as a scaffold for tissue reconstruction. Semin Cell Dev Biol 2002;13(5):377–83.

[11] Norsworthy GD. Closure of difficult surgical defects using an extracellular matrix bioscaffold. Vet Forum 2005;22(7):35–41.

[12] Gomez JH, Schumacher J, Lauten SD, et al. Effects of 3 biologic dressings on healing of cutaneous wounds on the limbs of horses. Can J Vet Res 2004;68(1):49–55.

[13] Canapp SO Jr, Farese JP, Schultz GS, et al. The effect of topical tripeptide-copper complex on healing of ischemic open wounds. Vet Surg 2003;32(6):515–23.

[14] Mulder GD, Patt LM, Sanders L, et al. Enhanced healing of ulcers in patients with diabetes by topical treatment with glycyl-L-histidyl-L-lysine copper. Wound Repair Regen 1994;2:259–69.

[15] Swaim SF, Bradley DM, Spano JS, et al. Evaluation of multipeptide-copper complex medications on open wound healing in dogs. J Am Anim Hosp Assoc 1993;29:519–25.

[16] Dart AJ, Dowling BA, Smith CL. Topical treatments in equine wound management. Vet Clin North Am Equine Pract 2005;21(1):77–89.

[17] Swaim SF, Riddell KP, McGuire JA. Effects of topical medications on the healing of open pad wounds in dogs. J Am Anim Hosp Assoc 1992;28(6):499–502.

[18] Thomas DR, Goode PS, LaMaster K, et al. Acemannan hydrogel dressing versus saline dressing for pressure ulcers. A randomized, controlled trial. Adv Wound Care 1998;11(6):273–6.

[19] McFadden EA. Multidex gel for use in wound care. J Pediatr Nurs 1997;12(2):125.

[20] Knighton DR, Ciresi K, Fiegel VD, et al. Stimulation of repair in chronic, nonhealing, cutaneous ulcers using platelet-derived wound healing formula. Surg Gynecol Obstet 1990;170(1):56–60.

[21] Carter CA, Jolly DG, Worden CE Sr, et al. Platelet-rich plasma gel promotes differentiation and regeneration during equine wound healing. Exp Mol Pathol 2003;74(3):244–55.

[22] Ueno H, Mori T, Fujinaga T. Topical formulations and wound healing applications of chitosan. Adv Drug Deliv Rev 2001;52(2):105–15.

[23] Brockman DJ, Pardo AD, Conzemius MG, et al. Omentum-enhanced reconstruction of chronic nonhealing wounds in cats: techniques and clinical use. Vet Surg 1996;25(2): 99–104.

[24] Hosgood G. The omentum—the forgotten organ: physiology and potential surgical applications in dogs and cats. Compend Contin Educ Pract Vet 1990;12(1):45–50.

[25] Matthews KA, Binnington AG. Wound management using honey. Compend Contin Educ Pract Vet 2002;24(1):53–60.

[26] Molan PC. The rate of honey in the management of wounds. J Wound Care 1999;8(8): 415–8.

[27] Subrahmanyam M. A prospective randomized clinical and histological study of superficial burn wound healing with honey and silver sulfadiazine. Burns 1998;24(2):157–61.

[28] Chirife J, Scarmato G, Herszage L. Scientific basis for use of granulated sugar in treatment of infected wounds. Lancet 1982;1(8271):560–1.

[29] Kamat N. Use of sugar in infected wounds. Trop Doct 1993;23(4):185–8.

[30] Matthews KA, Binnington AG. Wound management using sugar. Compend Contin Educ Pract Vet 2002;24(1):41–52.

[31] Schultz GS, Sibbald RG, Falanga V, et al. Wound bed preparation: a systematic approach to wound management. Wound Repair Regen 2003;11(2 Suppl):1–28.

[32] Eldor R, Raz I, Ben Yehuda A, et al. New and experimental approaches to treatment of diabetic foot ulcers: a comprehensive review of emerging treatment strategies. Diabet Med 2004;21(11):1161–73.

[33] Bowler PG, Duerden BI, Armstrong DG. Wound microbiology and associated approaches to wound management. Clin Microbiol Rev 2001;14(2):244–69.

[34] Fries RB, Wallace WA, Roy S, et al. Dermal excisional wound healing in pigs following treatment with topically applied pure oxygen. Mutat Res 2005;579(1–2):172–81.

[35] Jonsson K, Jensen JA, Goodson WH III, et al. Tissue oxygenation, anemia, and perfusion in relation to wound healing in surgical patients. Ann Surg 1991;214(5):605–13.

[36] Tibbles PM, Edelsberg JS. Hyperbaric-oxygen therapy. N Engl J Med 1996;334(25): 1642–8.

[37] Pryor KO, Fahey TJ III, Lien CA, et al. Surgical site infection and the routine use of perioperative hyperoxia in a general surgical population—a randomized controlled trial. JAMA 2004;291(1):79–87.

[38] Cronjé FJ. Oxygen therapy and wound healing—topical oxygen is not hyperbaric oxygen therapy. S Afr Med J 2005;95(11):840.

[39] Kalliainen LK, Gordillo GM, Schlanger R, et al. Topical oxygen as an adjunct to wound healing: a clinical case series. Pathophysiology 2003;9(2):81–7.

[40] Silva JCE, Lacava ZGM, Kuckelhaus S, et al. Evaluation of the use of low level laser and photosensitizer drugs in healing. Lasers Surg Med 2004;34(5):451–7.

[41] Samson D, Lefevre F, Aronson N. Wound healing technologies: Low-level laser and vacuum-assisted closure. Evid Rep Technol Assess (Summ) 2004;111:1–6.

[42] Scardino MS, Swaim SF, Sartin EA, et al. Evaluation of treatment with a pulsed electromagnetic field on wound healing, clinicopathologic variables, and central nervous system activity of dogs. Am J Vet Res 1998;59(9):1177–81.

[43] Lambert KV, Hayes P, McCarthy M. Vacuum assisted closure: a review of development and current applications. Eur J Endovasc Surg 2005;29(3):219–26.

[44] Caniano DA, Ruth B, Teich S. Wound management with vacuum-assisted closure: experience in 51 pediatric patients. J Pediatr Surg 2005;40(1):128–32.

[45] Lantis JC, Carr KL, Grabowy R, et al. Microwave applications in clinical medicine. Surg Endosc 1998;12:170–6.

[46] Xu KD, McFeters GA, Stewart PS. Biofilm resistance to antimicrobial agents. Microbiol 2000;146(3):547–9.

[47] Doughty D. Dressings and more: guidelines for topical wound management. Nurs Clin North Am 2005;40(2):217–31.

[48] Howell-Jones RS, Wilson MJ, Hill KE, et al. A review of the microbiology, antibiotic usage and resistance in chronic skin wounds. J Antimicrob Chemother 2005;55(2):143–9.

[49] Waldron DR, Zimmerman-Pope N. Superficial skin wounds. In: Slatter D, editor. Textbook of small animal surgery. 3rd edition. Philadelphia: WB Saunders; 2003. p. 259–73.

[50] Swaim SF, Henderson RA Jr. Wound management. In: Swaim SF, Henderson RA Jr, editors. Small animal wound management. 2nd edition. Baltimore (MD): Williams & Wilkins; 1997. p. 13–51.

[51] DiPiro JT, Edmiston CE, Bohnen JMA. Pharmacodynamics of antimicrobial therapy in surgery. Am J Surg 1996;171(6):615–22.

[52] Robson MC, Edstrom LE, Krizek TJ, et al. The efficacy of systemic antibiotics in the treatment of granulating wounds. J Surg Res 1974;16(4):299–306.

[53] Robson MC. Wound infection. A failure of wound healing caused by an imbalance of bacteria. Surg Clin North Am 1997;77(3):637–50.

[54] Hedlund CS. Surgery of the integumentary system. In: Fossum TW, editor. Small animal surgery. 2nd edition. St. Louis (MO): Mosby; 2002. p. 136–50.

[55] Lee AH, Swaim SF, Yang ST, et al. Effects of gentamicin solution and cream on the healing of open wounds. Am J Vet Res 1984;45(8):1487–92.

[56] Ashworth CD, Nelson DR. Antimicrobial potentiation of irrigation solutions containing Tris-[hydroxymethyl] aminomethane-EDTA. J Am Vet Med Assoc 1990;197(11):1513–4.

[57] Stubbs WP, Bellah JR, Vermaas-Hekman D, et al. Chlorhexidine gluconate versus chloroxylenol for preoperative skin preparation in dogs. Vet Surg 1996;25(6):487–94.

[58] Klohnen A, Wilson DG, Hendrickson DA, et al. Effects of potentiated chlorhexidine on bacteria and tarsocrural joints in ponies. Am J Vet Res 1996;57(5):756–61.

[59] Beitz JM. Wound debridement: therapeutic options and care considerations. Nurs Clin North Am 2005;40(2):233–49.

[60] Falanga V. Classifications for wound bed preparation and stimulation of chronic wounds. Wound Rep Reg 2000;8(5):347–52.

[61] Swaim SF, Henderson RA Jr. Wound dressing materials and topical medications. In: Swaim SF, Henderson RA Jr, editors. Small animal wound management. 2nd edition. Baltimore (MD): Williams & Wilkins; 1997. p. 53–85.

[62] Mekkes JR, Zeegelaar JE, Westerhof W. Quantitative and objective evaluation of wound debriding properties of collagenase and fibrinolysin/desoxyribonuclease in a necrotic ulcer animal model. Arch Dermatol Res 1998;290(3):152–7.

[63] Sherman RA. Maggot versus conservative debridement therapy for the treatment of pressure ulcers. Wound Repair Regen 2002;10(4):208–14.

[64] Sherman RA, Shimoda KJ. Presurgical maggot debridement of soft tissue wounds is associated with decreased rates of postoperative infection. Clin Infect Dis 2004;39(7):1067–70.

Vet Clin Small Anim 36 (2006) 759–791

VETERINARY CLINICS
SMALL ANIMAL PRACTICE

ELSEVIER
SAUNDERS

Dressings, Bandages, and Splints for Wound Management in Dogs and Cats

Bonnie Grambow Campbell, DVM, PhD

Department of Veterinary Clinical Science, College of Veterinary Medicine, Washington State University, Pullman, WA 99164, USA

PURPOSES OF A BANDAGE

Bandages play an important role in overall wound management. Unbandaged wounds desiccate, leading to healing delays and higher incidence of infection and scarring. Clinically, wounds exposed to air are more inflamed, painful, and pruritic, have thicker crusts, and are more likely to scar [1]. Veterinary patients are likely to lick exposed wounds, further compromising healing. In addition, unbandaged wounds are unaesthetic to pet owners. The ideal bandage protects the wound from contamination and mechanical forces exerted by the external environment or the patient, manages wound exudate, provides support and comfort, and creates a wound environment that actively promotes healing.

BUILDING THE BANDAGE: PRIMARY LAYER

The primary layer of the bandage, also called the contact layer or dressing, is the material directly in contact with the wound. This layer should be sterile [2]. The primary layer can protect, débride, absorb exudate, deliver topical medications, and promote healing. Primary dressings vary widely in their properties, two of the most important being occlusiveness and absorption. The contact layer is critical to establishing a wound environment that supports healing. It is important to select a primary dressing that is appropriate to the wound in its current state and to change the type of dressing used as healing progresses.

Basic Techniques
Wet-to-dry and dry-to-dry
Wet-to-dry and dry-to-dry bandages have been a standard means of debriding wounds. In the wet-to-dry technique, a primary dressing of gauze moistened with sterile saline, lactated Ringer solution, or 0.05% chlorhexidine diacetate

E-mail address: bjgc@vetmed.wsu.edu

0195-5616/06/$ – see front matter
doi:10.1016/j.cvsm.2006.03.002

solution is used for wounds with viscous exudate or necrotic tissues. Exudates are diluted and absorbed into outer bandage layers. The fluid evaporates and the bandage dries and adheres to the wound. In the dry-to-dry technique, wounds with low-viscosity exudate are dressed with dry gauze [3]. Exudate is absorbed, evaporates from outer bandage layers, and the dressing becomes dry, adhering to the wound. Gauze is absorptive and nonocclusive. Fibrin adheres the gauze to the wound bed as the wound dries, and adherent tissue is pulled away when the dry gauze is removed. Although wet-to-dry and dry-to-dry bandages are effective in removing necrotic tissue, these methods of mechanical debridement have several disadvantages: (1) Because both healthy and unhealthy tissues stick to the gauze and are removed with the dressing, debridement is nonselective. Healing is delayed by repeated removal of healthy tissue, such as new granulation tissue and epithelial cells [4]. (2) A dry environment does not support the function of the cells or proteases involved in cleanup and repair of the wound [5]. (3) Bacteria penetrate moistened gauze much more readily than occlusive dressings, increasing the risk for infection [6]. (4) Dry gauze disperses more bacteria into the air than moisture-retentive dressings (MRDs) during a bandage change, contaminating the treatment area and increasing risk for cross-contamination between wounds [7]. (5) Fibers from the adhered gauze may remain in the wound bed, acting as a nidus for inflammation [8]. (6) As reported by human patients, wet-to-dry and dry-to-dry bandages are painful to wear and to remove [9]. (7) Although gauze is cheaper than occlusive dressings, human studies consistently have found higher costs for wet-to-dry and dry-to-dry methods because of the need for more frequent bandage changes, increased use of sedation during each bandage change, and slower healing rates [4,10,11]. (8) By removing wound fluid, frequent bandage changes reduce availability of growth factors and cytokines that are essential for healing [12]. For all of these reasons, wet-to-dry and dry-to-dry bandages no longer are considered to meet the standard of care in human medicine, and their use should be limited in veterinary medicine now that so many other more effective options are available.

Moist wound healing

Moist wound healing is a technique being used to a greater extent in wound management. Moisture is retained over a wound by a bandage to enhance healing. The process is related to moisture vapor transmission rate (MVTR). Transepidermal water loss (TEWL), a measure of the movement of water through skin, is 4 to 9 $g/m^2/hr$ for intact skin [8]. TEWL increases to 80 to 90 $g/m^2/hr$ in partial and full-thickness wounds [8]. In a similar way, occlusiveness of bandage material is measured by the MVTR. Low MVTR strongly correlates with positive wound healing outcome, and is predictive of healing when all other variables are held constant [13]. Infection rates tend to be lower under dressings with lower MVTR [14]. When comparing dressings of the same type (eg, hydrocolloids), MVTR is predictive of dressing performance [13]. Dressings with an MVTR of lesser than 35 $g/m^2/hr$ are considered to be moisture retentive. The average MVTR (in $g/m^2/hr$) of hydrocolloid is 11.2, polyurethane film 13.7, polyurethane foam 33.4, and gauze 67.0 [13]. The MVTR of hydrocolloid and polyurethane film are close to the TEWL of skin. MVTR of a dressing may be decreased by the addition of petrolatum or antibiotic ointment or by accumulation of fibrin and other tissue debris on the dressing [6].

Moist wound healing is the process of creating a wound environment that optimizes the body's inherent wound-healing abilities. Cell proliferation and function in the inflammatory and repair phases of healing are enhanced in the warm, moist environment provided by an occlusive MRD (Table 1). Wound fluid provides a physiologic ratio of proteases, protease inhibitors, growth factors, and cytokines at each stage of wound healing. It is important to recognize the value of wound fluid. "To remove exudate solely because it is present does not constitute good practice" [15].

Under an MRD, white blood cells stay in the wound (rather than migrating up into the open weave of gauze) and perform selective autolytic debridement, specifically targeting necrotic tissue and leaving healthy tissue unharmed. The incidence of infection is lower in wounds kept moist by an occlusive dressing for several reasons, including the presence of a barrier to exogenous bacteria, prevention of tissue desiccation and necrosis, improved concentration of systemically administered antibiotics in the wound, and perhaps most importantly, increased viability and activity of white blood cells and their enzymes [8,10,13,16,17]. The low oxygen tension under an occlusive dressing lowers pH, which deters bacterial growth and favors collagen synthesis and angiogenesis [18,19]. Low oxygen tension also is a chemoattractant for white blood cells [18,20]. Occlusive dressings maintain the wound bed at physiological temperatures, supporting the functions of cells, proteases, and growth factors involved in wound repair [21]. People report that MRDs are more comfortable than nonocclusive dressings; this is believed to be because of the soothing effect of wound fluid covering exposed nerve endings [5,11]. MRDs do not adhere to the wound surface, so removal of the dressing is not painful. They are waterproof, preventing entry of urine or other fluids from the environment. Because MRDs allow longer intervals between bandage changes (by preventing desiccation) and result in faster healing, the number of bandage changes and cost of care are decreased [4,10,11]. Additional benefits of maintaining a proper level of moisture at the wound bed include limited expansion of tissue necrosis caused by desiccation [13], lower incidence of scarring [20], and less aerosolization of bacteria during bandage changes [22].

Excess exudate can damage peri-wound skin and the wound bed by way of maceration (softening caused by moisture trapped against the tissue) or excoriation (damage caused by excessive proteolytic enzymes, as found in chronic wound fluid) [23]. Care must be taken to ensure that the wound is kept moist while the surrounding skin remains dry. The clinician's goal is to select a primary dressing that maintains the proper moisture balance, whereby the wound is bathed but not drenched in wound fluid.

Table 1
Properties of primary dressings used for open wounds

Dressing	Level of wound exudate	Fluid management	Forms a gel	Debridement	Other wound effects
Highly Absorptive					
Hypertonic saline	High	Absorbs	–	Desiccation; nonselective	Increases wound perfusion, provides aggressive debridement
Calcium alginate	Moderate to high	Absorbs	+	Autolytic	Hemostatic, promotes granulation and supports epithelialization
Copolymer starch	Moderate to high	Absorbs	+	Autolytic	Supports granulation and epithelialization
Gauze	Moderate to high	Absorbs	–	Mechanical if dries, autolytic if kept moist	Adherence damages healthy tissue, use as 2° absorptive layer in highly exudative wounds
Moisture Retentive[a]					
Polyurethane foam	Moderate	Absorbs; can donate if premoistened	–	Autolytic	Promotes epithelialization, may inhibit exuberant granulation, can deliver moisture or medication
Hydrocolloid	Low to moderate	Absorbs	+	Autolytic	Promotes granulation and epithelialization, adhesion to peri-wound skin may delay contraction, may use as occlusive layer over other dressings
Hydrogel	None to low	Donates or absorbs	+	Autolytic	Supports granulation & epithelialization variable affect on contraction, rehydrates dry wounds

		Nonabsorbent		Autolytic	
Polyurethane film	None to minimal	—	—	—	Promotes epithelialization, do not adhere to fragile peri-wound skin, may use as occlusive layer over other dressings
Porous Non- or Low-Adherent					
Dry	Low	Transfers to 2° layer	—	Minimal	Supports granulation and epithelialization if stays moist
Petrolatum-impregnated	None to low	Transfers to 2° layer	—	Minimal	Granulation tissue can invade gauze, some inhibit epithelialization
Extracellular Matrix Derived					
Bovine collagen	Low	Cover with 1° dressing appropriate for exudate	—	None	Chemotactic, hydrophilic, promotes granulation, can induce inflammatory reaction if not hydrolyzed
Small intestine or bladder submucosa	Low (fenestrate if more)	Cover with 1° dressing appropriate for exudate	—	None	Chemotactic, antibacterial, promotes granulation, replaced by site-specific tissue

Assumes dressings are used with appropriate level of exudate in order to avoid maceration, excoriation, or desiccation. Properties listed are those most common for the dressing type indicated.

aMoisture retentive is defined as MVTR <35 g/m²/hr.

Primary Dressing Materials

One reason that medical and veterinary clinicians may be reluctant to adopt moist wound healing practices when first learning of them is the confusion generated by the plethora of dressing materials available [24] and their composition and properties [5]. When veterinarians were educated on newer bandage materials and provided with an opportunity to use them on clinical patients, they responded with enthusiasm for the products and their ability to improve the rate of wound healing [25].

In the following discussion, primary dressings are categorized into highly absorptive dressings, MRDs, porous low- or nonadherent dressings, and antimicrobial dressings. Extracellular matrix materials also are discussed. Information about each dressing is presented, with a summary in Table 1. Guidelines for dressing selection based on the type of wound and amount of exudate are provided in Fig. 1. Veterinarians are encouraged to become familiar with the use of one or two products for each dressing type in Table 1, and to consult the manufacturer's information for details about the specific characteristics of a particular product.

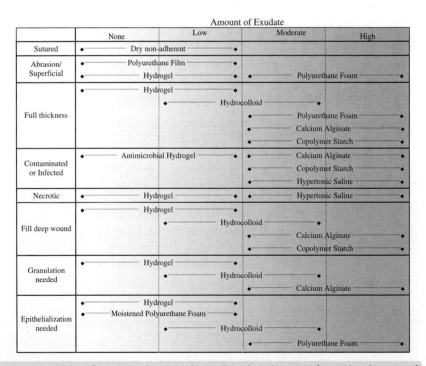

Fig. 1. Guidelines for primary dressing selection based on character of wound and amount of wound exudate.

Highly absorptive dressings

Hypertonic saline. Hypertonic saline dressings are 20% sodium chloride. Their osmotic effect draws fluid from the wound and into the dressing. Mobilization of fluid decreases interstitial edema, decreasing pressure on capillaries and ultimately increasing wound perfusion [26]. The osmotic action also desiccates tissue and bacteria, making hypertonic saline a good choice for infected or necrotic, heavily exudative wounds that need aggressive debridement. Osmotic debridement is nonselective (ie, both healthy and necrotic tissues are removed), and thus close monitoring is required to avoid damage to repair tissue. Hypertonic saline dressings are changed every 1 to 2 days until necrosis and infection are under control, at which time the wound often is ready for a calcium alginate dressing [21]. People report that the osmotic effect of hypertonic saline dressings is uncomfortable once exudate decreases [26].

Calcium alginate. Able to absorb 20 to 30 times its weight in exudate, a hydrophilic calcium alginate dressing is ideal for a highly exudative wound [7]. Calcium alginate dressings are derived from calcium and sodium salts of alginic acid, a polymer found in seaweed [27]. This dressing comes in sheet or rope form and is placed in the wound dry. Sodium ions in the wound fluid are exchanged with calcium ions in the dressing, converting the felt-like material into a hydrophilic gel that molds to the contour of the wound bed and maintains a moist wound environment [7,21,28].

Calcium alginate dressings help wounds transition from the inflammatory to repair phase by promoting autolytic debridement and granulation tissue formation (Fig. 2). They are a good choice in degloving wounds [7,24]. If granulation

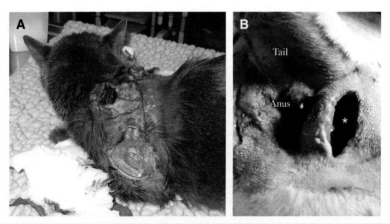

Fig. 2. Indications for calcium alginate dressings—wounds with irregular contours needing autolytic debridement and granulation tissue formation through moist wound healing. (*A*) Interscapular and left forelimb wounds with purulent exudate in a cat secondary to holistic Blood Root injections into a fibrosarcoma. (*B*) Large cavitary right perianal wound (*asterisk*) in a Dalmatian after dehiscence of an anal sacculectomy site.

tissue formation is needed in a wound without excessive exudate, the calcium alginate dressing can be premoistened with sterile saline [10,21,24]. Calcium ions released from the alginate activate prothrombin in the clotting cascade, promoting hemostasis [29]. Alginate dressings supplemented with zinc augment this hemostatic effect and also promote epithelialization [21,29]. Bacteria may become trapped in the alginate gel, decreasing the risk for infection [17,30]. After proper management with a calcium alginate dressing, the wound often is ready for a polyurethane foam contact layer [21].

Calcium alginate sheets are cut to the size and shape of the wound. The rope form is useful for filling deep wounds. The alginate should not be packed tightly into a cavity because this reduces its absorptive ability and because the material swells as exudate is absorbed [27]. To help maintain a moist wound environment, the alginate dressing can be overlaid with a vapor-permeable polyurethane film, or if a significant amount of exudate is escaping, an absorptive foam dressing can be used [31]. Complete gel formation of the alginate can take a few days, so premature removal may disrupt granulation tissue [31]. Alginates are changed when exudate starts to strike through, which may take up to 7 days [8,10]. Soft alginates are removed by lavage with sterile saline, whereas firmer gelled alginates are removed in one piece [32]. The alginate gel may have a foul odor and purulent appearance, but these findings are a normal property of the material and should not be mistaken as evidence of infection [10]. Alginate dressings may be used in infected wounds if they are changed daily [8,27]. Fragments of alginate left in the wound are broken down into Ca^{+2} and simple sugars, so they do not elicit a foreign body reaction [32]. People report that wounds packed with calcium alginate are comfortable [7].

The strong vertical wicking ability of calcium alginate decreases the risk for maceration of peri-wound skin [21], but it is still important to avoid extension of the dressing beyond the wound bed [27]. Because they are so absorptive, calcium alginate dressings can dehydrate a wound as exudate production decreases [7]. People report a burning sensation when alginates are used in sensitive areas or in wounds with low levels of exudate [9]. If left in a wound too long, dehydrated alginate hardens into a calcium alginate eschar that is difficult to take out [17,27]. Rehydration back to a gel with saline may aid in removal [31]. Wounds that are more than 25% necrotic should not be treated with calcium alginate [7].

Copolymer starch. Like calcium alginate, starch copolymers are able to absorb approximately 20 times their weight and are indicated for moderate to highly exudative wounds. Their amorphous shape makes them well suited for filling a deep, uneven wound. Starch copolymers support autolytic debridement and are suitable for necrotic or infected wounds with significant exudate. They also can be used in granulating and epithelializing wounds provided there is significant exudate [33]. Caution is taken to avoid overlaying the copolymer starch on normal peri-wound skin, because maceration can occur [7]. Copolymer starches can be overlaid with a hydrocolloid if an occlusive cover is needed

[34]. The polymer is removed by way of lavage when exudate strikes through [7], or daily if infection is present [8]. If exudate levels are too low the polymer adheres to the wound, causing damage when it is removed and potentially leaving behind dressing fragments that incite inflammation [8]. As with alginates, it is important to monitor wounds closely for decreases in the exudate level when using such a highly absorptive dressing.

Gauze. Gauze can absorb its own weight in exudate [7]. The MVTR of moistened gauze is not low enough for it to be considered an MRD [35]. The detriments of allowing the gauze to dry out on the wound were discussed previously (wet-to-dry bandages). To avoid wound desiccation, saline-soaked gauze may need to be remoistened every 4 hours or more, which is impractical [13].

Although wet-to-dry and dry-to-dry bandages are an older technique of bandaging, gauze continues to be useful in some bandages. In wounds with an extremely high amount of exudate, it may be more cost-effective to use gauze as the primary dressing initially when absorptive bandage changes are needed multiple times a day [8]. Gauze also is useful as a secondary absorptive dressing over wound fillers in exudative wounds [8,32].

Wrapped packages of sterile gauze sponges often are opened on a nonsterile surface. Sterile saline then is poured on the sponges to moisten them before placing them in the wound. Within 30 seconds of adding saline, the sponges become contaminated with small numbers of environmental organisms, regardless of whether the wrapper is coated or uncoated [36]. To decrease the risk for nosocomial infection, sterile gauze sponges should be moistened in a sterile, waterproof container or while held with sterile gloves [36].

Moisture-retentive dressings

Polyurethane foam. Foams are composed of polymers (usually polyurethane). They come in sheets of variable thicknesses, and have a soft, compressible texture (Fig. 3). Moisture vapor transmission rates of foams vary widely (from 33–208 $g/m^2/hr$) [8], so it is important to check the manufacturer's information on specific foam properties. Most foams have an MVTR in the moisture-retentive range. They are highly absorptive and thus are designed for wounds with moderate to high levels of exudate. Foam dressings maintain their structure. A wicking action draws exudate into the foam dressing. This property is useful in removing dampness from peri-wound skin macerated from excessive moisture left by less-absorptive dressings [7].

Foams support moist wound healing either by absorbing excessive exudate or, if pre-moistened, by delivering fluid to the wound bed [28]. Foams are suitable for necrotic wounds needing autolytic debridement. They are not as effective at debridement as alginates or hydrocolloids, however [32]. Foams promote epithelialization, so they are a good choice after a granulation bed has formed and epithelial coverage is needed (Fig. 3) [21]. In people and horses there is some suggestion that foams may help decrease formation of exuberant granulation tissue [8,21]. These compressible dressings decrease the impact of friction on the wound bed, but do not provide enough padding to protect bony

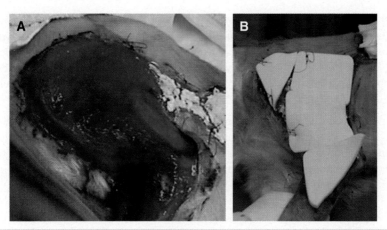

Fig. 3. Polyurethane foam dressing. (A) The degloving wound over the scapula and left fore-limb of this dog has a good granulation bed with a moderate amount of exudate and is in need of epithelialization. (Cranial is to the left, point of the elbow is in the lower right). (B) Polyure-thane foam dressing has been cut to fit the wound.

prominences from pressure [8]. Foams may be used over other wound fillers to provide additional absorptive capacity [8]. Polyurethane foam is used as the contact layer for vacuum-assisted wound closure [7] and as a moistened wound cover for softening and removing eschar (D.J. Krahwinkel, DVM, MS, DCVS, DACVA, DAVECC, personal communication, 2006).

After being cut to the shape of the wound, foam dressings are placed as is on exudative wounds or premoistened with sterile saline or liquid medication before placement on dry wounds (Fig. 3). They are changed every 3 to 7 days or when strikethrough comes within 1 inch of the foam edge, whichever is sooner [8,21]. Foams can be used in infected wounds if changed daily [8]. Foams should not be allowed to dry out because they then can become incorporated into the wound bed, making removal difficult and traumatic [10].

Hydrocolloid. Hydrocolloids are made from a combination of absorbent and elastomeric components that interact with wound fluid to form a gel, resulting in a thermally insulated, moist environment. Hydrocolloid sheets typically are translucent and are backed with a film that is impermeable to fluid, gas, and bacteria [8,33]. Paste, granular, and powdered forms of hydrocolloid lack an impermeable backing; they form a gel that readily fills deep and irregular wounds [34]. The average MVTR of hydrocolloids is less than 12.5 $g/m^2/hr$, similar to skin, meaning they essentially are impermeable to water vapor [8]. Their absorptive ability is suitable for low to moderate levels of exudate.

Hydrocolloids promote autolytic debridement provided there is enough ex-udate to ensure they do not dry out [7]. In the repair phase, hydrocolloids stimulate angiogenesis and collagen synthesis and enhance epithelialization, making them suitable for use in granulating wounds [10,37]. Hydrocolloids also protect the wound from friction, block entry of exogenous bacteria, and reduce wound pain [8]. In deep, highly exudative wounds, hydrocolloid sheets can be used on top of an absorptive wound filler to provide an occlusive component to the bandage [8]. Their occlusive nature also makes hydrocolloids a good choice in areas subject to contamination by urine and feces [7].

Before opening the package, the hydrocolloid sheet is warmed in the hands to soften it and make it moldable [3]. It then is cut to a size and shape slightly larger than the wound. The hydrocolloid is tacky and able to adhere to wet and dry tissues [24]. Light pressure is applied where the hydrocolloid overlaps the peri-wound skin until it adheres [3]. Clipping hair around the wound makes it easier to remove the gel from the skin during bandage changes [38]. The wound bed is not traumatized when the hydrocolloid is removed because the dressing dissolves into a gel on the moist wound surface [24]. The gel may have a mild odor and yellow, purulent appearance; these characteristics should not be misinterpreted as infection [8]. The hydrocolloid sheet is changed when it feels like a fluid-filled blister (2 to 7 days), before fluid leaks out from around the edges. After removing the dressing, remaining gel is lavaged or gently wiped away from the wound or the skin, respectively [3]. This gel usually is more tenacious than that associated with hydrogel dressings.

Hydrocolloids should not be the primary dressing in wounds with a large amount of exudate, because this can lead to maceration or excoriation [9]. The hypoxic environment they create also may favor growth of anaerobes [37]. Bacteria colony counts often are increased under hydrocolloids, but this does not slow healing or increase infection rates [10]. Hydrocolloids should not be used in infected wounds, however. There is some evidence that the hydrocolloids adhered to peri-wound skin may delay wound contraction, so they should be used with caution in the later repair phase [38].

Hydrogel. True to their name, hydrogels are water in a gel form. A fiber network of polymers and humectants is combined with 90% to 95% water to form a sheet or amorphous hydrogel [28,39]. Because they are able to donate moisture and rehydrate tissue, hydrogels are beneficial in dry wounds. Eschars or dry sloughing tissues can be rehydrated with hydrogels sheets, easing their removal [33]. Amorphous hydrogels are available in a semisolid form that can be used to fill deep, dry wounds.

Hydrogels aid necrotic wounds by promoting autolytic debridement and aid granulating wounds by maintaining a moist environment and possibly enhancing fibroblast activity (Fig. 4) [4,34]. Some hydrogels are able to absorb considerable fluid, so they can be used in exudative wounds [10]. Hydrogels are flexible and able to fill in dead space [34]. People report that hydrogels are soothing and cooling, making them a good choice in painful wounds [8,10]. Canine studies found that hydrogels increased contraction of limb wounds [40], but delayed contraction of trunk wounds [41].

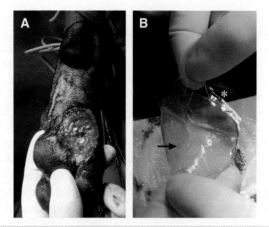

Fig. 4. Indications for a hydrogel dressing—low level of exudate and need for autolytic de-bridement and granulation tissue. (*A*) Debrided chronic ulcer surrounding a draining tract on the palmolateral surface of the paw. (*B*) Using aseptic technique, the hydrogel was cut to the shape of the wound and the backing (*arrow*) was peeled off, exposing the transparent dressing (*asterisk*) to be placed in the wound bed.

Hydrogels containing acemannan (see elsewhere in this issue) may be useful in slow-healing wounds [28]. Those made with alginate, collagen, or starch polymer provide some absorptive capability [8]. Hydrogels containing metronidazole or silver sulfadiazine release their antimicrobial agent into the wound [24].

It is important for the hydrogel to be in contact with the wound surface [7]. To ensure that moisture from the hydrogel is transferred to the wound and not to the rest of the bandage, it is covered with a secondary dressing with a low absorptive capacity, such as a nonadherent dressing or a vapor-permeable polyurethane film [42]. Hydrogel sheets may have this secondary cover built in [43]. Hydrogel sheets are cut to the shape of the wound and placed on the wound bed after peeling off the thin cover (Fig. 4) [24]. They should not overlap skin, because maceration could result [34]. The hydrogel is removed from the wound with gentle saline irrigation at dressing change. In noninfected, full-thickness wounds, hydrogels are changed when they start to get dry, typically every 3 days [7]. In abrasions with minimal exudate, hydrogels may be left in place for 4 to 7 days [8]. Amorphous hydrogels can be used in dry infected wounds if changed daily [43]. Hydrogel sheets are not recommended in the face of infection because of their occlusive nature.

Polyurethane film. Polyurethane films are thin, flexible, and semiocclusive (permeable to gas but not water or bacteria), allowing water vapor to escape [44]. They are nonabsorptive, and thus are indicated for use in wounds with no or minimal exudate. The MVTR of polyurethane film typically ranges from 12.5 to

$33 \text{ g/m}^2/\text{hr}$, so they are moisture retentive and support autolytic debridement. Some films are made with a thin layer of hydrocolloid that provides some absorbency and further decreases MVTR [45]. Films are transparent, allowing visualization of the wound, and have an adhesive perimeter. Unfortunately, hair growth in animals can interfere with adherence to the peri-wound skin. Close clipping of hair is recommended before use of a film dressing.

When used as a primary dressing, films are suited best for dry, shallow wounds or dry abrasions [33]. For this application, they are useful in the repair stage of healing, in which they promote epithelialization [10]. Films are also commonly placed over other contact layers to support moisture retention and provide a bacteria- and waterproof cover. For example, a film may be placed over an amorphous hydrogel to speed autolytic debridement of an eschar, or over a wound filled with calcium alginate to prevent the filler from drying while still allowing excess moisture to evaporate [8,46].

Before applying the film, a backing must be removed. The film should not be applied under tension, because this can damage the peri-wound skin to which it adheres [46]. In people, it is recommended to cover at least 1 in of peri-wound skin with the film to assure good adherence and to change the film when exudate starts to leak onto intact skin, typically every 3 to 7 days [7,8]. It is normal for the exudate accumulating under a film to appear cloudy white or yellow; this should not be misinterpreted as infection [34]. When used over another contact layer, the adhesive perimeter of the film is stuck to peri-wound skin, holding the underlying wound dressing in a picture frame manner [44]. To minimize patient discomfort and skin damage when removing the film, hold the film with one hand, lift up a corner, and stretch the film parallel to the skin to break the adhesive seal [44].

Because it is nonabsorptive, care must be taken to ensure the film does not entrap moisture over intact skin, causing maceration [7]. Polyurethane films do not provide the benefit of thermal insulation [32]. Polyurethane films made for wounds should not be confused with transparent films made for use over intravenous catheters; the former have a low MVTR and create a moist environment that promotes wound healing whereas the latter have a high MVTR and create a dry environment for the catheter site [44]. Polyurethane films are contraindicated in wounds that have high levels of exudate, are infected, or have fragile peri-wound skin [8]. They should not be used over exposed muscle, tendon, or bone, or on third-degree burns [46].

Nonadherent semiocclusive dressings

Nonadherent semiocclusive dressings have low absorptive capacities. They are porous, allowing fluid to move through them into the remainder of the bandage [21]. They should be covered with an absorptive secondary layer and a tertiary layer that allows fluid to evaporate [3]. The porous nature of these dressings also means that they may be penetrated by environmental bacteria [24]. Although often labeled as nonadherent, many of these dressings are actually low-adherent [47]. The chance of adherence is greater when the wound dries because exudate can dry in the pores of the pad [47]. If the pore size is large enough, new granulation or epithelial tissue can grow up into the dressing, resulting in adherence and damage to the repair tissue when the dressing is removed [48,49]. If adhesion has occurred, the bandage should be changed more frequently or the contact layer should be switched to a material that will not adhere [47]. Porous low- or nonadherent semiocclusive dressings come in petrolatum-impregnated and dry forms.

Petrolatum-impregnated gauze is an example of a semiocclusive dressing and is most suitable for the early repair phase. The wide mesh of the gauze is able to absorb the viscous exudate common at this time, whereas the petrolatum minimizes adhesion and damage to new repair tissue [3]. The MVTR of petrolatum-impregnated gauze is not low enough for it to be moisture retentive. These dressings must be changed often enough to prevent incorporation of the dressing into granulation tissue because of growth of capillary loops up into the gauze (Fig. 5) [48]. In a stack of autoclaved petrolatum-impregnated gauze, those at the top may have less petrolatum than those at the bottom, and therefore be less occlusive [48]. Irrigation with saline is of little help with removal of the dried dressing because petrolatum is hydrophobic [49]. Some types of petrolatum slow the rate of epithelialization [48,50], so such dressings should be avoided once epithelialization has begun.

Dry, porous, semiocclusive, nonadherent dressings consist of a layer of absorbent material encased in a perforated sleeve. The sleeve minimizes adhesion, whereas the perforations allow exudate to pass from the wound into the absorbent center. Dry nonadherent dressings are suitable for superficial wounds with low to moderate levels of exudate. They are often used in the later stages of the repair phase when exudate levels are low. Under these

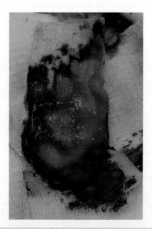

Fig. 5. Petrolatum-impregnated gauze removed from a granulating wound. Granulation tissue grew into the dressing (discoloration on dressing), resulting in loss of healthy tissue when the gauze was removed.

conditions, dry nonadherent dressings retain a moisture balance in the wound that promotes epithelialization while preventing maceration [3]. They are also well suited for covering a sutured wound. Dry nonadherent dressings are changed before strike-through. Viscous exudate may not be able to migrate through the small perforations in the dry nonadherent dressing and can become trapped underneath, resulting in maceration and excoriation.

Antimicrobial dressings

Porous materials like gauze and nonadherent dressings allow fluid to pass through to the secondary bandage layer, but also can be penetrated by bacteria traveling from the external environment into the wound. To counteract this problem, antimicrobial agents, such as iodine, silver, and polyhexamethylene biguanide (PHMB) have been built into dressings. Antimicrobial dressings are indicated for infected wounds or wounds at risk for infection, especially around areas like a joint where infection may be catastrophic. It is important to treat the patient appropriately with systemic antibiotics also, and not rely solely on an antimicrobial dressing in the face of infection (see elsewhere in this issue). Because many antimicrobial dressings are not moisture retentive, covering with polyurethane film may keep the dressing from drying out.

Dressings containing cadexomer iodine absorb wound fluid and subsequently release iodine into the wound. Such dressings maintain a moist wound environment and provide antimicrobial action without affecting wound cells negatively [7,8]. Caution should be used in large wounds, where there is a risk for iodine toxicity from excessive coverage with these dressings [7].

Dressings that release silver ions into the wound can be effective against otherwise antibiotic-resistant organisms, such as *Staphylococcus, Pseudomonas, Enterococcus,* and *Candidiasis* [1,7]. Silver ions also may decrease inflammation by limiting matrix metalloproteinase activity [8]. Silver-releasing dressings are available in gauze, gauze roll, low-adherent, hydrocolloid, hydrogel, and alginate forms [51–53].

PHMB is a cationic surface-active agent related to chlorhexidine that destabilizes bacterial cytoplasmic membranes irreversibly. Bacteria thus cannot develop resistance to this broad-spectrum compound [21]. In an in vitro study, PHMB-impregnated dressings decreased or eliminated proliferation of bacterial pathogens (isolated from patients in a small animal veterinary teaching hospital) within and underneath the dressing [54].

Dressings derived from extracellular matrix

Bovine collagen. Extracellular matrix (ECM) components or a complete matrix bioscaffold may be used underneath a primary dressing to provide a biologic boost to granulation and epithelialization. Bovine collagen provides a ready-made template of organized fibrils that serves as a substrate for fibroblast, endothelial, and epithelial cell migration [55]. Collagen also is chemotactic for white blood cells and fibroblasts [56]. Because the implanted collagen matrix is mature, collagen deposited by host fibroblasts is organized quickly in an appropriate three-dimensional ultrastructure, accelerating the formation of granulation tissue [57]. Powdered hydrolyzed bovine collagen is hydrophilic and draws fluid up through the wound, keeping the wound clean and providing a moist environment. This hydrophilic property may explain the enhancement of early epithelialization found in experimental full-thickness canine wounds covered with hydrolyzed bovine collagen powder [58]. Bovine collagen is recommended for the late inflammatory and repair phases of healing in support of granulation tissue formation and epithelialization [28]. In people, bovine collagen placed in full-thickness scalp defects provided a means to create a receptive site for skin grafting approximately 4 weeks later [59]. Inflammatory reactions to bovine collagen have been observed in horses and in dogs (Steven Swaim, DVM, MS, personal communication, 2006) [60] with experimental wounds covered with porous bovine collagen membranes. Healing was not delayed in horses, however [60].

Extracellular matrix bioscaffolds. Extracellular matrix bioscaffolds are acellular, biodegradable, sterilized sheets. They are most commonly made from porcine small intestinal submucosa (SIS) or porcine urinary bladder submucosa matrix (UBM). The ECMs of these tissues are rich in growth factors and have pre-existing vascular and lymphatic channels [61]. Implantation of an ECM bioscaffold provides structural proteins, growth factors, cytokines, and their inhibitors in physiologic proportions and in a native three-dimensional ultrastructure [62]. When an ECM scaffold is placed in a wound, it is invaded by polymorphonuclear and mononuclear cells [62]. By day three, the cell population is primarily mononuclear, and new blood vessels begin moving into the scaffold. Over the next 2 weeks, mononuclear cells break down the scaffold and deposit a site-specific matrix. Neovascularization during this time is intense. Degradation of the scaffold releases cytokines and growth factors, which further promote healing. The degradation products of the ECM itself are chemotactic for repair cells, stimulate angiogenesis, and have antibacterial properties [39,63,64]. In 30 to 90 days the entire bioscaffold is replaced by site-specific tissue that is capable of handling local mechanical and environmental stresses [62]. Most of the endothelial cells and fibroblasts involved in bioscaffold remodeling are derived from the bone marrow [65]. Healing occurs without infection, necrosis, scarring, or immune rejection [62,64].

ECM bioscaffolds may be indicated when there is a need for granulation tissue. Before implanting SIS or UBS, the recipient site must be thoroughly debrided, free of all topical medications, cleansing agents, and exudates, and infection should be eliminated or well controlled. The ECM sheet is cut to a size slightly larger than the wound and placed in sterile saline for a few minutes to rehydrate. The scaffold is tucked underneath the edges of the wound and sutured in place (Fig. 6). It is important to establish good contact with the wound bed so that host cells can move into the bioscaffold [66]. The sheet can be fenestrated if significant exudate is expected. Based on the level of exudate, the surgery site is covered with a hydrating gel and nonadhesive dressing

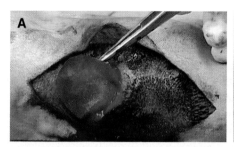 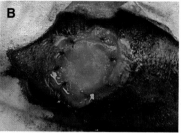

Fig. 6. Indication for extracellular matrix bioscaffold dressing—promote granulation tissue and epithelialization. (A) Extracellular matrix bioscaffold derived from porcine small intestinal submucosa is placed in a nonhealing wound on the carpus of a dog. The bioscaffold was cut slightly larger than the defect and moistened in sterile saline for a few minutes. (B) The bioscaffold was tucked under the edges of the debrided wound and sutured to the skin edges to ensure contact with the wound bed.

or an absorptive MRD. Similar to a free skin graft, motion (including initial bandage changes) at the surgery site is minimized until the bioscaffold is incorporated into the wound. A yellow or brown, almost purulent appearance is normal at the time of the first bandage change on day three or four, and is not an indication for removing the bioscaffold [66]. Outer layers of the bandage are changed; however, the ECM bioscaffold, which is being remodeled within the wound, is left in place. A fresh layer of ECM bioscaffold is placed over the previous ECM, and the next bandage change is performed 4 to 7 days later, depending on the amount of exudate present. After two to three applications a healthy granulation bed typically is present, and no additional ECM bioscaffold needs to be added [66]. Wound management continues with appropriate bandaging for a granulating wound. The cost of ECM bioscaffolds is higher than most other wound dressings, so they are not used routinely in wounds that are healing well.

BUILDING THE BANDAGE: SECONDARY AND TERTIARY LAYERS

Together, the secondary and tertiary layers determine the amount of pressure (used for support, elimination of dead space, or hemostasis), protection, and immobilization provided by the bandage. The thickness of the secondary layer is determined by the amount of wound exudate it is expected to absorb, the occlusivity of the primary dressing, and the amount of protection and support needed [67]. Specific loose-weave, absorbent secondary wrap materials, cast padding, and absorbent bulk roll cotton are available for the secondary layer. It is difficult to apply the latter two materials too tightly because they tear under low levels of extension. The secondary layer is applied in a spiral manner around the affected area, overlapping the bandage material by 50% with each wrap. On limbs, application proceeds from distal to proximal and spans from joint to joint to avoid a tourniquet effect [68]. Self-adherent gauze roll or tubular gauze is placed over the padding to increase support and rigidity by compression of this layer [67]. Multiple layers help distribute differentials in pressure caused by any one layer and provide additional support [68]. Multilayer bandages are also appropriate in patients that cannot be evaluated daily, because they are more likely to stay in place and manage exudate better [68]. The secondary layer should be in contact with the primary layer, but not wrapped so tightly that pressure limits absorption by the primary layer [2]. The secondary layer is changed before exudate soaks through to the tertiary layer [2]. PHMB-impregnated cotton roll gauze can be used in the secondary layer to reduce penetration of bacteria from the environment to the wound and colonization of the gauze itself as exudate is absorbed [24].

Common materials used for the tertiary layer are porous surgical adhesive tape, elastic adherent or self-adherent material, and stockinette. The tertiary layer should be in contact with the secondary layer but not wrapped so tightly that it limits absorption by the secondary layer [2]. Fluid absorbed by the secondary layer can evaporate if the tertiary layer is porous and if a non- or semi-occlusive primary layer has been used [17]. Evaporation concentrates the exudate in the bandage, decreasing bacterial growth [3,17]. Waterproof tape should be used with caution because it may lead to excess moisture retention and the need for more frequent bandage changes [67]. This is true especially for paw bandages in which sweat from the pads added to wound exudate could result in considerable moisture. Any liquid that gets into a bandage covered with waterproof material stays there.

BUILDING THE BANDAGE: SPECIAL CONSIDERATIONS
Bandaging Surgically Closed Wounds
Surgically closed wounds typically have minimal to no drainage. Nonetheless, such wounds may require a bandage to provide hemostasis, decrease seroma or hematoma formation, absorb exudate from the wound or from a surgically placed drain, support surrounding tissue, or protect the wound from self-mutilation or from the environment. A dry, nonadherent, semiocclusive dressing is placed over the surgically closed wound, followed by standard secondary and tertiary layers. In a nondraining wound, the main role of the secondary layer is protective rather than absorptive [69]. The nonadherent dressing absorbs small amounts of exudate, blood, or serum that do develop. If cast padding has been used as the secondary layer, the nonadherent dressing also prevents the padding from getting caught on skin sutures or staples. Moisture-retentive dressings should be avoided because they can lead to maceration when placed over intact skin if some exudate is present. If a Penrose drain is in the wound, the exposed portion of the drain is covered with a nonadherent dressing followed by multiple layers of sterile wide-mesh gauze or laparotomy pads to absorb the discharge and protect from environmental contaminants that could ascend the drain. Collection of discharge in the bandage also allows the clinician to assess the quantity and quality of the drainage fluid and determine when removal of the drain is indicated [69].

Anchoring the Bandage

Stirrups are used to prevent limb bandages from slipping distally. Segments of cotton or cast padding are placed in the interdigital and interpad area to absorb moisture. Then, starting approximately at the level of the carpus or tarsus, two strips of adhesive tape are placed along the longitudinal axis of the limb with half of each strip extending distal to the toes. A tongue depressor is positioned between the two ends of the tape for ease of handling while the primary and secondary layers of the bandage are placed. The tongue depressor then is removed, each strip of tape is twisted 180 degrees at the level of the digits, and the strips are folded proximally to adhere to the secondary layer of the bandage. Hair from the digits that is being pulled by the tape is cut or freed, because this constant pull is uncomfortable for the patient. The tertiary layer of the bandage is then put in place. When the bandage is changed the segments of the stirrups originally extending beyond the toes are cut and removed with the old bandage. New stirrups are placed on top of the segments of the initial stirrups, which remain adhered to the skin. This process avoids pain and damage to the skin caused by repeated removal of the tape stirrups with each bandage change.

Stirrups may not be suitable when the wound involves the paw or distal limb. An alternative method for preventing slippage of a limb bandage is to place a piece of tape so that one half overlaps the dorsal extent of the tertiary layer of the bandage and the other half is on the skin. The tape should not be placed tightly. By holding the tape against the patient's skin for a short period, the heat of the hand and of the patient's body soften the tape adhesive, making it more adherent [70]. Spraying the skin with an acrylate polymer in a hexamethyldisiloxane solution (Cavilon, 3M Animal Care Products) further assures tape adherence and also prevents stripping of the epidermis when the tape is removed [70].

Front or hind limb bandages that extend high on the limb may also be held up with straps that extend over and around the thorax or abdomen, respectively. The straps should be padded appropriately. Abdominal straps must not interfere with urination in male dogs.

Thoracic or abdominal wall bandages tend to slip caudally because of narrowing of the body caudal to the thorax. Thoracic bandages are anchored by a figure eight of bandage material that goes between the front limbs dorsal to the manubrium. To prevent the portion of the figure eight cranial to the shoulders from slipping down, the two straps are taped together where they cross each other dorsal to the manubrium. To prevent caudal slippage of an abdominal bandage, an anchor band of adhesive tape is placed on healthy skin just cranial to the cranial termination of the bandage. As discussed above, the skin can be sprayed with an acrylate polymer in a hexamethyldisiloxane solution before placing the anchor band. The bandage is taped to the anchor band rather than to the skin itself using a piece of wide tape positioned half on the bandage and half on the anchor band as it encircles the body (Fig. 7). When the bandage is changed, the anchor band is left in place, avoiding trauma to the skin caused by repeated removal of tape. The author has also used anchor bands at the proximal end of limb bandages to prevent distal slippage.

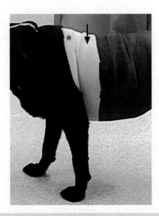

Fig. 7. Labrador Retriever with abdominal wrap. Before placing the abdominal wrap, a piece of elastic adhesive tape was placed around the body just caudal to the forelimbs to serve as the bandage anchor (*asterisk*). After completing the abdominal wrap, a second piece of tape (*arrow*) was placed half on the abdominal bandage and half on the anchor tape so that the abdominal wrap could not slide caudally.

Tie-over bandages are useful for wounds located in regions that are not amenable to traditional bandages (eg, perineum, inguinal region, shoulder) (Fig. 8) [71]. Multiple loose simple interrupted 0 or 2-0 sutures are placed in healthy peri-wound skin, forming loops. The primary dressing is placed on the wound and overlaid with an absorbent layer, such as polyurethane foam, multiple open weave sterile gauze sponges, or sterile laparotomy pads. An occlusive layer, such as polyurethane film, also may be used over the primary dressing

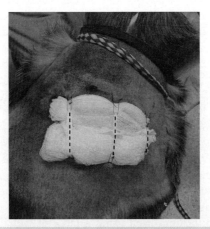

Fig. 8. Tie-over bandage for several puncture wounds over the right shoulder of a Blue Heeler. Suture loops were placed in the peri-wound skin. The primary dressing was covered with multiple gauze sponges. Pieces of umbilical tape (*dashed lines*) were passed through the suture loops and tied to secure the bandage material.

if indicated. Umbilical tape or elastic bandage strips are laced through the suture loops and tied down over the bandage material to secure it in place and provide tension toward the wound's center. When the bandage needs to be changed, the umbilical tape or elastic strips are untied or cut, the wound is cared for, and the suture loops are reused to secure the next bandage (see elsewhere in this issue).

Immobilization with Splints and Casts

Splints commonly are used when wounds are present over joints, because constant motion interferes with wound healing. Splinting also is important after placing a free mesh skin graft or ECM bioscaffold in a mobile area, because any movement of the graft or bioscaffold relative to the wound bed shears off new vessels growing into the graft or bioscaffold. To prepare for a splint or cast, the appropriate primary dressing is covered with a secondary layer of cast padding. Compared with cast padding placed over bony prominences, cast padding placed on either side of bony prominences, and no cast padding, cast padding applied over the whole limb was the best method to prevent pressure injuries over bony prominences on casted limbs [72]. The central two toes are left accessible if possible. More slender areas of the limb are built up to a diameter equal to thicker areas to give the bandage an even cylindrical shape, avoiding a concentration of pressure at sites where the limb narrows proximally (see section on Excessive Pressure and Tissue Ischemia elsewhere in this article). Avoid excess padding underneath a splint, because this increases movement of the splint relative to the skin and decrease its effectiveness [73]. Padding should extend proximal and distal to the splint to avoid friction and pressure wounds on the skin from the splint edge. Commercial Mason metasplints are available in metal or plastic. Splints can be made to fit the patient with plaster of Paris, fiberglass, or thermomoldable plastic. Handmade splints can be reinforced by incorporating metal rods or by molding a longitudinal ridge into the material (Fig. 9). Movement of wounds involving the proximal

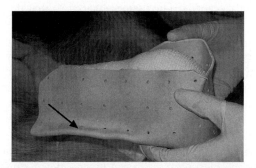

Fig. 9. A splint made from thermomoldable material is applied to the right hind limb of a German Shepherd dog after self- and surgical amputation of all digits because of a neurological injury affecting both hind limbs. A ridge (*arrow*) was made in the splint for reinforcement.

limbs may be minimized with a spica splint or a Velpeau or Ehmer sling. Slings should be applied and monitored carefully. Improper application of a Velpeau sling can lead to excessive compression and carpal hyperflexion, causing circulatory embarrassment because of pressure and a tourniquet effect [74,75]. When using an Ehmer sling, care must be taken to provide sufficient padding just proximal to the metatarsal pad to prevent pressure necrosis from the bandage [74,75].

When a musculoskeletal injury requiring rigid immobilization is present near a wound, a plaster or fiberglass cast can be placed on the patient and then cut longitudinally into two halves [75]. The resulting bivalved cast is removed readily when wound care is needed, and replaced readily after each bandage change. Note should be made of the amount of padding applied deep to the cast the first time so that the same number of layers can be replaced, ensuring a good fit when the cast is reapplied. As soft tissue swelling decreases, the number of cast padding layers may need to be increased. The bivalved cast is secured with a snugly applied circumferential wrap of tape or self-adherent material. A fully encasing cast is contraindicated in a newly traumatized limb with marked soft tissue damage because the limb may swell to the point that the cast compromises the blood supply to the limb [75].

Bandage windows permit examination of the wound and change of the primary dressing without removing the entire bandage, thus maintaining partial or full immobilization of the region. A window that is slightly larger than the wound is cut out of the bandage material, including cast or splint, that overlies the wound. The window site is then appropriately dressed with contact, absorptive, and tertiary layers. Care is taken not to create pressure points around the periphery of the window. Selecting a wound dressing appropriate for the amount of wound exudate may help avoid transport of exudate into the peri-window portion of the bandage, increasing the time interval needed between complete bandage changes.

Pressure-Relief Bandages

A donut bandage is used to relieve pressure on a bony prominence, such as the olecranon or tuber calcaneus. The donut is placed so that the hole is over the point of concern. The donut tends to slip if padding is placed underneath it, so holding it in place calls for creative bandaging. The donut can be taped to the skin, but the skin around the pressure point may not be healthy and tape can be irritating [76]. Stockinette can be taped in place after being fitted snugly over the donut and limb, but caution must be taken to avoid excessive pressure that compromises venous and lymphatic return or creates pressure sores. The donut also may be sewed inside snug-fitting commercial dog clothing (eg, http://www.dogleggs.com/) designed to stay in place.

An inexpensive donut pad that can be incorporated in bandages over convex surfaces, such as the olecranon, calcaneal tuberosity, or carpal pad, is made from rolled cast padding [69]. Several layers of the roll are folded together, making a 6- or 7-cm square pad. The square is temporarily folded in half while a hole is cut in the pad's center. The hole is placed over the convex surface to relieve pressure at the time the secondary and tertiary layers are applied. A do-nut also can be made by cutting a piece of large diameter foam pipe insulation with a transverse cut, or by tightly wrapping tape around a rolled up huck towel, laparotomy pad, or similar material [69].

To avoid pressure on limb lesions not amenable to a donut bandage, foam pipe insulation can be split lengthwise and incorporated into a bandage with a window over the lesion [76]. Several pieces of pipe insulation can be stacked and taped together to increase protection. When foam pipe insulation is used for lesions on the olecranon or calcaneus, it is important to pad the cranial as-pect of the joint while in extension [76].

Another technique for keeping pressure off wounds over the olecranon is to make an elbow loop splint [69]. Aluminum splint rod is bent into a rectangle and the ends of the rod are taped together to maintain this shape. Each long arm of the rectangle is bent in its center to conform to the natural cranial angle of the elbow joint. The short arms of the rectangle are bent in their centers to conform to the transverse curve of the cranial surface of the humerus or radius. After putting a thick bandage on the limb, the elbow loop splint is centered on the cranial aspect of the radial–humeral joint and taped in place to prevent flex-ion of the joint and to limit contact of the olecranon with the ground if the pa-tient should attempt to lie in sternal recumbency.

Wounds on weightbearing pads are subjected to spreading forces that coun-teract wound contraction and cause sutures to tear through wound edges [77]. Non-weightbearing slings may be best for the wound itself, but can cause other problems such as disuse atrophy, pressure sores, joint stiffness, and cartilage degeneration [77]. In a study of paw pad pressures exerted by different ban-dage configurations, extra padding over the metacarpal pad increased pressure on the pad during weight bearing, especially if a metal splint paw cup was used [77]. Pad pressure was relieved by the combination of a foam pad with a hole centered over the metacarpal pad and a metal splint paw cup placed outside the foam pad. A clamshell splint made from two metal splint paw cups extending approximately 2.5 cm distal to the digits further minimized pressure on all of the palmar pads and was recommended for severe pad wounds or after paw pad grafts or other major pad surgery. A piece of folded gauze taped over the ends of the splints provided traction when the dog walked.

Perineal wounds can be protected by side splints anchored to the torso and extending caudal to the tuber ischii, preventing the perineal area from contact-ing the ground when the animal sits [76].

CHANGING THE BANDAGE
Frequency of Bandage Change
The frequency of bandage changes generally decreases as wound healing prog-resses. During the inflammatory and débridement phase, exudate production tends to be at the highest point, requiring close monitoring for strikethrough. Highly absorptive MRDs (eg, calcium alginate, polyurethane foam) that

support autolytic debridement may be left in place for 1 to 3 days, whereas dressings with inadequate absorptive capacity or those prone to drying out (eg, gauze, nonadherent semiocclusive dressings) may need to be changed multiple times a day. Once a healthy granulation bed is established and exudate levels are low, the time between bandage changes often can be expanded to 3 to 4 days with nonadherent dressings and as long as 5 to 7 days with some MRDs. Indications for an unscheduled bandage change include slippage, strikethrough, wetness or damage to the bandage from the environment, odor, swelling or hypothermia in tissues adjacent to the bandage, and constant licking or chewing at the bandage by the patient [76].

Need for Sedation or Anesthesia During Bandage Change

Wound pain is caused by stimulation of nociceptors and damage to local nerves. The latter may lead to altered local sensations, shooting ectopic pain at a distance from the wound, or extreme wound sensitivity to seemingly insubstantial stimuli (eg, decrease in temperature when bandage is removed) [78]. Pain typically is increased in cases of infection or ischemia [78]. The level of pain actually experienced by the patient thus may be disproportionate to that predicted by the appearance of the wound. Appropriate analgesia should be provided to the patient during and between bandage changes.

Pain or discomfort caused by bandage changes can be decreased in several ways. Autolytic debridement with a nonadherent MRD is less painful than mechanical debridement with a wet-to-dry or dry-to-dry dressing. If these latter dressings are used, however, moistening the last layer of gauze on the wound with warm 2% lidocaine a few minutes before removal provides comfort [70]. Adhesive material is removed from the skin in the direction of hair growth, with countertraction provided by a hand on the skin; adhesives also may be loosened with ethanol or a commercial adhesive remover. Anchor bands and stirrups decrease the need for repeated removal and reapplication of adhesive material to the skin. Hexamethyldisiloxane solution can be sprayed on the skin before applying adhesive tape to prevent epidermal stripping when the tape is removed [70].

Sedation is required in some veterinary patients during bandage changes, especially early on in the process when serial lavage and debridement are still being done. Sedation and analgesia may be needed because of wound pain or because the animal resists restraint. Although sedation is an additional expense and risk, the benefits gained include having a tractable patient that allows proper wound management (thus potentially decreasing overall costs because of faster healing) and decrease in stress for the patient and the clinician. General anesthesia typically is required for aggressive surgical debridement, and may be needed for bandage changes when the wound is painful or the patient is particularly aggressive.

Risk for Contamination During Bandage Change

Every time the bandage is changed, the wound is at risk for contamination from the environment, and the environment is at risk for contamination from the wound. In human medicine, aseptic technique (including hand washing and the use of sterile gloves and instruments) is standard when changing a dressing on an open wound [79]. The risk for contamination of the wound and of the environment is increased in open wards and areas of high activity, so it is recommended that bandage changes be performed in well-cleaned, low-traffic areas [79]. After lavage, the peri-wound skin is dried before reapplying the bandage, because retention of moisture on intact skin can lead to maceration and increased risk for infection. The primary dressing is applied to an open wound in a sterile manner. If sterile gloves are not used, the primary dressing is handled by the edges that do not touch the wound.

Moisture-retentive dressings decrease the number of bandage changes needed, thus decreasing the opportunity for contamination. They also decrease bacterial aerosolization. Because all wounds are colonized by bacteria, bacteria are released into the air whenever a primary dressing is changed [22]. Half of the aerosolized bacteria still are present in the room 30 minutes later unless a special ventilation system is in place [22]. This presence puts the patient with multiple wounds at risk for transferring bacteria from one wound to another, and puts subsequent patients that occupy the room at risk for contracting wound bacteria. The number of bacteria released into the environment was 20% higher with removal of a gauze-type dressing than with removal of a MRD [22].

Risk for Damage to Wound Bed During Bandage Change

With removal of an adherent primary bandage layer, material that adheres to the wound bed can cause damage by injuring healthy tissue as the dressing is pulled away and by leaving fragments of material in the wound that incite an inflammatory foreign body reaction. Soaking an adherent contact layer with saline to ease its removal from the wound must be done with caution, because this may increase the risk for maceration of the wound and of peri-wound skin [9].

Cells and proteins involved in wound healing function best at physiologic temperatures and in a moist environment. Each time the wound is exposed to air evaporation occurs, decreasing the temperature and moisture content of the wound. Having all materials needed for wound care ready before unbandaging the wound and sedating the patient if needed to ensure cooperation minimizes the time during which the wound is uncovered. MRDs decrease the frequency of bandage changes, thus providing more uniform hydro- and thermoregulation.

Who Should Perform Bandage Changes?

Because of financial or time constraints, clients may be interested in performing bandage changes on their pet at home. It is advisable for the veterinarian to be involved with each bandage change, especially in the early phases of wound healing when exudate levels can change quickly and debridement is ongoing. Once a healthy granulation bed is established and the interval for bandage changes increases, client participation in wound care becomes more feasible.

The veterinarian or veterinary technician should instruct the client, ensuring he or she uses proper bandaging techniques and understands when veterinary attention is indicated. If a client purchases bandage material from somewhere other than the veterinary practice, the veterinarian should confirm that the material is suitable for the wound.

Cost of Open Wound Management

Clients may request nonsurgical wound management even when surgical options are available because of a false impression that this is certainly less expensive than surgical closure. In the author's experience, however, when the expense of material and professional time is taken into account for treatment of an open wound with serial debridement and bandage changes, costs can equal or exceed those of surgical closure. As discussed above, moist wound healing consistently is less expensive then wet-to-dry and dry-to-dry treatments in human studies [4,10,11].

PREVENTING BANDAGE COMPLICATIONS

Excessive Pressure and Tissue Ischemia

Pressure induced by a wraparound bandage material is determined by the tension of application, number of layers, degree of overlap between successive wraps, and radius of curvature (R) of the part being bandaged [80]. Because R generally increases as one moves proximally on the limb, the pressure exerted by a bandage steadily decreases in a distal to proximal direction [74]. Lower proximal pressure is beneficial in that venous and lymphatic return is not blocked. In anatomical regions where R is smaller proximally than distally (eg, just proximal to the carpus or tarsus or just proximal to the digits), however, an increase in proximal bandage pressure can lead to a tourniquet effect [74]. Padding is added to increase the effective limb radius in these areas to avoid this problem. Flexion and extension of a joint under a bandage puts tension on elastic bandage material and causes a spike in bandage pressure. Elastic cohesive (self-adherent) bandage material cannot move relative to itself to allow redistribution of the increased pressure, thus predisposing to pressure sores around the joint if padding is inadequate [74].

Unfortunately, even after removal of an overly tight bandage, the ischemic effect can be perpetuated by edema from the original injury plus secondary reperfusion injury as blood flow returns to the area [74]. Ischemic injuries from improper bandaging can be severe, resulting in the need for skin grafts, digit or limb amputation, loss of normal limb function, or even death [74]. If pressure bandages are used to control postoperative hemorrhage after onychectomy, extreme care should be used because overly tight bandages can cause ischemic necrosis of the paw [81].

Improper bandages cause signs of discomfort or pain [74]. People with ischemic injury report a burning sensation or numbness; these signs might lead to licking or chewing in dogs and cats [74]. It is important for the veterinary team to educate owners to watch for these signs and for swelling in any exposed digits, and to re-examine the patient if such signs are reported by the client. It is good practice to recheck a bandage within 24 hours after application, because most of the patients in one study developed ischemic injuries 24 to 48 hours after bandage application [74]. If an ischemic injury is suspected, the whole bandage is removed to allow complete evaluation of the limb [74].

Restriction of Joint Mobility

Bandages often are used to restrict motion that would place tension on a wound. The clinician should be aware that prolonged immobilization could lead to disuse atrophy, joint stiffness, pressure sores, and cartilage degeneration [77]. During bandage changes the clinician assesses the patient for joint problems caused by the bandage in addition to caring for the wound itself.

Joint mobility also influences healing of overlying wounds. Wounds on the flexion surface of a joint heal mainly by contraction when the joint is mobile and by epithelialization when the joint is immobilized [82]. Contraction is preferred because it brings full-thickness, haired skin to the area. If there is an adequate amount of peri-wound skin such that the edges can be comfortably brought together it should be sutured; however, if left to heal by second intention the area should be bandaged in such a way as to allow joint movement and healing by contraction [82]. If the wound edges can be brought together only by flexing the joint, the site is at risk for a deforming contracture and the area should be casted to favor epithelialization [82]. Healing of wounds over immobile areas is not influenced by mobility or immobility of nearby joints [82]

Maceration and Excoriation

When the skin remains in contact with wound exudate for a prolonged period, keratinocytes absorb several times their weight in liquid to the point of overhydration [83]. This phenomenon in turn compromises the skin's barrier function and may incite release of proinflammatory mediators; this process is termed maceration [15,83]. Barrier function also is damaged by excoriations, which are abrasions caused by high levels of matrix metalloproteinases (as found in exudate of chronic wounds) [9]. To avoid maceration and excoriation, a contact layer is chosen that is appropriate for the amount of exudate being produced. Wound fluid promotes healing, and the goal is to achieve a moist, not wet, wound environment [15]. Appropriate treatment of bacterial infections further reduces the risk for maceration (see elsewhere in this issue) [15]. Caution must be used when using saline to try to release an adherent dressing from the wound, because soaking the dressing may increase the risk for maceration and tissue trauma [9]. Peri-wound skin may be protected by zinc oxide cream or a barrier film [15], or by cutting the MRD to the size and shape of the wound so that it does not overlap onto healthy skin.

Under an appropriate MRD, newly formed epithelium may appear pale white and be mistaken for maceration. If the clinician consequently switches to a gauze contact layer, the fragile new epithelium dries and dies, reinforcing the clinician's misperception that maceration was occurring [13,15]. When this pale white tissue is seen it is advisable to wait 24 to 48 hours to see if the tissue becomes pale pink, indicating healthy epithelium. True maceration or necrosis stays white or turns a pale yellow [13].

Protecting the Bandage from the Patient and the Environment

An Elizabethan collar (E-collar) is the most common means of protecting a bandage from chewing by the patient. Transparent E-collars allow retention of peripheral vision as compared with opaque models, and in the author's experience are better tolerated by the patient. Commercially available rigid neck collars held in place with Velcro straps prevent flexion of the neck and may restrict access to certain wounds better than an E-collar. Body splints incorporate rigid metal rods that prevent an animal from bending the spine laterally. They are used to immobilize a wound on the body wall or to prevent an animal from bending around to lick or chew at a wound. Muzzles can prevent chewing but may not prevent licking. Cage muzzles are recommended over solid muzzles because their open design helps avoid hyperthermia by allowing airflow and panting. The patient can drink and sometimes eat with the cage muzzle on, and if the patient vomits while wearing the muzzle the risk for aspiration is decreased.

In general, cats are not as tolerant of bandages as dogs. Some cats become aggravated by a bandage, flipping around, trying to shake it free, or even attacking it. Other cats act as if they are uncoordinated or paralyzed when a body bandage is placed. Minimizing the bulk and weight of bandages placed on cats can help mitigate their resistance to the bandage. Good pain control with or without light sedation also may help the patient adjust to the presence of the bandage.

Bandages must be protected from the environment and outside moisture, such as rain, snow, urine, and feces. The weightbearing surface of limb bandages can be reinforced with additional tape to increase durability. When outside in inclement weather, distal limb bandages can be protected with plastic grocery bags or better yet, empty intravenous (IV) bags, which are more durable (Fig. 10). Bandages also can be protected with Saran-wrap type plastic wrap that adheres to itself, or with waterproof diaper pads that are taped in place. Waterproof barriers should be removed once the patient is indoors, because humidity within the bandage can build to the point at which there is risk for maceration.

Specially designed commercial dog and cat products can be used to protect bandages. Canine footgear provides traction and a cushioned surface that protect distal limb wounds (eg, http://www.therapaw.net/). Washable polypropylene covers secured by Velcro are available for hard-to-bandage regions, such as the canine head, hip, shoulder, elbow, and hock (eg, http://www.dogleggs.com/, www.vsmllc.com). Lycra body suits (eg, http://www.k9topcoat.com/) provide a breathable cover (Fig. 11). Diapers designed for dogs and cats with incontinence

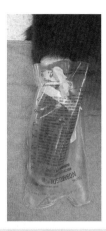

Fig. 10. Distal limb bandage protected with an IV bag before walking the dog outside in inclement weather. The edge of the IV bag containing the entry port was cut off and several holes were punched around the open end of the bag. Roll gauze was threaded through the holes, the bag was slipped over the foot, and the gauze was tied to hold it in place.

or during estrus can help protect wounds in the perineal and inguinal regions (eg, http://www.joybies.com/). In people, clothing has been shown to decrease transmission of water vapor from the bandage to the environment [6]. This decreased transmission may not be as big of a concern in dogs because of differences in sweat glands, but care should be taken to make sure pet clothing does not lead to excessive moisture retention.

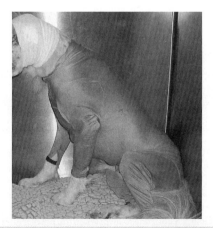

Fig. 11. A lycra body suit used to help hold bandages in place on the thorax, abdomen, and limbs, and to prevent the patient from chewing at the underlying tie-over bandages.

SUMMARY

As our understanding of the cellular and molecular biology of wound healing has grown in recent years, the materials available for bandaging wounds have expanded considerably. No longer limited to a choice between passive adherent or nonadherent dressings, clinicians now can select from an array of materials that interact with wound fluid actively to promote or participate in the wound-healing process. The wound is a dynamic environment. It is important to tailor bandage composition and structure to the specific needs of the wound at each phase of the healing process. Proper selection and application of bandage materials lead to faster wound healing, lower risk for infection, less frequent bandage changes, lower treatment cost, and improved patient comfort.

References

[1] Papen J. Moist wound healing. In: Proceedings of the Society of Veterinary Soft Tissue Surgery. Breckenridge (CO): Society of Veterinary Soft Tissue Surgery; 2003. p. 1–13.
[2] Simpson AM, Beale BS, Radlinsky M. Bandaging in dogs and cats: basic principles. Comp Cont Educ 2001;23(1):12–6.
[3] Swaim SF. Bandages and topical agents. Vet Clin N Amer Sm Anim Prac 1990;20(1):47–65.
[4] Capasso VA, Munro BH. The cost and efficacy of two wound treatments. AORN J 2003; 77(5):984–92, 995–7.
[5] Mureebe L, Kerstein MD. Wound infection: a physician's perspective. Ostomy Wound Manage 1998;44(8):56–60, 62, 63.
[6] Lawrence JC. Moist wound healing: critique I. J Wound Care 1995;4(8):368–70.
[7] Campton-Johnson S, Wilson J. Infected wound management: advanced technologies, moisture-retentive dressings, and die-hard methods. Crit Care Nurs Q 2001;24(2):64–77.
[8] Seaman S. Dressing selection in chronic wound management. J Am Podiatr Med Assoc 2002;92(1):24–33.
[9] Hollinworth H, Collier M. Nurses' views about pain and trauma at dressing changes: results of a national survey. J Wound Care 2000;9(8):369–73.
[10] Kannon GA, Garrett AB. Moist wound healing with occlusive dressings: a clinical review. Dermatol Surg 1995;21(7):583–90.
[11] Kerstein MD. Moist wound healing: the clinical perspective. Ostomy Wound Manage 1995;41(Suppl 7A):37S–44S [discussion 45S].
[12] Cutting KF. Wound exudate: composition and functions. Br J Community Nurs 2003; 8(Suppl 9):S4–9.
[13] Bolton LL, Monte K, Pirone LA. Moisture and healing: beyond the jargon. Ostomy Wound Manage 2000;46(Suppl 1A):51S–62S.
[14] Hutchinson JJ, Lawrence JC. Wound infection under occlusive dressings. J Hosp Infect 1991;17(2):83–94.
[15] Cutting KF, White RJ. Avoidance and management of peri-wound maceration of the skin. Prof Nurse 2002;18(1):35–6.
[16] Hutchinson JJ. Prevalence of wound infection under occlusive dressings: a collective survey of reported research. Wounds 1989;1(2):123–33.
[17] Swaim S. What's new in bandaging wounds. In: Proceedings of the 88th Annual Conference for Veterinarians, College of Veterinary Medicine, Cornell University. Ithaca (NY): Cornell University; 1996. p. 15–8.
[18] Varghese M, Balin AK, Carter DM, et al. Local environment of chronic wounds under synthetic dressings. Arch Dermatol 1986;122:52–7.
[19] Henry M, Byrne P, Dinn E. Pilot study to investigate the pH of exudate on varicose ulcers under DuoDERM. In: Ryan TJ, editor. Beyond occlusion: wound care proceedings. London: Royal Society of Medicine; 1988. p. 67–70.

[20] Jones J. Winter's concept of moist wound healing: a review of the evidence and impact on clinical practice. J Wound Care 2005;14(6):273–6.

[21] Hendrickson DA. Not your ordinary bandage: equine wound care for the 21st century. DVM Best Practices 2002;Feb:7–10. Available at: http://www.dvmnews.com/dvm/issue/issuelist.jsp?id=30.

[22] Lawrence JC. Dressings and wound infection. Am J Surg 1994;167(1A):21S–4S.

[23] Fletcher J. Managing wound exudate. Nurs Times 2003;99(5):51–2.

[24] Stashak TS, Farstvedt E, Othic A. Update on wound dressings: indications and best use. Clin Tech Equine Pract 2004;3(2):148–63.

[25] Cockbill SME, Turner TD. Management of veterinary wounds. Vet Rec 1995;136(14):362–5.

[26] Watret L, White R. Surgical wound management: the role of dressings. Surg Wound Management 2001;15(44):59–69.

[27] Fletcher J. Understanding wound dressings: alginates. Nurs Times 2005;101(16):53–4.

[28] Swaim SF, Gillette RL. An update on wound medications and dressings. Comp Cont Educ 1998;20(10):1133–45.

[29] Segal HC, Hunt BJ, Gilding K. The effects of alginate and non-alginate wound dressings on blood coagulation and platelet activation. J Biomater Appl 1998;12(3):249–57.

[30] Zhai H, Maibach HI. Occlusion vs. skin barrier function. Skin Res Tech 2002;8(1):1–6.

[31] Pudner R. Alginate and hydrofibre dressings in wound management. J Comm Nurs Online 2001;15(5). Available at: http://www.jcn.co.uk/journal.asp?MonthNum=05&YearNum=2001&Type=search&ArticleID=355. Accessed November 14, 2005.

[32] Casey G. Modern wound dressings. Nurs Stand 2000;15(5):47–51.

[33] Eaglstein WH. Moist wound healing with occlusive dressings: a clinical focus. Dermatol Surg 2001;27(2):175–81.

[34] Walker D. Back to basics: Choosing the correct wound dressing. Am J Nurs 1996;96(9):35–9.

[35] Rijswijk L, Harding K, Bacilious N, et al. Issues and clinical implications. Ostomy Wound Manage 2000;46(1A):59S.

[36] Popovich DM, Alexander D, Rittman M, et al. Strike-through contamination in saturated sterile dressings: A clinical analysis. Clin Nurs Res 1995;4(2):195–207.

[37] Pudner R. Hydrocolloid dressings in wound management. J Comm Nurs Online 2001;15(4). Available at: http://www.jcn.co.uk/journal.asp?MonthNum=04&YearNum=2001&Type=search&ArticleID=343. Accessed November 14, 2005.

[38] McGlennon NJ. The role of bandaging in the management of open wounds. Vet Rec 1988;122(26):630–3.

[39] Sarikaya A, Record R, Wu CC, et al. Antimicrobial activity associated with extracellular matrices. Tissue Eng 2002;8(1):63–71.

[40] Morgan PW, Binnington AG, Miller CW, et al. The effect of occlusive and semi-occlusive dressings on the healing of acute full-thickness skin wounds on the forelimbs of dogs. Vet Surg 1994;23(6):494–502.

[41] Ramsey DT, Pope ER, Wagner-Mann C, et al. Effects of three occlusive dressing materials on healing of full-thickness skin wounds in dogs. Am J Vet Res 1995;56(7):941–9.

[42] Thomas S. A structured approach to the selection of dressings. Available at: http://www.worldwidewounds.com/1997/july/Thomas-Guide/Dress-Select.html. Accessed November 14, 2005.

[43] Pudner R. Amorphous hydrogel dressings in wound management. J Comm Nurs Online 2001;15(6). Available at: http://www.jcn.co.uk/journal.asp?MonthNum=06&YearNum=2001&Type=search&ArticleID=365. Accessed November 14, 2005.

[44] Fletcher J. Using film dressings. Nurs Times 2003;99(25):57–8.

[45] Thomas S. Vapour-permeable film dressings. J Wound Care 1996;5(6):271–4.

[46] Pudner R. Vapour-permeable film dressings in wound management. J Comm Nurs Online 2001;15(12). Available at: http://www.jcn.co.uk/journal.asp?MonthNum=12&YearNum=2001&Type=search&ArticleID=422. Accessed November 14, 2005.

[47] Pudner R. Low/non-adherent dressings in wound management. J Comm Nurs Online 2001;15(8). Available at: http://www.jcn.co.uk/journal.asp?MonthNum=08&YearNum=2001&Type=search&ArticleID=380. Accessed November 14, 2005.

[48] Lee AH, Swaim SF, McGuire JA, et al. Effects of nonadherent dressing materials on the healing of open wounds in dogs. J Am Vet Med Assoc 1987;190(4):416–22.

[49] Edwards J. Telfa Clear. J Comm Nurs Online 2002;16(5). Available at: http://www.jcn.co.uk/journal.asp?MonthNum=05&YearNum=2002&Type=search&ArticleID=467. Accessed November 14, 2005.

[50] Eaglstein WH, Mertz PM. "Inert" vehicles do affect wound healing. J Invest Dermatol 1980;74(2):90–1.

[51] Lansdown AB, Jensen K, Jensen MQ. Contreet Foam and Contreet Hydrocolloid: an insight into two new silver-containing dressings. J Wound Care 2003;2(6):205–10.

[52] Dowsett C. The use of silver-based dressings in wound care. Nurs Stand 2004;19(7): 56–60.

[53] Meaume S, Vallet D, Morere MN, et al. Evaluation of a silver-releasing hydroalginate dressing in chronic wounds with signs of local infection. J Wound Care 2005;14(9): 411–9.

[54] Lee WR, Tobias KM, Bemis DA, et al. In vitro efficacy of a polyhexamethylene biguanide-impregnated gauze dressing against bacteria found in veterinary patients. Vet Surg 2004;33(4):404–11.

[55] Smith KJ, Skelton HG, Barrett TL, et al. Histologic and immunohistochemical features in biopsy sites in which bovine collagen matrix was used for hemostasis. J Am Acad Dermatol 1996;34(3):434–8.

[56] Bello TR. Practical treatment of body and open leg wounds of horses with bovine collagen, biosynthetic wound dressing and cyanoacrylate. J Equine Vet Sci 2002;22(4): 157–64.

[57] Doillon CJ, Whyne CF, Berg RA, et al. Fibroblast-collagen sponge interactions and the spatial deposition of newly synthesized collagen fibers in vitro and in vivo. Scan Electron Microsc 1984;Pt 3:1313–20.

[58] Swaim SF, Gillette RL, Sartin EA, et al. Effects of a hydrolyzed collagen dressing on the healing of open wounds in dogs. Am J Vet Res 2000;61(12):1574–8.

[59] Wilensky JS, Rosenthal AH, Bradford CR, et al. The use of a bovine collagen construct for reconstruction of full-thickness scalp defects in the elderly patient with cutaneous malignancy. Ann Plast Surg 2005;54(3):297–301.

[60] Yvorchuk-St Jean K, Gaughan E, St Jean G, et al. Evaluation of a porous bovine collagen membrane bandage for management of wounds in horses. Am J Vet Res 1995;56(12): 1663–7.

[61] Prevel CD, Eppley BL, Summerlin DJ, et al. Small intestinal submucosa: utilization for repair of rodent abdominal wall defects. Ann Plast Surg 1995;35(4):374–80.

[62] Badylak SF. The extracellular matrix as a scaffold for tissue reconstruction. Semin Cell Dev Biol 2002;13(5):377–83.

[63] Badylak SF, Coffey AC, Lantz GC, et al. Comparison of the resistance to infection of intestinal submucosa arterial autografts versus polytetrafluoroethylene arterial prostheses in a dog model. J Vasc Surg 1994;19(3):465–72.

[64] Badylak SF. Xenogeneic extracellular matrix as a scaffold for tissue reconstruction. Transpl Immunol 2004;12(3–4):367–77.

[65] Badylak SF, Park K, Peppas N, et al. Marrow-derived cells populate scaffolds composed of xenogeneic extracellular matrix. Exp Hematol 2001;29(11):1310–8.

[66] Wood JD. Regenerative medicine: new approaches to old problems. In: Veterinary Wound Management Society Newsletter 2004; Spring:1, 4.

[67] Pavletic MM. Drains, dressings, and bandages. In: Proceedings of the 89th Annual Conference for Veterinarians, College of Veterinary Medicine, Cornell University. Ithaca (NY): Cornell University; 1997, p. 7–10.

[68] Baxter H, Ballard K. Bandaging: a vital skill. Nurs Times 2001;97(28):57–60.
[69] Swaim SF. Bandaging and splinting techniques. In: Bistner SI, Ford RB, Raffe MR, editors. Handbook of veterinary procedures and emergency treatment. 7th edition. Philadelphia: WB Saunders; 2000. p. 549–71.
[70] Swaim SF, Henderson RA. Wound dressing materials and topical medications. In: Small animal wound management. 2nd edition. Baltimore: Williams and Wilkins; 1997. p. 53–86.
[71] Seim HB. Tie-over bandage. In: Proceedings of the Atlantic Coast Veterinary Conference. Atlantic City: Atlantic Coast Veterinary Conference; 2003.
[72] Swaim SF, Vaughn DM, Spalding PJ, et al. Evaluation of the dermal effects of cast padding in coaptation casts on dogs. Am J Vet Res 1992;53(7):1266–72.
[73] Simpson AM, Beale BS, Radlinsky MA. Bandaging in dogs and cats: external coaptation. Comp Cont Educ 2001;23(2):157–63.
[74] Anderson DM, White RAS. Ischemic bandage injuries: A case series and review of the literature. Vet Surg 2000;29(6):488–98.
[75] DeCamp CE. External coaptation. In: Slatter DS, editor. Textbook of small animal surgery, vol. 2. 3rd edition. Philadelphia: WB Saunders; 2002. p. 1835–48.
[76] Swaim SF, Hanson RR, Coates JR. Pressure wounds in animals. Comp Cont Educ 1996;19(3):203–18.
[77] Swaim SF, Marghitu DB, Rumph PF, et al. Effects of bandage configuration on paw pad pressure in dogs: a preliminary study. J Am Anim Hosp Assoc 2003;29(2):209–16.
[78] Briggs M, Torra i Bou JE, EWM Association. Understanding the origin of wound pain during dressing change. Ostomy Wound Manage 2003;49(2):10–2.
[79] Xavier G. Asepsis. Nurs Stand 1999;13(36):49–53.
[80] Swaim SF. The effects of dressings and bandages on wound healing. Semin Vet Med Surg (Small Anim) 1989;4(4):274–80.
[81] Hedlund CS. Surgery of the digits and footpads. In: Fossum TW, editor. Small animal surgery. 2nd edition. St. Louis: Mosby; 2002. p. 202–9.
[82] Swaim SF, Lee AH, Henderson RA. Mobility versus immobility in the healing of open wounds. J Am Anim Hosp Assoc 1989;25(1):91–6.
[83] Fletcher J. Exudate theory and the clinical management of exuding wounds. Prof Nurse 2002;17(8):475–8.

Vet Clin Small Anim 36 (2006) 793–817

VETERINARY CLINICS
SMALL ANIMAL PRACTICE

Head and Facial Wounds in Dogs and Cats

Eric R. Pope, DVM, MS

University of Missouri, A302 Clydesdale Hall, 379 E. Campus Drive, Columbia, MO 65211, USA

There are many potential causes for wounds on the head and neck. Commonly encountered causes are blunt and sharp trauma, such as lip avulsion, traumatic cleft palate, and maxillary and mandibular fractures. Wounds left by excision of masses, iatrogenic injuries, such as complications of extensive surgeries or radiation therapy, and burns attributable to chewing electrical cords and contact with caustic substances are other wound sources.

In some instances the cause of the wound may affect the approach to its management. Various benign and malignant tumors of soft tissues occur on the head. A thorough diagnostic workup is essential to determine the type and extent of the tumor because this information may affect treatment recommendations. Burn lesions of the mouth from chewing on electrical cords typically present as blanched, pale gray or tan lesions with marked edema. The extent of the injury may not be demarcated clearly for up to 2 to 3 weeks, however [1,2]. The presence of pulmonary edema, which is a common sequela of electrical shock, should be monitored and treated as necessary because it can be a life-threatening complication of these wounds.

Surgical repair of the oral lesions is delayed until the full extent of injury can be determined. Minor lesions can be allowed to heal by second intention. In young animals, injuries that occur along the dental arcade and are allowed to heal by second intention can result in deviation of the teeth, especially if an adjacent oronasal fistula is present. Oronasal fistulas, unless small and asymptomatic, are surgically repaired. Fistulas in the rostral palate tend to be less troublesome to repair than those located more caudally in the mouth. Second intention healing of lip injuries, particularly those involving the commissures, can limit opening of the mouth [2]. Chronic exposure and drying of teeth and gingiva predispose to periodontal disease. Cheiloplasty is indicated to correct these problems.

PRINCIPLES OF SKIN FLAP DESIGN AND TRANSFER

The extensive blood supply and abundance of skin on the head and in the cervical area provide various options for reconstructing wounds on the head and

E-mail address: Popee@missouri.edu

0195-5616/06/$ – see front matter
doi:10.1016/j.cvsm.2006.03.001

neck. Most defects can be reconstructed using single pedicle advancement flaps, transposition flaps, rotations flaps, axial pattern flaps, or combinations of these procedures. (Details of flap design are discussed in the article by Hedlund elsewhere in this issue.) Microvascular transfer of skin or composite flaps occasionally may be indicated, as detailed in the article by Fowler elsewhere in this issue. Selection of a particular procedure or combination of procedures is influenced by the location of the defect, size of the defect, and availability of local tissue, which is influenced by the patient's species, breed, and individual conformation. For example, defects in dogs with large lips and cheeks, such as the Mastiff, can be reconstructed more easily than in breeds such as the greyhound. As a general rule, tissue is moved from caudal to rostral for facial and head reconstruction.

The single pedicle, transposition, and rotation flaps typically used on the head or the head and neck are subdermal plexus flaps. The blood supply to these flaps does not contain a dominant artery but rather is from branches of the direct cutaneous vessels that run superficial and deep to the cutaneous muscles of the head and neck. There are no reliable formulas for determining length–width ratios to ensure adequate blood supply to subdermal plexus flaps, so clinical judgment (experience) is important in planning procedures. Making a subdermal plexus flap wider increases the likelihood of including one of the larger branches of a direct cutaneous artery but generally decreases the mobility of the flap. Because of the robust blood supply in the head and neck region these flaps usually can be made longer than similarly sized flaps in other areas, such as on the extremities. The goal always should be to make the flap only as long as necessary and with the widest base possible. For this reason, the author typically makes the incisions for creating single pedicle and rotational flaps incrementally until the flap can be moved easily into the recipient site without excessive tension. For transposition flaps, preoperative measurements are needed to help ensure adequate flap length. These flaps always should be elevated in the loose areolar tissue below the cutaneous muscle to minimize trauma to the subdermal plexus vessels and reduce the risk for damaging major blood vessels, nerves, and other important structures, such as salivary ducts. Axial pattern flaps, which incorporate direct cutaneous vessels, allow the veterinary surgeon to develop and transfer large flaps in one setting.

Selection of a particular technique is influenced by the location of the wound and the availability of donor skin. Occasionally only one type of flap is applicable but in most instances more than one option is available. Some wounds may require a combination of flaps. Preoperative planning includes manipulation of the skin at potential donor sites to determine which technique provides adequate tissues for closing the defect while facilitating closure of the donor site with the least interference in function and cosmesis at both sites. If more than one technique still is applicable, choose the one that is easiest to perform with the greatest chance of success. For example, a wound on the midline between the eyes likely could be closed with either a single pedicle advancement flap or transposition flap from the top of the head, depending on the length of the wound. Shorter wounds usually can be closed with single pedicle advancement flaps with little tension on the flap and minimal problems at the donor site, whereas longer defects generally are more amenable to closure with a transposition flap.

LIP AVULSION

Traumatic lip avulsions most commonly involve the mandible but occasionally occur on the upper lip. Injury usually is limited to the premaxillary area, but more extensive injuries can be seen. Avulsion of the lower lip can vary from small rostral injuries to complete separation of the lower lip from the mandible to the level of the commissures. Lip avulsion usually is the result of automobile accidents or falls from heights. In most instances the avulsion occurs along the mucogingival line leaving only the gingiva and mucosa in the interdental space for reattaching the lip. Suturing to the gingiva on the labial (buccal) surface of the teeth is difficult because the gingiva is attached tightly to the underlying bone, and sutures often tear out. Suturing through just the mucosa in the interdental space may not provide enough support to hold the tissue in apposition until adequate healing has occurred. Tissue swelling increases the weight of the lip, placing even more stress on simple suture repairs [3–5].

These wounds often are contaminated and should be thoroughly debrided and lavaged before reconstruction is attempted. Successful repair usually can be obtained by combining direct apposition of the gingiva through the interdental papilla with sutures placed through the mandible (Fig. 1). To place sutures through the mandible a small Kirschner wire is used to drill paired holes through the mandible, avoiding the roots of the teeth. A hypodermic needle can be passed directly through the soft bone rostral to the canine teeth. The lip is held in its normal position and then a hypodermic needle is placed from lateral to medial through the lip and a hole in the mandible. A strand of 2-0 nylon or stainless steel suture is passed through the hypodermic needle from the lingual side of the mandible (point to hub). The needle is withdrawn and placed through the lip and next hole in the mandible. The other end of the suture material is passed through the needle (point to hub) so that the suture is tied on the outside of the mouth. The number of these supporting sutures placed depends on the length of the jaw and extent of the avulsion. All of the supporting sutures are preplaced before any are tied. A Penrose drain can be placed through a stab incision in the intermandibular space before tying the supporting sutures. The supporting sutures are tied just tight enough to hold the lip tissue against the bone. Buttons or plastic tubing can be used to prevent excessive pressure on the skin as the knots are tied. The gingiva is apposed at the interdental papilla using 3-0 or 4-0 absorbable sutures. The drain is removed in 3 to 4 days and the supporting sutures in 10 to 14 days [3,5]. Direct suture apposition of the oral mucosa usually is sufficient for upper lip avulsions, but if additional support is needed interrupted sutures can be placed through the bone between the incisors [5].

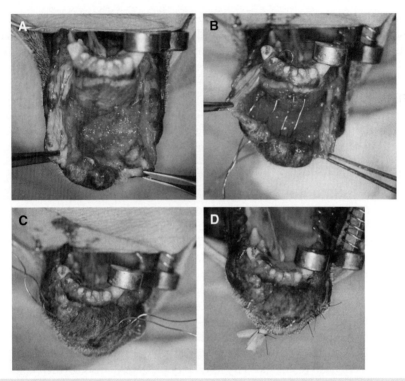

Fig. 1. Dehisced rostral mandibular labial avulsion in a dog after primary suture repair. (A) Appearance of the wound after debridement. (B) Stainless steel sutures passed between tooth roots to support repair. (C) Wire sutures have been pulled snug but not tied. Lip held in close approximation to mandible. (D) The oral mucosa has been sutured. A Penrose drain was placed in the intermandibular space before final tightening of the wires.

LABIAL RECONSTRUCTION

Labial reconstruction is needed following lip lacerations, electrical burn wounds, chemical burns, tumor removal, and tissue loss secondary to injuries, such as gunshot wounds, snake bites, and so forth. Closure of the lip is relatively simple by apposition of the edges following standard wound management. The ability to perform full-thickness resection of masses on the lip and then achieve direct apposition of the tissue varies greatly, however. Marginal excision of benign tumors is appropriate, but excision of malignant tumors should include at least 1 to 2 cm of normal tissue. Simple closure of labial defects in cats and breeds of dogs with relatively tight lips may result in excessive tension or interference with function. Conversely, it may be possible to resect one third to one half of the lip in dogs with large pendulous lips and then directly appose the wound edges without resulting in significant deformity or interference with function.

Wedge Resection

Wedge resection may be appropriate for smaller masses near the lip margin but can result in removal of excessive tissue when the lesion is located away from the lip margin. More lip margin can be preserved in these cases when the incision lines are made to include the margin of normal tissue desired dorsally and laterally and then continued ventrally to the lip margin more or less parallel to the lateral margins of the excision (Fig. 2). After hemorrhage is controlled the oral mucosa is apposed with a simple continuous suture pattern using absorbable material. Inversion of the oral mucosa is avoided because this can interfere with healing. In cats and small dogs the author closes the muscle and oral mucosa as a single layer. A submucosal suture pattern that excludes the mucosa can be used to help assure the mucosa is not inverted. In larger dogs with thicker lips the author prefers to close the muscle as a separate layer. The skin is sutured with a simple interrupted or cruciate suture pattern using monofilament nonabsorbable suture material. Place the first skin suture at the mucocutaneous junction to assure precise alignment of the lip margin.

Lip Flaps

The large and often pendulous lips of dogs allow many major lip and nasal skin defects to be closed using labial advancement and buccal rotation flaps. As a rule of thumb, the labial advancement flap can be used to reconstruct defects

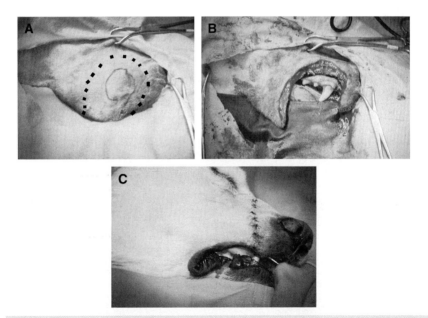

Fig. 2. Lip tumor excision. (A) Solid line outlines a soft tissue sarcoma in the lip. Broken lines indicate wide conforming line of excision. (B) Appearance of the wound after full-thickness resection of the lip. (C) The defect has been closed by direct apposition of the wound edges.

of the rostral one third to one half of the lip. Larger lesions or lesions also involving the skin over the nasal bones likely will require a buccal rotation flap.

Labial advancement flap

To mobilize a labial advancement flap, incise the skin and muscle down to the level of the oral mucosa back to the level of the oral commissure (Fig. 3) [4,5,7]. Incise the oral mucosa at least 5 mm from the mucogingival line to facilitate closure of the oral mucosa incision. As the incision continues caudally look for and preserve the parotid duct papilla if possible. The parotid duct can be cannulated with a lacrimal needle over the needle catheter or suture material to aid in its identification. If the parotid duct cannot be preserved, it should be ligated proximal to the lesion. If necessary the skin incision can be lengthened. The lip must be mobilized to the point that the flap can be advanced over the defect without tension. If tension is present, palpate the base of the flap for any restricting bands in the subcutaneous or submucosal tissue and muscle. If present, carefully divide them to mobilize the flap further. Closure is facilitated by closing the oral mucosa first. Suture the oral mucosa with a simple continuous or interrupted pattern using absorbable suture material. Next, re-establish the lip margin with a cruciate suture (or other tension-relieving suture) at the mucocutaneous junction. Suture the muscle and subcutaneous tissues with interrupted absorbable sutures. The author typically closes the skin with cruciate sutures using monofilament nonabsorbable suture.

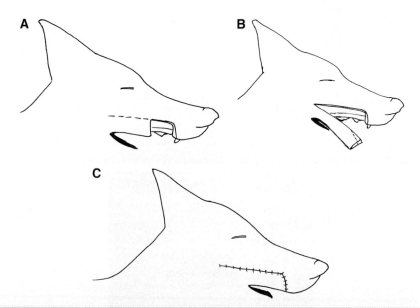

Fig. 3. Labial advancement flap. (A) Diagram of a wound on rostral upper lip. (B) Full-thickness lip incision parallel to the lip margin. Corner of leading edge can be removed (*broken lines*) to reduce vascular compromise. (C) Labial flap advanced and sutured in place to close defect.

Buccal rotation flap

The buccal rotation flap is indicated when there is insufficient tissue to use a labial advancement flap [5–7]. This technique takes advantage of the abundant cheek pouch present in many dogs. It is performed similar to a labial advancement flap except that caudal to the lip commissure the incision curves caudally and ventrally to mobilize the skin and oral mucosa of the cheek pouch (Fig. 4).

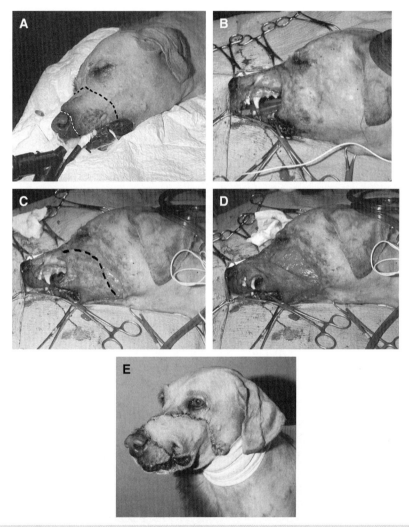

Fig. 4. Buccal rotation flap. (*A*) Diffuse dermal mass located in rostral lip, between broken lines. (*B*) Complete excision necessitated removal of the rostral two thirds of the lip. (*C*) Large buccal skin rotation flap being elevated. (*D*) The flap has been advanced into position. Note the first two sutures were placed at the most distant point of the flap and at the lip margin. (*E*) Appearance of the reconstruction 5 days after surgery.

By continuing the skin incision down onto the cervical area, a skin flap large enough to cover the entire hemimaxilla can be elevated in most dogs. The opening of the parotid salivary duct may need to be relocated or the duct can be ligated.

Lip commissure reconstruction

Resection or loss of tissue near the commissure may leave insufficient oral mucosa for closure. Although the skin defects often can be closed by elevating a skin flap, failure to reconstruct the oral mucosa underneath may lead to saliva trapping, excessive contraction of the skin flap, and a less than optimal result. Two options that can be considered are creation of an inverse tubed skin flap to replace the missing mucosa or use of an acellular matrix material such as porcine intestinal submucosa (VET BIOSIST, Global Veterinary Products, Inc).

The author has used biologic substitutes in several instances in place of the inverse tubed skin flap. After elevating the skin flap to cover the defect, a piece of the acellular matrix material that will span the mucosal defect is cut and sutured to the edges of the oral mucosa. The material also is sutured to the underside of the skin flap with tacking sutures as it is advanced across the defect. The tacking sutures help to eliminate dead space and maintain contact between the material and the underside of the skin flap. The material is eventually replaced with oral mucosa. This technique is easier than the inverse tubed skin flap and has been reasonably effective in limiting contraction of the skin flap.

NASAL PLANUM AND PREMAXILLA

Resection of the nasal planum or premaxilla is indicated most commonly in the management of neoplasia, particularly squamous cell carcinoma. Animals also occasionally are presented following traumatic amputation of these structures. Small superficial lesions may be amenable to conservative resection, but larger and deeper lesions usually are managed by complete resection of the nasal planum or premaxilla. Preoperative CT studies often are helpful in assessing the extent of the lesion and in developing the operative plan. Lesions involving the ventral portion of the nasal planum may necessitate premaxillectomy in addition to nasal planum resection to achieve adequate surgical margins.

Nasal Planum Resection

Nasal planum resection is accomplished by incising the skin circumferentially around the external nares [8,9]. As much of the nasal cartilage and turbinates as necessary is resected to achieve surgical margins. Blood loss can be significant and should be monitored, especially in smaller patients. Using CO_2 laser radiosurgery or electrosurgery helps to minimize blood loss. Direct closure of the skin and nasal mucosa is not necessary in cats. Placing a purse-string suture in the skin and tightening it until the skin edge is brought into close proximity with the nasal cavity provides adequate closure in many cases (Fig. 5). Alternatively, a few interrupted sutures can be placed around the periphery if the defect is not circular. The remaining wound is allowed to heal by second intention. Small dogs can be managed similar to cats. In larger dogs the author

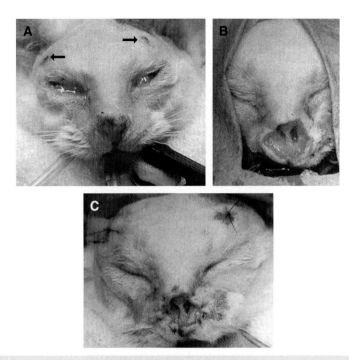

Fig. 5. Nasal planum resection for squamous cell carcinoma in a cat. (A) Preoperative appearance. Excisional biopsy of two lesions on the forehead (*arrows*) also was performed with nasal planum resection. (B) Appearance after nasal planum excision. (C) Immediate postoperative appearance with purse-string suture placed.

prefers to suture the nasal mucosa to the skin dorsally and laterally (Fig. 6). This procedure seems to hold the nasal apertures open and decrease the amount of contraction and stenosis postoperatively. Making small releasing incisions in the lip ventrally makes reconstruction of the lip easier. Continued contraction of the wound sometimes leads to complete stenosis of the reconstructed nares.

Nasal Planum Resection and Premaxillectomy

Nasal planum resection with premaxillectomy starts with incision of the skin dorsally and laterally on the nose [10]. The incision is continued ventrally through the full thickness of the lip and then through the oral mucosa so that the nasal planum and premaxilla can be removed en bloc. The premaxilla can be cut with an osteotome and mallet or sagittal saw. Closure of the defect in the premaxilla is by elevating full-thickness labial advancement flaps bilaterally. Be sure to make the advancement flaps sufficiently long so that tension on the closure is eliminated and dehiscence is less likely to occur. If necessary the labial flaps can be split partially along the dorsal border to facilitate closure of the mucosal defect. The oral mucosa of the flap is sutured either to the mucosa of

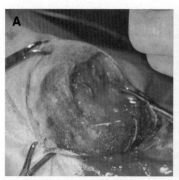 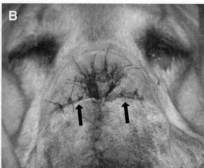

Fig. 6. Extensive nasal planum squamous cell carcinoma removal and reconstruction. (*A*) Appearance of excision of the nasal planum, a portion of the nasal turbinates, and skin ventrally. (*B*) Immediate postoperative appearance. Note sutures from nasal skin to mucosa dorsally to maintain opening of nasal aperture. Horizontal releasing incisions were made in the lip bilaterally to facilitate closure of the skin ventrally (*arrows*).

the premaxilla or to the palatal mucoperiosteum if premaxillectomy was performed. Closure is facilitated by suturing the mucosal layer first as the flaps are advanced toward the midline rostrally. Suture the leading edges of the labial flaps to each other. Suture the muscle and subcutaneous tissue as a single layer using monofilament absorbable suture material. Usually a continuous pattern is used in the oral mucosa and interrupted sutures in the muscle and skin layers. The nasal planum is managed as described above after the lip continuity has been re-established.

Owners generally find the cosmetic appearance of cats after nasal planum resection acceptable. The appearance of dogs after nasal planum resection usually is not as good as cats but is still acceptable to most owners. Nasal planum resection with premaxillectomy obviously causes more significant alteration of cosmetic appearance. Owners should be educated adequately about the postoperative appearance before surgery. Showing owners pictures of previous cases preoperatively can help them appreciate how their pet might look after surgery.

DORSAL NASAL MIDLINE AND FRONTAL SINUS DEFECTS

This area can be one of the more difficult to reconstruct depending on the size and cause of the wound. Some of the most challenging cases the author has managed have been wounds in this area that developed as a complication of radiation therapy, particularly when radiation therapy followed rhinotomy with removal of the nasal bones. These wounds heal poorly and can be challenging because of the degenerative changes that occur in the skin and blood vessels surrounding the wound. Options for reconstruction include the use of nasolabial flaps, single pedicle advancement, or transposition flaps from the dorsum of the head. Indirect tube flaps from the cranial cervical area, axial pattern flaps, and microvascular transfer of skin or composite flaps also can be used.

Nasolabial, inverted hinge, single pedicle, and transposition flaps

Nasolabial transposition flaps are useful for reconstructing rostral dorsal midline defects (Fig. 7 A–E). These flaps take advantage of the abundant lip tissue. The flaps can be constructed using skin only, or a composite flap including the skin and oral mucosa can be used. The latter technique can be used when a bone defect is present. It provides mucosa in the nasal cavity with skin on the outside in hopes of achieving an airtight seal and more stable closure to reduce the risk for dehiscence. These flaps typically are based below the eyes so that they easily can be transposed dorsally to fill the defect. They can be created unilaterally or bilaterally. The donor site is closed easily by direct apposition of the tissues. (See description of the lip-to-lid flap for more details.)

For full-thickness midline defects above the eyes, bilateral hinge inverted flaps can be rotated 180° and sutured together, thus giving a skin lining to the nasal cavity and frontal sinuses. Care must be taken when elevating these flaps to avoid disrupting the blood supply entering the base of the flaps from the nasal mucosa. A single pedicle advancement flap or transposition flap from the dorsum of the head (see later discussion) is used to cover the subcutaneous surfaces of the hinge flaps (Fig. 7 F–G). Tubed skin flaps may be indicated for large defects extending rostrally. Because these procedures typically require multiple surgeries, single pedicle advancement flaps and transposition flaps are used whenever possible.

Single pedicle advancement flaps and transposition flaps from the dorsum of the head can be used to close midline defects between the orbits and to reconstruct the upper eyelids, especially when the conjunctiva can be preserved. Which flap to use is determined by manipulating the potential donor tissue to see which procedure will provide the amount of tissue needed to close the defect while resulting in the least effect on function and cosmetic appearance at the donor site. Because these flaps often are long and narrow they should be as thick as possible (ie, undermined directly off the muscle fascia) so that the subdermal plexus blood supply is compromised as little as possible. The thicker flap also provides the option of performing a two-layer closure when communication with nasal cavity is present and the use of inverted hinge flaps or nasolabial flaps is not possible. If possible, make the flap wide enough that the suture lines lie over the nasal bones and not directly over the nasal bone defect. This position aids in achieving an airtight closure and also minimizes movement at the suture line with respiration. Using monofilament absorbable suture material the subcutaneous tissue of the flap is sutured to fascia or subcutaneous tissue surrounding the defect as the first layer. The skin is closed as the second layer using monofilament nonabsorbable suture material.

WOUNDS ON THE DORSUM OF THE HEAD

Single pedicle advancement flaps, transposition flaps, and the caudal auricular axial pattern flap from the cervical area are useful for reconstructing wounds on the dorsum of the head, including those on the pinna of the ear.

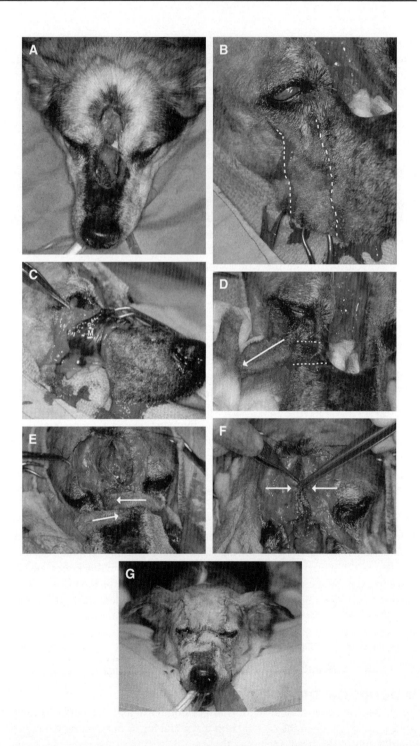

Subdermal Plexus Flaps

Single pedicle advancement flaps take advantage of the loose skin in the cranial cervical area [5]. In most instances the veterinary surgeon can determine if this technique will yield enough skin simply by measuring the length of the defect and then pinching up the skin on the neck. If there are concerns as to whether or not this technique will work, consider using a transposition flap instead [5]. Large transposition flaps usually can be elevated with minimal morbidity at the donor site because of the abundant loose skin the cervical area (Fig. 8). If the base of the flap cannot be incorporated into the edge of the defect, a bridging incision between the edge of the wound and base of the flap is made so that the flap can be sutured completely in place. This procedure avoids tubing the skin flap over an area of intact skin. If necessary, a strip of skin is excised along the bridging incision so that the flap lies flat. A closed suction drain can be placed under the flaps, particularly in the donor area, because seromas are common because of the movement in the cervical area.

Caudal Auricular Artery Axial Pattern Flap

The caudal auricular artery axial pattern flap is a type of transposition flap that incorporates the sternocleidomastoid branches of the caudal auricular artery and vein [11]. Inclusion of these direct cutaneous vessels allows development of longer flaps than the standard transposition flaps based on the subdermal plexus. This flap is based at the caudal aspect of the ear and its length can extend to the cranial or midscapular area. The further the flap extends toward the scapula, however, the greater the chances of failure of its end.

Patient positioning is important to avoid distortion of the cervical skin and underlying anatomic landmarks. Center the base of the flap over the lateral wing of the atlas. Make parallel skin incisions dorsally and ventrally in the central one third of the lateral cervical profile. The flaps can be wider if necessary. Extend the incision far enough caudally to provide a flap that can be transposed to fill the defect without tension. The length of flap needed can be determined preoperatively using a strip of cloth laid over the donor site and then rotated over the defect. Connect the dorsal and ventral incisions caudally. Elevate the flap from caudal to cranial beneath the sphincter colli superficialis muscles. As dissection continues cranially toward the wing of the atlas care

Fig. 7. Dorsal nasal reconstruction. (A) Massive defect after surgical and radiation therapy for a nasal tumor. (B) Initial incisions (*dotted lines*) to elevate a full-thickness nasolabial transposition flap. (C) Flap lifted up to show oral mucosa (M). (D) Bridging incisions between the edge of the flap and the defect (*dotted lines*). Nasolabial flap is indicated by long arrow. The skin and scar tissue were excised. (E) Bilateral nasolabial flaps (*arrows*) transposed into defect. (F) Bilateral hinge flaps based on the edge of the defect (*arrows*) were rolled back toward the midline to reconstruct the nasal mucosa side of the defect. (G) Final appearance after a single pedicle advancement from the top of the head was used to close the remaining skin defect. (*Courtesy of* the University of Tennessee College of Veterinary Medicine, Knoxville, TN; with permission.)

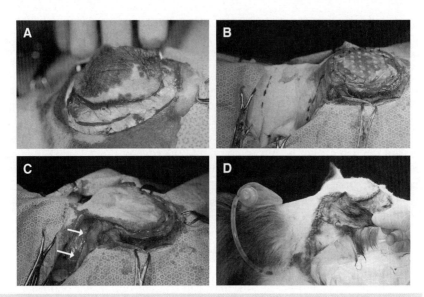

Fig. 8. Dorsal head wound reconstruction by transposition flap. (A) Excision of a large sarcoma including a portion of the temporalis muscle and skull from the top of the head (nose is to the right). (B) The outline for a transposition flap has been made on the cervical skin (*broken line*). Prosthetic implant was placed over the dura. (C) The flap has been transposed to the recipient site. Note how transposition of the flap has facilitated closure of the donor site (*arrows*). (D) Immediate postoperative appearance.

is taken to preserve the vessels entering the base of the flap. Rotate the flap to cover the defect. Placement of a closed suction drain is recommended. The flap and donor site are closed routinely.

EYELID RECONSTRUCTION
The primary objectives during eyelid reconstruction are to maintain a normal palpebral fissure, maintain lid function, and prevent damage to the cornea from exposure and mechanical trauma. Small defects in the upper eyelid usually can be corrected using single pedicle advancement flaps (Fig. 9) while transposition flaps often are necessary for larger defects. The lid margin and conjunctiva are maintained whenever possible, especially on the upper lid because it is primarily responsible for the blink reflex. The same techniques can be used on the lower lid but full-thickness defects also can be reconstructed using composite transposition flaps from the upper lip (lip-to-lid flap).

Single Pedicle Advancement Flaps
The single pedicle advancement flap is designed to match the length and width of the defect [5,12]. A skin marker can be used to draw the intended incision lines on the skin as for almost all flap procedures. The sides of the flap are

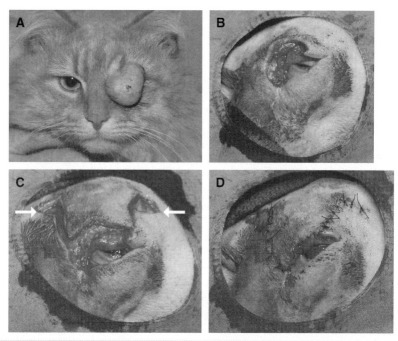

Fig. 9. Single pedicle advancement flap for eyelid reconstruction. (*A*) Large fibroma on the upper eyelid of a cat. (*B*) Defect left after the mass is excised. (*C*) Single pedicle advancement flap. Note excision of Bürow's triangles at the base of the flap (*arrows*). (*D*) Immediate postoperative appearance. (*Courtesy of* the University of Tennessee College of Veterinary Medicine, Knoxville, TN; with permission.)

incised down to the level of the fascia. Beginning at the leading edge, the flap is undermined from the deep fascia. If the flap cannot easily be advanced to cover the defect, the incisions are extended on each side incrementally and the flap undermined further until the tissue is mobilized adequately. The technique of excising Bürow's triangles from base of the lateral borders of the flap is done to decrease dog ear formation and also to decrease the tendency of the flap to retract if subcutaneous sutures are placed into the underlying fascia. The first two sutures are placed at the corners of the leading edge of the flap to re-establish the lid margin. The next two sutures are placed at the base of the flap where the Bürow's triangles have been removed. Sutures should be placed from the dermis down into the underlying fascia to help hold the flap in its advanced position until healing occurs. Additional tacking sutures can be placed if there is adequate exposure. The leading edge of the flap is sutured to the conjunctiva with a simple continuous pattern using absorbable suture material, making sure the suture material does not rub on the cornea. Additional subcutaneous and skin sutures are placed on each side of the flap to complete the procedure. The hair may have to be trimmed periodically to prevent it from rolling in and abrading the cornea.

Transposition Flaps

When a larger defect is present (eg, the defect extends further than the eyelid proper) reconstruction may be accomplished more appropriately with a transposition flap or rotation flap [4,5]. Selecting the best location for the base of the flap is influenced by the location of the defect and manipulation of the surrounding skin. For the upper lid, flaps from the top of the head work well for defects on the medial half of the lid. Defects of the lateral half of the lid may be corrected more easily with flaps from the side of the head. There generally is adequate skin in these areas to allow closure of the donor site with minimal difficulty. If the conjunctiva is excised, it can be replaced with an oral mucosal graft sutured to the underside of the skin flap before the flap is sutured into place. The thin oral mucosa on the frenulum of the tongue is a good source for the graft. Care is exercised to avoid damaging the salivary ducts at the base of the frenulum.

Lip-to-Lid Flap

An advantage of using transposition flaps on the lower lid is the ability to create lip-to-lid mucocutaneous composite flaps to reconstruct full-thickness lid defects. The base of the flap usually is positioned ventrolateral to the lateral canthus on the side of the face to facilitate rotation of the flap into the defect [4,12] This positioning also helps to minimize the flap length. The length and width of flap needed is measured and transferred to the donor site. The flap is harvested from the caudal aspect of the upper lip near the commissure, starting the skin incisions at the mucocutaneous junction. The incisions continue down through the full thickness of the lip to include the oral mucosa for a distance equal to the length of the defect in the conjunctiva. The mucosal incisions are connected, being careful to incise only the mucosa to avoid compromising the vascular supply of the flap. From this point, the flap is undermined as a subdermal plexus flap beneath the platysma muscle. Care is used to avoid damaging the parotid duct, facial vessels, and buccal nerve. The skin incisions are continued until the flap is of adequate length to reach the recipient site. If necessary, a bridging incision may be made between the base the flap and base of the defect. The flap is transposed into position with suturing beginning at the oral mucosa to the conjunctiva at the base of the defect with fine absorbable suture material. Mucosal suturing is continued to the conjunctiva along the sides of the flap up to the mucocutaneous junction. The first skin suture is placed at the lid margin with continued suturing down each side toward the base of the flap. The donor site is closed by first apposing the oral mucosa and then the skin. No attempt is made to correct puckers at the initial surgery. Many times they flatten over time. If necessary, large puckers can be corrected after the flap has completely healed. For more information on blepharoplasty, the reader is referred to ophthalmology texts or chapters in other texts.

AURAL HEMATOMAS

Aural hematomas are the result of scratching or head shaking that causes rupture of the great auricular vessels, with atopy, otitis, and ear mites being underlying factors. Bleeding starts within the cartilage plate of the ear and may extend to either or both sides, but hematomas usually appear to involve only the concave surface of the ear. No one management seems to be successful universally, so treatment largely is based on personal preference and experience. Treatment options include aspiration of the hematoma followed by the application of a pressure bandage, aspiration followed by instillation of steroids or systemic steroids, drainage and insertion of a drain with or without postoperative bandaging, and incisional drainage with or without suturing and bandage application [13,14]. The ear must be evaluated thoroughly and underlying ear disease aggressively treated with antimicrobials and systemic corticosteroids as indicated.

Conservative Therapy

Currently, the author tries aspiration followed by instillation of steroids (for example, triamcinolone) as the first treatment for most patients. If there is improvement but resolution is incomplete, a second treatment usually is attempted. Surgery is recommended if this treatment is unsuccessful.

Drainage

Larger chronic hematomas and recurrent hematomas usually are treated by drainage with drain insertion, or open curettage followed by suturing. A wide variety of drain materials have been used, including silastic tubing, intravenous catheters, red rubber catheters, Penrose drains, and teat cannulas. In most instances drains can be placed using local anesthesia or mild sedation plus local anesthetics. Stab incisions are made at the proximal and distal extents of the hematoma. The hematoma is drained and clots massaged out. Lavaging the cavity with sterile saline may help evacuate the cavity totally. Forceps can be used to pull the drain through the hematoma cavity. The drain is secured at both ends with sutures, leaving adequate space around the drain at emergence sites to allow drainage. Teat tubes are inserted through a single tab incision. The drain is left in place until the hematoma cavity is obliterated, which may take as long as 2 to 3 weeks. The ear can be bandaged over the head if there is considerable drainage or if the animal shakes its head excessively. Otherwise, the author prefers not to bandage the ear. If the drain has a single exit site and the ear will be bandaged, make sure the drain is in a dependent location when the ear is bandaged. Bandages are changed at 5-day intervals unless the drainage soaks through or the bandage becomes wet. This technique is particularly useful in animals that are poor anesthetic risks.

Incision and Suturing

Large hematomas with well-organized clots are treated best by surgical incision, removal of all clot, and suturing. Various types of incisions, including linear, S-shaped, and X-shaped, have been used to open hematomas. A narrow strip of tissue (3–5 mm wide) can be removed from one side of the incision to ensure that the pocket heals before the skin closes. After curetting and lavaging the hematoma cavity, through-and-through mattress sutures are placed to obliterate dead space. The sutures are placed parallel to the major arteries with the knots on the convex surface. The knots should not be tied tightly or postoperative swelling will cause them to cut into the tissue. Stents or other materials can be used to support the sutures and decrease the likelihood of the sutures cutting into the tissues. A bandage is applied to immobilize the ear postoperatively. The bandage should be changed at 3- to 5-day intervals depending on the amount of drainage. If the drainage soaks the bandage or if the bandage gets wet it should be changed immediately. Sutures should be left in until the ear has healed, typically about 14 days, but possibly longer.

EAR RECONSTRUCTION

Lacerations

The initial management of ear lacerations is the same regardless of the severity of the injury. The wound should be cleansed thoroughly, debrided, and protected from secondary infection. Whether or not surgical management is necessary depends on the severity and depth of the laceration. Linear lacerations through one skin surface with the underlying cartilage and contralateral skin intact may be managed as open wounds, although suturing generally produces a better cosmetic result [5,13]. If the laceration has resulted in the formation of a two- or three-sided skin flap, the ear should be sutured to prevent retraction of the skin flap leaving a large defect to heal by second intention. This retraction could result in an epithelialized wound without hair covering or deformation of the ear from wound contraction.

Partial-thickness lacerations

Lacerations through one skin surface and through the cartilage should be sutured to prevent malalignment of the cartilage as the wound heals. These wounds are best sutured with vertical mattress sutures, placing the deep bite to align the cartilage and the superficial bite to appose the skin edges. Simple interrupted sutures also may be used.

Full-thickness lacerations

Full-thickness (perforating) lacerations of the ear should be sutured for best results, especially when the helical border is involved. The laceration may be sutured with simple interrupted sutures through each skin surface or with a simple interrupted pattern in one skin surface and a vertical mattress pattern to align the cartilage and contralateral skin surface as previously described.

Pinna Replacement

Partial or complete loss of the pinna may occur secondary to trauma, frostbite, and vascular impairment because of such things as improper ear bandaging, application of hair bands, and so forth. Partial or complete amputation of the pinna may be necessary in the management of tumors on the pinna. Techniques for replacing lost pinna tissue have been described [5,13], but in most instances the cosmetic appearance is acceptable after amputation.

WOUNDS ON THE VENTRUM OF THE HEAD

Wounds on the ventrum of the head often involve the intermandibular space. Tissue must be moved from caudal to rostral for reconstruction. This reconstruction may be done by a single pedicle advancement flap or caudal auricular artery axial pattern flap [5,15].

Single Pedicle Advancement Flap

The single pedicle advancement flap is designed such that the caudal border of the defect is the rostral edge of the flap [5]. The sides of the flap are incised incrementally following the angulation of the mandibles until the flap is long enough to advance and cover the defect. Walking sutures can be used to advance the flap into position, followed by suturing the flap edges [5].

Caudal Auricular Artery Axial Pattern Flap

The caudal auricular artery axial pattern can also be used to reconstruct large defects in the intermandibular space. The flap is designed as described (see section on Wounds on the Dorsum of the Head elsewhere in this article). Once the flap has been elevated from the donor site, it is transposed ventrally into the intermandibular area. The pedicle of the flap can be tubed, with excision of the tube in 14 to 21 days, or it can be sutured to the edges of a bridging incision. The procedure would be most applicable in brachycephalic breeds of dogs or in cats [15].

ORONASAL FISTULA

Oronasal fistulas most commonly result from dental disease or its treatment (ie, poor extraction technique) but may also be caused by trauma, electrical burns, complications of maxillary fracture, excision of nonneoplastic masses involving the hard palate, and as a complication of surgery, radiation, or hyperthermia treatment of maxillary neoplasia. Common clinical signs of oronasal fistula include sneezing and serous, serosanguineous, or purulent nasal discharge. Food particles occasionally are seen in the nose. The diagnosis often is obvious during physical examination. Oronasal fistula because of periodontal disease or periapical infection usually is diagnosed by periodontal probing or radiography. The palatal surface of the maxillary canine teeth is a common site of oronasal fistula in small breeds of dogs.

The goals for optimal oronasal fistula repair are a well-supported, double-layered, airtight closure that is free of tension. The options for surgical closure of oronasal fistulas are determined by the size, location, and chronicity of the fistula.

Small Alveolar Ridge Fistulas

The technique used for repairing oronasal fistulas located along the dental alveolar ridge is determined primarily by the size and chronicity of the defect. Small fistulas resulting from advanced periodontal disease or tooth extraction are closed with a one- or two-layer technique depending on whether the fistula is acute or chronic. Acute fistulas are corrected with single pedicle advancement or transposition flaps from the buccal mucosa.

Single pedicle advancement flap

In preparation for a small flap, a 2- to 3-mm wide rim of mucosa is excised from the palatal, rostral, and caudal edges of the fistula so that the suture line lies over bone [16]. This placement helps to stabilize the flap against movement and aids in the formation of an airtight seal. If healthy bone is not present or if there is concern that removal of additional tissue will cause excessive tension, the edges of the flap can be sutured to the mucoperiosteum with two layers of sutures after flap creation. The first layer of sutures apposes the deep connective tissue and the second layer apposes the oral mucosa of the flap with the mucosa of the palate.

Necrotic tissue and sharp bone edges are debrided and the area is lavaged thoroughly. A single pedicle advancement flap is used unless it will restrict lip movement excessively. Slightly diverging incisions are made in the gingival and labial mucosa starting at the rostral and caudal borders of the fistula and extending laterally. The labial mucosa–submucosa between the incisions is elevated by sharp and blunt dissection from the underlying bone. If a longer flap is needed, the dissection is continued toward the lip margin separating the layers of the lip. The flap should be sufficiently long that it can be advanced across the defect without tension. The flap is sutured with interrupted cruciate or vertical mattress sutures using 3-0 to 4-0 synthetic absorbable suture material.

Transposition flap

If it is likely that the single pedicle flap will restrict movement of the lip, a transposition flap of labial mucosa is used to repair the fistula [16]. Because of the abundance of cheek tissue in most breeds of dogs, the flap usually is based on the rostral extent of the fistula and developed caudally. The first incision begins at the caudal-most point of the lateral border of the fistula and continues caudally, and the flap is made long enough that it can be transposed over the fistula without tension. The second incision is parallel to the first one so that the width of the flap is equal to the width of the defect. Incisions are connected caudally. The flap is undermined by sharp and blunt dissection, making the flap as thick as possible. It is transposed over the fistula and sutured in place as described previously. The donor site is closed with an interrupted or simple continuous pattern.

Double mucosal flap

Chronic fistulas, in which the oral and nasal mucosa have healed together, can be repaired using a double-flap closure technique that provides a mucosal surface on the oral and nasal sides of the fistula (Fig. 10) [16]. The first step is to create one or two single pedicle hinge flaps based on the edge of the fistula that are inverted back over the fistula so that the mucosal surface is on the nasal side. If a single flap is used it usually is raised from the hard palate mucosa and inverted back to the labial (buccal) side of the fistula. The alternative is to create two opposing flaps, one from the hard palate and the other from the labial (buccal) gingiva, that are inverted back over the fistula. The flaps

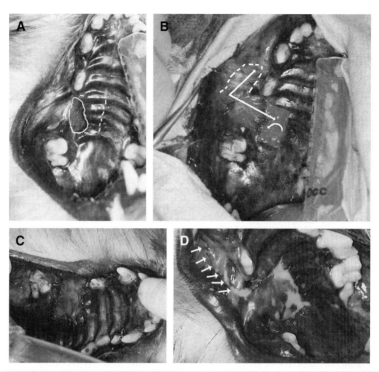

Fig. 10. (A) Oronasal fistula after excision of the upper fourth premolar (*solid line*). Broken lines delineate hinge flap from hard palate to be used as the first layer of closure. (B) Hinge flap has been inverted back over defect to close nasal side of defect (*curved arrow*). Broken line outlines buccal mucosal flap transposed to cover the hinge flap (*straight arrows*). (C) Immediate postoperative appearance. (D) Appearance of flap and donor site at 14 days after surgery. Arrows indicate healed buccal mucosa donor site.

must be undermined carefully to avoid damaging the blood supply entering the flap at the edge of fistula. The hinge flap is sutured to the nasal mucosa laterally (if a single flap has been used) or to each other at the center of the defect (if two flaps have been used) and to the rostral and caudal edges of the fistula with interrupted sutures using 3-0 to 5-0 synthetic absorbable suture material. The second step is to create a flap from the buccal mucosa to cover completely the first layer of closure and the donor site on the hard palate. Either a single pedicle advancement flap or transposition flap is used depending on the size of the defect and availability of lip tissue. If the fistula is large, intact mucosa will remain along the rostral and caudal edges of the fistula. This intact mucosa is incised to create flaps for the nasal and oral sides of the reconstruction.

Large Alveolar Ridge Fistulas

Large oronasal fistulas, as might result from the excision of neoplasms, are repaired with labial mucosa–submucosa single pedicle advancement flaps.

Diverging incisions are made in the labial (buccal) mucosa–submucosa extending toward the lip margin as far as necessary to allow closure of the defect without tension. The flap is created by undermining the mucosa–submucosa between the incisions by sharp and blunt dissection. The thickness of the lip can be split to mobilize the flap further. If the lip is split, the portion with the oral mucosa should be made thicker. The flap is advanced and sutured to the hard palate mucosa in two layers using synthetic absorbable suture material. The first suture layer apposes the submucosa of the labial flap with the mucoperiosteum of the hard palate. Sutures are placed so that the knots lie in the nasal cavity. The second layer of sutures apposes the flap and hard palate mucosa with the knots in the oral cavity. Cruciate or vertical mattress sutures may be used in this area.

Central Hard Palate Fistulas

Oronasal fistulas in the central portion of the hard palate are more of a challenge because reconstruction with labial (buccal) flaps is not an option because of the dental arcade. Oronasal fistulas rostral to the upper fourth premolar are amenable to closure with hard palate mucoperiosteal transposition flaps. Central hard palate oronasal fistulas at the level of the upper fourth premolar or more caudal can often be closed more easily with a partial-thickness transposition flap or hinge flap from the soft palate. The angularis oris flap is another potential technique for reconstructing defects in this area [17]. Large central hard palate fistulas also can be repaired using microvascular transfer of tissue [18].

Fistulas rostral to the fourth premolar

The mucoperiosteum contains little elastic tissue so the pliability of flaps created from this tissue is limited. Also, these flaps will not stretch so it is essential that the caudally based flap be made long enough to avoid tension as the flap is transposed into the defect. The flap is planned so that one edge of the defect is one edge of the flap [16]. If the fistula is chronic, freshen the edges. Laterally, an incision is made parallel to the defect so that the flap is 2 to 3 mm wider than the defect, if possible. The transverse diagonal (distance between the most lateral extent of the base of the flap and the rostral edge of the fistula) is measured. The diagonal of the flap will be this length. Once the dimensions of the flap have been determined, the mucoperiosteum is incised. Side incisions are made first and the rostral incision last. The rostral incision is made using alternating short incisions starting at the lateral and medial edges so that the major palatine artery can be identified and clamped with hemostats before transection. Although some veterinary surgeons just sever the vessel as the rostral incision is made, retraction of the vessel rostrally may make grasping it for ligation difficult. A periosteal elevator is used to elevate the flap, taking care not to injure the origin of the major palatine artery or the base of the flap at the edge of the fistula. The flap is transposed to cover the defect. In some instances removing a triangular-shaped segment of mucoperiosteum from the caudal aspect of the fistula to the base of the flap is necessary to facilitate transposition of the flap over the defect. Because there is no soft tissue to which the flap can be secured on one side of the fistula (the side adjacent to the donor site), drill holes are made in the hard palate bone with a small Kirschner wire to allow preplacement of sutures to secure the flap along the edge of the fistula. The remainder of the flap is sutured in one or two layers with synthetic absorbable suture material. The exposed bone of the donor site is allowed to heal by second intention.

Fistulas caudal to the fourth premolar

Fistulas located more caudally can be reconstructed using a partial-thickness flap from the soft palate. Design the transposition flap to incorporate the edge of the defect into one side of the flap. Incise the oral mucosa of the soft palate and elevate a partial-thickness flap using sharp and blunt dissection. Again, it is important to make the flap of sufficient length to avoid tension on the closure. The edges of the fistula are freshened and the flap is moved over the defect and sutured in place with the synthetic absorbable suture material. The donor site is allowed to heal by second intention. An acrylic dental appliance wired to the teeth can be used to protect the site from trauma during healing.

Postoperative Care

The pharyngeal area should be examined and any blood suctioned before extubation. Most patients are allowed nothing by mouth overnight. A soft diet is recommended for 3 to 4 weeks. Patients should not be allowed to chew on toys and other hard objects during this time. A pharyngostomy or esophagostomy tube can be placed to avoid oral feeding. In most instances problems with healing will become evident within the first week. If dehiscence occurs, the feeding tube can be maintained until another repair is attempted in 3 to 4 weeks. Tube feeding decreases the amount of material that can enter the nose and worsen the inflammatory response. Most complications can be avoided by gentle tissue handling, achieving a tension-free closure, and accurate suture placement. Although most fistulas can be successfully closed, there are instances of failure even after multiple attempts at surgical correction. The best chance of success is with the first surgery. Several different types of obturators have been used to create a barrier to movement of materials into the nasal cavity [19,20]. A simple technique that has been used successfully uses a nasal septal button to achieve obturation [19]. The device is self-retaining but can be removed if necessary.

TRAUMATIC CLEFT PALATE

Traumatic cleft palates most commonly occur in cats that are hit by cars or jump from high places. Other oral trauma, such as mandibular symphyseal separation, also may be present. Although many of these injuries heal spontaneously, the author prefers to correct them surgically while the edges are fresh and can be apposed easily. If conservative management fails, the resulting oronasal fistula is much more difficult to repair.

With the patient anesthetized, blood clots and exudate are suctioned from the nasal cavity. If the cleft is narrow and the edges of the mucoperiosteum can be apposed without tension, the mucoperiosteum is sutured with absorbable suture material using an interrupted suture pattern, such as the cruciate suture pattern. If the defect is wider or the edges of the mucoperiosteum tend to separate again after being manually apposed, apposition can be maintained by passing a small Steinmann pin across the floor of the nasal cavity between the second and third premolars while the fracture is manually reduced and then placing a figure-of-eight wire around the pin ends to achieve compression. The mucoperiosteum is sutured with interrupted absorbable sutures as described above. The pin and wire usually can be removed in 2 to 3 weeks.

References

[1] Pope ER. Thermal, electrical and chemical burns and cold injuries. In: Slatter DH, editor. Textbook of small animal surgery. 3rd edition. Philadelphia: Saunders; 2003. p. 356–72.
[2] Kolata RJ, Burrows CF. The clinical features of injury by chewing electrical cords in dogs and cats. J Am Anim Hosp Assoc 1981;17:219.
[3] Miller WW, Swaim SF, Pope ER. Labial avulsion repair in the dog and cat. J Am Anim Hosp Assoc 1985;21:435–8.
[4] Pavletic MM. Atlas of small animal reconstructive surgery. 2nd edition. Philadelphia: WB Saunders Co.; 1999.
[5] Swaim SF, Henderson RA. Small animal wound management. 2nd edition. Baltimore: Williams and Wilkins; 1997.
[6] Smeak DD. Lower labial pedicle rotation flap for reconstruction of large upper lip defects in two dogs. J Am Anim Hosp Assoc 1992;28:565–9.
[7] Pavletic MM. Reconstructive surgery of the lips and cheeks. Vet Clin N Amer: Small Anim Pract 1990;20:201–26.
[8] Withrow SJ, Straw RC. Resection of the nasal planum in nine cats and five dogs. J Am Anim Hosp Assoc 1990;26:219–22.
[9] Straw RC. Resection of the nasal planum. In: Bojrab MM, editor. Current techniques in small animal surgery. 4th edition. Baltimore: Williams & Wilkins; 1998. p. 343–6.
[10] Kirpensteijn J, Withrow SJ, Straw RC. Combined resection of the nasal planum and premaxilla in three dogs. Vet Surg 1994;23:341–6.
[11] Smith MM, Payne JT, Moon ML, et al. Axial pattern flap based on the caudal auricular artery in dogs. Am J Vet Res 1991;52:922.
[12] MacLaughlin SA, Whitley RD. Eyelid wounds. In: Swaim SF, Henderson RA, editors. Small animal wound management. 2nd edition. Baltimore: Williams and Wilkins; 1997. p. 403–30.
[13] Henderson RA, Horne R. Pinna. In: Slatter DH, editor. Textbook of small animal surgery. 3rd edition. Philadelphia: Saunders; 2003. p. 1737–46.
[14] Bojrab MJ, Constantinescu GM. Sutureless technique for repair of aural hematoma. In: Bojrab MM, editor. Current techniques in small animal surgery. 4th edition. Baltimore: Williams & Wilkins; 1998. p. 97–8.
[15] Aber SL, Amalsadvala T, Brown JE, et al. Using a caudal auricular axial pattern flap to close a mandibular skin defect in a cat. Vet Med 2002;(Sept):666–71.
[16] Pope ER. Repair of oronasal fistula. In: Bojrab MM, editor. Current techniques in small animal surgery. 4th edition. Baltimore: Williams & Wilkins; 1998. p. 120–4.
[17] Bryant KJ, Moore K, McAnulty JF. Angularis oris axial pattern buccal flap for reconstruction of recurrent fistulae of the palate. Vet Surg 2003;32(2):113–9.
[18] Lanz OI. Free tissue transfer of the rectus abdominis myoperitoneal flap for oral reconstruction in a dog. J Vet Dent 2001;18(4):187–92.

[19] Smith MM, Rockhill AD. Prosthodontic appliance for repair of an oronasal fistula in a cat. J Am Vet Med Assoc 1996;208:1410–2.

[20] de Souza HJ, Amorim FV, Corgozinho KB, et al. Management of the traumatic oronasal fistula in the cat with a conical silastic prosthetic device. J Feline Med Surg 2005;7(2): 129–33.

Vet Clin Small Anim 36 (2006) 819–845

VETERINARY CLINICS
SMALL ANIMAL PRACTICE

Distal Limb and Paw Injuries

David Fowler, DVM, MVetSc

Western Veterinary Specialist Centre, 1635 17th Avenue SW, Calgary, Alberta T2T 0E5, Canada

D istal limb reconstruction is complicated by the paucity of local tissues and the frequent association of orthopedic injury with cutaneous loss. Second-intention healing or skin stretching techniques are used for wounds involving less than a 30% circumference of the limb. Skin grafts are recommended for reconstruction of larger superficial wounds after establishing a bed of granulation tissue or for immediate reconstruction of clean wounds overlying healthy muscle. Wounds complicated by orthopedic injury benefit from early reconstruction using vascularized tissue. Weight-bearing surface reconstruction and management of partial amputation injuries are functionally difficult because of the environmental stress placed on the paw pads. Paw pad grafts, paw pad transposition techniques, centralization of digits, and microvascular free tissue transfer of paw pads can be considered for weight-bearing surface reconstruction. Definitive guidelines describing when each of these techniques should be used have not been established.

INJURIES OF THE DISTAL LIMB AND NON–WEIGHT-BEARING SURFACE OF THE PAW
Evaluation of Wounds
Causes

There are numerous causes of distal limb and paw wounds. An encounter with an automobile tire is a common source of injury. Other sources of wounds include tumor removal, snake and insect bites, perivascular injection of irritating medications, leg hold trap injuries, chronic interdigital pyoderma, burns, gunshot wounds, and animal interaction wounds.

Awareness of materials and methods

An awareness of newer wound management medications, bandage materials, and surgical techniques is essential for proper management of all wounds. Each technique, material, or product has specific indications and contraindications depending on the type of wound and the stage of wound healing. Knowledge of wound healing phases and of the effects of each of these factors on

E-mail address: dave2@shawcable.com

0195-5616/06/$ – see front matter
doi:10.1016/j.cvsm.2006.02.004
vetsmall.theclinics.com

wound healing is necessary for optimal treatment of wounds. These issues are covered in detail in other articles elsewhere in this issue.

Classification of wounds

Wounds of the distal extremities should be classified according to the level of contamination, cause, extent of vascular injury, and presence or absence of deep tissue or orthopedic trauma. Wound classifications have profound meaning with respect to proper management and, if overlooked, can lead to the development of nonhealing wounds or systemic complications. The reader is referred to Dr. Dernell's article on initial wound management elsewhere in this issue for detailed information on wound classification.

An understanding of wound biology leads to the conclusion that several factors beyond the level of contamination have a profound effect on the progression of wound healing. The damaged vascularity of the wound and the presence and amount of foreign material must be considered for their potential to enhance tissue necrosis. These, along with necrosis, are associated with the cause of the wound. Underlying orthopedic injury also affects wound severity.

Laceration implies a wound created by sharp incision. Cutting the footpad on a piece of glass is one example. The zone of injury associated with lacerations is limited to the immediate wound environment, and there is little potential for ongoing necrosis. Most lacerations can be converted to a clean-contaminated status with appropriate single-stage debridement and lavage.

Crush-avulsion refers to a wound that is created by severe shear stresses, such as those occurring in a degloving injury. The zone of injury extends well beyond the physical limits of the wound because of extensive vascular trauma, contamination, foreign material (dirt), and underlying orthopedic damage. The extent of vascular injury is often not obvious for 5 to 7 days after injury. Bites are a specific form of crush-avulsion injury and warrant independent classification because of the severity of bacterial contamination. Crush-avulsion injuries require a period of open-wound management, with repeated evaluation, debridement, and lavage, before achieving a clean-contaminated status. At this point, the wound can be managed open or by delayed closure.

Pressure wounds develop because of prolonged impairment of vascular supply to regional tissues. They may be associated with an ill-fitting distal limb splint or cast. Tissues surrounding pressure wounds are usually poorly perfused because of pressure occlusion and biochemical tissue changes. Successful treatment of pressure sores requires appreciation and modification of the environmental factors that contributed to initial wound development (ie, relief of pressure by modifying cast or splint application procedures).

Orthopedic injury complicates many traumatic distal extremity wounds. Shear wounds often extend into joints, with a classic example being a degloving injury to the medial aspect of the tarsus with loss of the medial malleolus and medial collateral ligament and exposure of the tibiotarsal articulation. Open fractures of the distal extremities, particularly the tibia, are common. Tendon, ligament, and bone injuries are frequently associated with severe injuries of the paw.

Although the basic tenant of converting to a clean-contaminated status prevails when treating wounds complicated by orthopedic injury, the presence of bone injury adds an additional factor when considering the timing and method of reconstruction. Early reconstruction using well-vascularized tissues is of paramount importance in such injuries. Early vascular reconstruction of wounds associated with fractures has been associated with earlier and more robust fracture healing as well as a lower complication rate during fracture healing [1].

Options for Reconstruction
Cascade of reconstructive techniques
There has been a plethora of reconstructive techniques introduced to veterinary surgery over the past 2 decades, ranging from simple to advanced. All have advantages, disadvantages, applications, and contraindications. As a general rule, it is preferred to use the simplest method to achieve effective wound reconstruction. It is imperative, however, that the surgeon understand that the simplest method of wound management is not necessarily the most economic or the most effective in terms of total healing time, function, and cosmesis. Second-intention healing is arguably the simplest method of wound healing. Prolonged open management of a large-extremity wound, however, is likely to be more expensive and yield poorer cosmetic and functional results than would a skin graft or flap. Reconstructive options as a cascade listed from simplest to most complex include direct closure, incisional plasties, subdermal plexus flaps, skin grafts, axial pattern skin flaps, pedicled muscle flaps, and microvascular free tissue transfer.

The primary factors in determining the reconstructive technique of choice include inherent vascularity of the wound, exposure of vital structures (eg, joints, fractures), anatomic location, and size of the wound. These factors mandate the urgency of reconstruction (ie, can the wound be managed open for prolonged periods, or is early reconstruction mandatory?). Likewise, the necessity of introducing a new vascular supply to the wound and the availability of regional tissues to facilitate reconstruction are determined by these factors.

Smaller superficial extremity wounds are at little risk for developing complications, such as infection or contracture, as a consequence of a prolonged healing time. In some cases, adequate tissue may be available for direct closure. If not, second-intention wound healing or delayed reconstruction after the appearance of granulation tissue in the wound is appropriate. Conversely, large superficial wounds, especially those overlying joints, have a greater risk of causing contracture or a fragile epithelial scar if left to heal by second intention. Early reconstruction, however, is not mandatory to prevent these complications. Reconstruction using local flaps, where available, or skin grafts after the appearance of granulation tissue in the wound is appropriate.

Wounds with exposed fractures, open joints, or compromised vascular supply benefit from early reconstruction using tissues with a vascular supply independent of the wound, such as axial pattern skin flaps, pedicled muscle flaps, or microvascular free tissue transfer. These reconstructive techniques introduce a new vascular supply to the wound, decrease the risk of subsequent wound infection, and augment healing of deeper injuries [1].

Techniques

Second-intention healing. Second-intention healing can be considered for superficial wounds involving less than a 30% circumference of the limb. Initially, staged debridement is performed to rid the wound of foreign debris and necrotic tissue and to limit the inflammatory phase of wound healing. Topical medications and dressings are applied to the wound. Atraumatic contact dressings that provide a moist wound environment and allow gas exchange are most appropriate once the wound enters the repair phase of healing. Using such treatment, the wound is allowed to heal by contraction and epithelialization. Specific medications, dressings, and healing by second intention are addressed in articles by Krahwinkel and Booth, Campbell, and Hosgood elsewhere in this issue.

Skin relaxing and stretching

Presuturing. Skin has viscoelastic properties that can be used to advantage with advanced planning of wound reconstruction. When placed under tension, skin initially deforms to accommodate the new stresses to which it is exposed. Skin rapidly accommodates to these new stresses via a process of mechanical creep and stress relaxation [2]. Within 12 hours of application of tension, a marked reduction in resistance to tensile forces is noted. When planning reconstruction of an anticipated wound (eg, tumor or scar excision), this process can be used to advantage. Tension is placed on skin surrounding the wound via application of preplaced Lembert sutures for 72 to 96 hours before surgery (Fig. 1). At the time of surgery, tensioning sutures are removed and excision of the lesion is completed. Remaining skin surrounding the wound is then advanced toward the center of the wound with far less tension than had prior skin stretching not been used.

Multiple punctuate relaxing incisions. Multiple punctuate relaxing incisions, or mesh expansion, involve placing staggered parallel rows of stab incisions through skin surrounding the wound to facilitate advancement of skin margins over the wound. In essence, this technique converts a single large wound into multiple small wounds that heal much more rapidly by second intention. Skin is first undermined, and an attempt is made to advance margins over the wound. The first row of punctuate incisions is made as a continuous, intradermal, absorbable suture is placed and tightened. Incisions are made parallel to and approximately 1 to 2 cm from the skin margins on both sides of the wound. They are approximately 1 cm in length and are spaced 1 to 2 cm apart. The skin is advanced over the wound as the suture is tightened. If excessive tension persists while the suture is being tightened, a second row of punctuate incisions is made. The second row is placed approximately 1 to 2 cm from the first row with incisions again parallel to the skin margins but staggered in

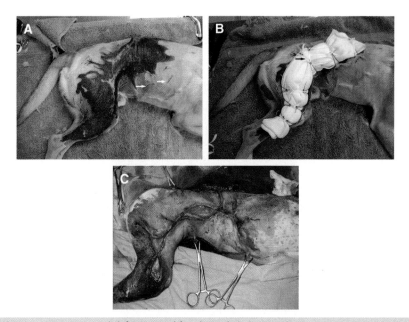

Fig. 1. (A) Contractural deformity and fragile epithelial scar subsequent to a severe burn injury are shown. Mattress sutures are placed over stents (*arrows*) circumferentially around the wound. (B) Mattress sutures are placed under tension using an umbilical tape lace placed over a padded bandage (*arrow*). (C) Full-thickness resection and beginning of reconstruction after skin stretching is complete.

position relative to those in the first row. Simple interrupted or cruciate skin sutures complete the closure (Fig. 2). Staggering of relaxing incisions helps to ensure vascularity of skin margins. Making the incisions as the suture is placed helps to avoid making more incisions than necessary, which might compromise blood supply in surrounding skin. After reconstruction, contact dressings and protective bandages are applied until the expanded punctuate incisions have healed by contraction and epithelialization.

Z-plasty. A Z-plasty adjacent to a wound may also be helpful in providing relaxation for closure [3]. The "Z" is designed adjacent to the wound with the central limb going in the direction in which relaxation is needed. Generally, the arms of the Z are designed off the ends of the central limb at 60°. After making the Z-shaped incision and undermining its flaps and the skin between the Z and the wound, the wound is sutured. The flaps of the Z-plasty automatically transpose into their new position, into which they are sutured. The principle of a Z-plasty is to take skin from one plane and move it into a perpendicular plane so it can be used for wound closure. Thus, it is wise to manipulate skin adjacent to the wound to determine its availability for the procedure. The size of Z-plasty angles and length of its components govern the amount of relaxation attained.

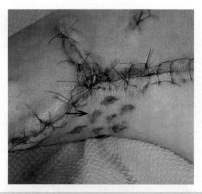

Fig. 2. Multiple punctate relaxing incisions (*arrow*) have been used to decrease tension on the primary incision during three-point closure of a wound.

V-to-Y plasty. A V-to-Y plasty can be considered when a small amount of relaxation is needed [3]. A V-shaped incision is made adjacent to the wound with the point of the "V" going away from the wound. After undermining the skin between the V and the wound, the wound is closed. One technique for closure of the V is to begin at the ends of the arms, placing sutures alternately back and forth between the arms. When tension begins to develop in closure, the remaining area is closed to form the stem on the Y.

Adjustable horizontal mattress sutures. Adjustable horizontal mattress sutures are used to facilitate wound contraction [4]. This technique is, in essence, a form of progressive skin stretching and is appropriate primarily for wounds involving less than 30% circumference of the limb and situated away from flexion and extension surfaces (eg, those that are otherwise appropriate for second-intention healing). A monofilament nonabsorbable suture is placed along the length of the wound using a continuous horizontal mattress or continuous intradermal suture pattern. One free end of the suture is passed through a button (or similar device) to distribute pressure on underlying skin, and the end of the suture is clamped in a split-shot fishing weight. The opposite suture end is then placed under tension, advancing skin margins partially over the wound. This end of the suture is then passed through a second button and is also secured using a split-shot fishing weight. The wound is dressed as for second-intention healing. After 24 hours, the dressing is removed, the suture is retightened from both ends, and new split-shot anchors are placed (Fig. 3). This process is repeated at 24-hour intervals until skin margins are apposed at the center of the wound. This technique capitalizes on progressive skin stretching over time and is effective in reducing healing time.

Tissue expanders. Tissue expanders have an inflatable bag and reservoir made of silicone elastomer. They are placed and inflated in subcutaneous tissues to stretch the overlying skin, allowing creation of larger flaps for closing defects [5–7]. Although expensive, they are available in various sizes and shapes (eg, Radovan

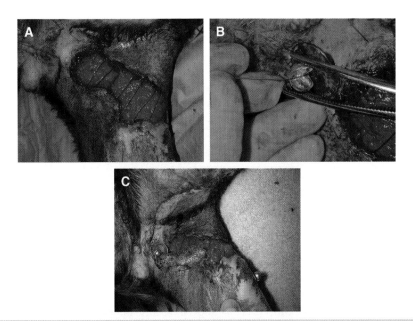

Fig. 3. (A) Continuous intradermal suture pattern using a monofilament suture has been placed along the length of this wound after establishment of granulation tissue. (B) Ends of the suture are placed under tension and are secured using a split-shot fishing weight. The suture is first passed through a button to distribute tension at the suture ends. (C) Immediate reduction in wound size is noted.

Tissue Expander; Mentor Corporation, Santa Barbara, California). Careful planning is required for optimum expansion and reconstruction. The base of the expander should approximate the size of the donor site. The incision for insertion of the expander should be made parallel to tension lines at the leading edge of the future flap, or skin adjacent to the site is likely to be inappropriately stretched. The device is placed subcutaneously and inflated with saline. Rapid expansion requires intermittent intraoperative short-term inflation of the expander. It involves inflating the expander for 2 to 3 minutes, deflating, and letting the tissue rest for 3 to 4 minutes and then repeating the cycle two or three times before creating a flap. Gradual expansion involves injecting to a given pressure or volume at intervals spanning days to weeks (every 2–7 days usually). Inflation at injection is continued until the skin feels tense or looks blanched or discomfort is perceived. When the tissue is sufficiently stretched to allow reconstruction, the device is removed and a skin flap is created to close the defect. Complications of tissue expanders include pain, seroma formation, scar widening, infection, dehiscence, skin necrosis, and implant failure, and they should not be used in previously irradiated tissues.

Skin grafts. Skin grafts are segments of epidermis and dermis that are completely detached from the donor site and transferred to a recipient site. Survival of skin grafts depends on early fluid absorption, followed by revascularization and development of a fibrous attachment at the recipient site. Thus, skin grafts are highly dependent on a healthy, well-vascularized, and stable wound environment. The sole purpose of skin grafting is to re-establish an intact cutaneous barrier in an otherwise reasonably healthy open wound.

Skin grafts should be considered for reconstruction of open wounds on the distal extremity when (1) the wound is of sufficient size or in an anatomic area that precludes direct closure via mobilization of surrounding skin, (2) the recipient site is characterized by a healthy granulation bed or a minimally contaminated and well-vascularized fresh tissue bed that is capable of providing early vascularization to the graft, and (3) there is an adequate quantity and quality of donor skin available for harvest.

Classification of skin grafts. Virtually all skin grafts used in small animals are autogenous (derived from the same animal). Skin allografts (same species, different individual) and xenografts (different species) have been described and used for specific applications in wound reconstruction but have little role in the routine management of open wounds in small animals.

Skin grafts are also classified as full or split thickness. Full-thickness skin grafts incorporate the entire dermis and epidermis. Split-thickness skin grafts may be further classified as thin, intermediate, or thick split-thickness grafts depending on the relative thickness of dermis incorporated into the graft. Full-thickness skin grafts are more easily harvested by surgeons without extensive experience in grafting techniques and without special equipment. Full-thickness grafts also carry a full complement of adnexal structures that provide a cosmetic and durable result. In the author's opinion, split-thickness grafts are rarely indicated in reconstruction of wounds in small animals.

Skin grafts are classified as sheet, mesh, strip, or seed depending on the configuration of the graft [3,8]. Sheet grafts are harvested as a single piece of skin that is cut to the shape of the recipient bed. Sheet grafts have a distinct disadvantage in that they do not allow the escape of serum, blood, and exudate, which may accumulate beneath the graft and inhibit revascularization. Sheet grafts thus have an increased failure rate and are not recommended.

Mesh grafts are formed by placing multiple staggered rows of parallel incisions through the graft (Fig. 4). These can be made by hand, using a scalpel blade, or with instrumentation specifically designed for this purpose. Meshed grafts can be expanded or nonexpanded when placed on the recipient bed. Expansion of a mesh graft allows wound reconstruction with less graft material and ensures adequate wound drainage. The open areas in an expanded mesh graft heal by contraction and epithelialization. All mesh grafts should be at least slightly expanded when placed on the recipient site to open the meshes, allowing escape of wound fluid or blood from beneath the graft and into the bandage. Full-thickness mesh grafts are preferred for most wound reconstructions based on their ease of use, success of graft take, and final cosmetic outcome.

Strip grafts involve the use of strips of skin of varying width placed in parallel rows of grooves in granulation tissue to cover the recipient site partially. Open

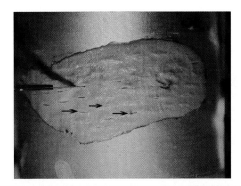

Fig. 4. Full-thickness skin grafts are meshed by placing multiple staggered rows of incisions (arrows).

areas interposed between the strip grafts heal through contraction and epithelialization [3]. Seed (pinch) grafts are similar to strip grafts but involve the harvest of multiple "plugs" of skin that are placed into slit-like pockets in the wound's granulation bed. Each pocket serves as a "bandage" to hold a graft in place as it heals. The purpose of seed and strip grafts is to provide multiple areas from which epithelialization can proceed. Cosmetic outcome after strip or seed grafting techniques is substantially poorer than with mesh grafts. Use of these types of grafts should be limited to situations in which massive skin loss precludes the harvest of adequate quantities of skin to reconstruct the recipient site completely. These grafts can also be used in areas that are difficult to bandage or immobilize. Each graft pocket serves to immobilize the graft as it heals in place.

Healing of skin grafts. Skin grafts are dependent on the recipient site for nourishment. Adequate contact and stability between the graft and the recipient bed are essential. After transfer, the graft initially adheres to the recipient bed via formation of a fibrin network. This fibrin network is easily disrupted by motion or traumatic handling of the graft within the first few days after grafting. The fibrin network is subsequently invaded by fibrovascular tissue (fibroblasts that produce collagen) to form a stable bond between the graft and recipient bed.

Immediately after transfer, the graft is nourished through a process termed *plasmatic imbibition.* Serum-like fluid moves between the graft and the recipient bed to provide nourishment to the graft cells. The graft appears slightly edematous and cyanotic during this phase of healing (ie, the first several days). Within the first few days after grafting, revascularization of the graft begins. New capillary buds from the wound bed can invade the dermis directly or form anastomoses with preexisting dermal vessels, a process termed *inosculation.* Grafts take on a dark red to purplish appearance during early vascular ingrowth (usually 3–5 days). Vascularization of the graft is relatively advanced within 7 to 10 days. Thus, successful grafts develop a progressively pink to red coloration between days 5 and 7. By day 10, grafts should appear relatively normal and early hair regrowth is often evident (Fig. 5).

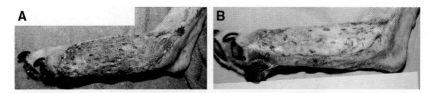

Fig. 5. (A) Full-thickness skin graft appearance at day 4 is shown. The graft has a deep red to purple appearance because of sluggish blood flow after early revascularization. (B) Graft gradually resumes a relatively normal appearance by day 10. Early hair regrowth is evident.

Recipient site selection and preparation. Because skin grafts are ultimately dependent on the recipient site for survival, the graft bed must comprise tissue that is capable of generating a vascular response. In addition, graft beds must be free of necrotic tissue, foreign material, and infection. A general rule of thumb is that a wound that would not support direct closure (given adequate surrounding skin) should not be grafted. Recipient beds may comprise granulation tissue or well-vascularized fresh tissue (Fig. 6). Wounds with granulation tissue should be scraped with a scalpel blade and bandaged with an antibiotic ointment on a wide mesh gauze sponge 12 to 24 hours before skin grafting to reduce topical wound flora. Immediate grafting is recommended in situations involving clean wounds that have been made in a controlled environment (eg, after tumor excision) and have a tissue bed capable of producing granulation tissue. Tissue that is limited in its ability to produce a vascular response, such as exposed bone, cartilage, or tendon, as well as chronic poor-quality granulation tissue does not support skin grafts (Fig. 7).

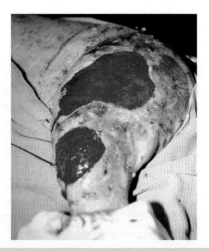

Fig. 6. Healthy granulation tissue with a strong vascular response serves as an excellent recipient site for full-thickness skin grafts.

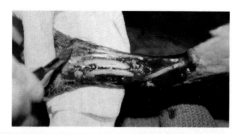

Fig. 7. Wounds with exposed bone, tendon, or other poorly vascularized tissues do not support full-thickness skin grafts.

Donor site selection and graft preparation. Considerations in the selection of an appropriate donor site include the ability to close the site primarily after graft harvest, the morbidity associated with harvesting the graft from a particular site, and the cosmetic match between the donor skin and the normal skin and hair at the recipient site. Every effort should be made to ensure as close a match as possible for hair color, length, and direction of growth between the donor and recipient sites. A template of the recipient bed is made before harvesting graft skin to assist in planning graft size and shape. For wounds with a granulation bed, the epithelium at the wound edge should be excised before creating the template.

Full-thickness skin is harvested from the donor site via simple excision, and the graft is then transferred onto a working surface. The graft is inverted so that the subcutaneous tissue is exposed, and the graft is stabilized under tension. Many techniques can be used, including tacking the graft to a sterile cork board or corrugated cardboard, suturing graft edges to a rigid surface, placing stay sutures around the graft and pulling them through slits in the edge of a piece of cardboard, or placing the graft over an inverted saline bowl. Subcutaneous tissue is then meticulously excised from the deep surface of the graft. Subcutaneous tissue blocks serum absorption and revascularization and increases the risk of graft failure. The deep surface of the finished skin graft should have a pebbled appearance, and the bottom of hair follicles should be visible (Fig. 8).

Graft inset. After preparation, the graft is transferred to the recipient site and positioned using a few interrupted sutures. Skin edges are then apposed using a simple continuous, simple interrupted, or cruciate suture pattern or skin staples (Fig. 9). The graft is placed under mild tension so that mesh incisions are slightly opened. Through-and-through tacking sutures can be placed between graft mesh holes to anchor the graft to the underlying tissue bed and especially to stabilize the graft over areas where it tends to lift from the wound bed. The graft is then covered with a nonadherent permeable contact dressing and stabilized under a padded bandage. Splints are applied if the wound is located over or near a flexion or extension surface.

Postoperative care and monitoring. The required frequency of postoperative bandage changes is somewhat contentious. Early and frequent bandage changes

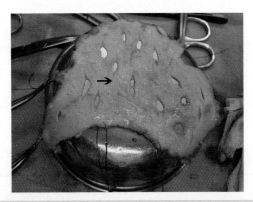

Fig. 8. This full-thickness skin graft has been placed under tension over an inverted saline bowl to facilitate dissection of subcutaneous tissue from its deep surface. The dermal surface of the graft has a pebbled appearance (*arrow*) after removal of subcutaneous tissue.

are potentially deleterious to graft survival, because early vascular ingrowth may be disturbed during the act of rebandaging. The author always examines skin grafts on the first postoperative day to assess graft adherence to the recipient bed. Uncooperative or anxious patients should be sedated during bandage changing. Pockets of fluid accumulation can be gently drained, if present, to reestablish graft-bed contact. Subsequent bandage changes are performed at 1- to 3-day intervals, depending on the amount of exudate present at the time of the initial bandage change. Successful grafts follow the coloration pattern previously described during their healing. A pale, progressively dark, or leathery appearance of the graft indicates impending failure. Partial-thickness take, or loss of superficial layers of the graft, is common, and areas of suspect devitalization should not be debrided too early or too aggressively (Fig. 10). It is often

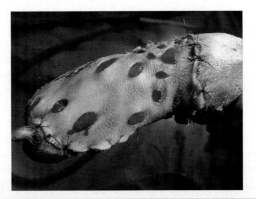

Fig. 9. Inset of a full-thickness slightly expanded mesh graft is shown. The graft has been sutured circumferentially using cruciate sutures.

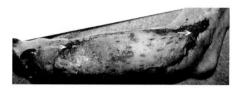

Fig. 10. Areas of partial graft failure are common (*arrows*).

difficult to determine the failure of a graft with certainty for 7 to 10 days. Protective bandaging is usually continued for 3 weeks after surgery.

Reverse saphenous conduit flap. The reverse saphenous conduit flap, although not truly an axial pattern flap, is dissected and behaves in a similar fashion to axial pattern flaps. The vascular supply to this flap arises from the medial saphenous vessels (Fig. 11) [9,10]. These vessels do not form a direct cutaneous vascular supply as in an axial pattern flap but, instead, give rise to numerous small cutaneous branches throughout their course; thus, they serve as a vascular conduit from which several small cutaneous angiosomes arise. This flap is extremely useful for reconstruction of wounds involving the tarsus and metatarsus. The only prerequisites for success of this flap are absence of trauma to the medial saphenous vascular system and absence of trauma to the deep vascular structures of the metatarsus and paw.

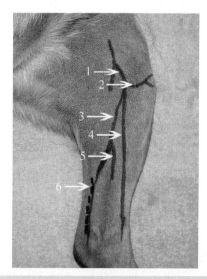

Fig. 11. Vascular anatomy of the reverse saphenous conduit flap is shown on the medial aspect of the thigh and crus: 1, medial saphenous artery; 2, medial genicular artery; 3, caudal branch of the medial saphenous artery; 4, cranial branch of the medial saphenous artery; 5, peroneal (fibular) branch; 6, tibial nerve (*broken line*).

Normally, the flow of arterial blood through the medial saphenous vessels passes from proximal to distal, and vice versa for venous flow. In forming the reverse saphenous flap, however, the medial saphenous artery and vein are ligated at their origin from the femoral artery and vein. Flow through the vessels becomes retrograde, arising from collateral communications between the saphenous vessels and other arteries and veins in the distal extremity; thus, the term *reverse saphenous conduit flap.*

The flap is formed by transversely incising the skin at the level of the origin of the medial saphenous vessels, which are subsequently ligated (Fig. 12A). Proximal dissection can be extended to the level of the inguinal crease if necessary. The flap is constructed with the saphenous vessels centered under the flap. Cranial and caudal incisions are extended to the level of the tarsus, taking care to include the cranial and caudal branches of the medial saphenous

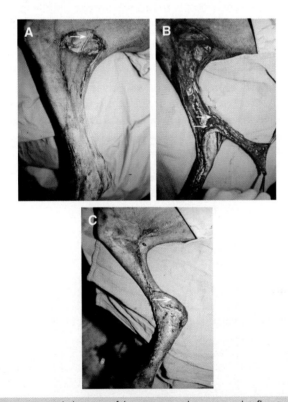

Fig. 12. (*A*) Dissection and elevation of the reverse saphenous conduit flap is shown. A proximal transverse skin incision has been made at the level of the origin of the medial saphenous artery and vein (*arrow*). The saphenous vessels are ligated and transected. (*B*) Cranial and caudal incisions are extended along the medial aspect of the tibia. Dissection is performed deep to the saphenous vessels, maintaining the saphenous vessels on the deep surface of the flap (*arrows*). (*C*) Elevated flap has been transposed via a bridging incision to reconstruct a defect over the calcaneus (*arrow*). The donor site is closed primarily.

vessels within the flap. A Doppler flow probe can be used to identify the position of the saphenous vessels if they are not visible through the skin. The flap is elevated deep to the saphenous vessels (see Fig. 12B). The genicular artery and vein are ligated and transected as they arise from the cranial branch of the saphenous vessels at the level of the stifle. At the midpoint of the tibia, a deep peroneal branch arises from the caudal branch of the saphenous vessels. The peroneal vessels are ligated and transected to facilitate further flap dissection. The tibial nerve joins the caudal branch of the saphenous artery at the level of the distal third of the tibia. The tibial nerve is carefully dissected from the caudal branch of the saphenous artery as flap dissection continues distally to the level of the tarsus. A distal skin pedicle is left intact, along with the underlying cranial and caudal branches of the saphenous artery and vein.

After flap elevation, a bridging incision is made between the donor and recipient sites and the flap is transposed into position. Alternatively to a bridging incision, the flap can be transposed over intact skin and inset at the recipient site. Flap skin that overlies intact skin is sutured into a tube that is excised in 14 days. The donor defect is closed primarily (see Fig. 12C). Venous flow is typically sluggish for the first few days, resulting in an edematous and cyanotic appearance to the flap. The appearance of the flap returns to normal over 5 to 7 days as venous and lymphatic outflow reforms.

Distant flaps. Hinge or pouch flaps are flaps created on the trunk. The distal limb or paw is moved to and affixed under the flap. The limb is immobilized against the body as the flap heals. After healing, the flap is freed from the body with its healed flap in place. Such flaps are occasionally used and work best on the forelimbs of cats and small dogs [3].

Microvascular free tissue transfer. Microvascular reconstructive surgery is any surgery involving the repair of small vessels, usually in the size range of 0.5 to 2 mm. This type of reconstruction involves the harvest of autogenous tissue(s) with a consistent vascular pedicle from a donor site, its transfer to a recipient site, and the re-establishment of vascular flow via microvascular anastomosis of the donor artery and vein to an artery and vein at the recipient site. Tissue transferred in this manner is called free tissue transfer, free flaps, or microvascular free flaps. The diversity of tissues available for microvascular transfer has led to their acceptance for a wide variety of reconstructive problems, especially including reconstruction of the distal limb and paw [11].

The success of a free flap depends on appropriate selection of donor tissues and proper microvascular surgical technique. Suitable donor tissues must have a consistent and reliable dominant vascular pedicle with a diameter and length appropriate for microsurgical reconstruction (generally at least 1 mm in diameter and 5 mm in length). Harvest of the donor tissue should result in minimal donor site morbidity. Regional tissue that is consistently perfused by a single-source artery and vein is termed the *angiosome* of the source vessel. Single or composite tissues may be included within a single angiosome depending on the specific source artery. All tissues contained within an angiosome may be included within a free flap and are expected to survive after microvascular repair of the source artery and vein.

Free flaps are defined by the tissue(s) that are transferred. Skin, muscle, and bone are commonly used as single tissue flaps. Complex defects often benefit from the use of composite flaps, such as myocutaneous (muscle and skin), myo-osseous (muscle and bone), fasciocutaneous (fascia and skin), or osteomusculocutaneous (skin, muscle, and bone) flaps. Free flaps are useful for one-stage reconstruction of difficult defects resulting from trauma or ablative cancer surgery, congenital defects, osteomyelitis and nonunion fractures, and segmental bone loss [11].

Advantages of free flaps include versatility, reliability, vascularity, and the ability to develop early one-stage corrective procedures for difficult reconstructive problems (Fig. 13). Tissues to be transferred microsurgically can be "matched" to a specific reconstructive requirement. Because free flaps are revascularized at the recipient site, they provide a new blood supply that can

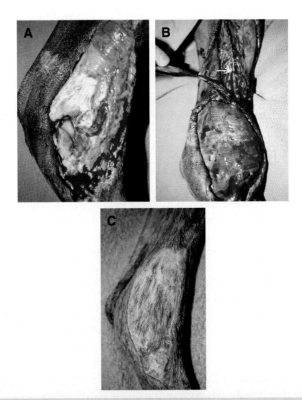

Fig. 13. (A) Medial degloving injury of the tarsus is shown immediately after initial debridement. (B) Free microvascular transfer (*arrow*) of a trapezius muscle flap has been performed to benefit healing of the underlying fractures. (C) Fourteen-day appearance of a full-thickness mesh graft that was placed on the muscle.

be used by the healing wound. This revascularization of the wound bed is advantageous in the treatment of ischemic diseases, such as osteomyelitis and postirradiation necrosis.

Free flaps have three primary disadvantages: they are time-consuming, they require expertise in microvascular technique, and they require specialized instrumentation. They have limited application in veterinary surgery. As techniques and indications for veterinary reconstructive microsurgery are further refined, however, increasing numbers of veterinary surgeons are likely to develop expertise in this area.

Clinically useful flaps. Skin, muscle, bone, and paw pads are used most frequently for distal extremity reconstruction. The medial saphenous flap is preferred for cutaneous reconstruction because it most closely matches recipient site characteristics on the distal extremity [12]. The trapezius muscle flap is used to provide robust vascular tissue over exposed bone [13]. This flap is then resurfaced using a full-thickness skin graft. Options for reconstruction of segmental bone loss include the saphenous vessel–based medial tibial flap [14], the scapular spine harvested as an extension of the trapezius muscle flap [15], and the distal ulna based on the caudal interosseous vessels [16]. Microvascular free transfer of the fifth digital paw pad of the pelvic limb and the carpal paw pad of the forelimb has been described [17,18].

Indications. The indications and contraindications of free tissue transfer in veterinary reconstructive surgery remain to be defined fully. It is important to recognize that the major advantage of microvascular reconstruction is early and complete reconstruction of difficult defects and rapid rehabilitation of unhealthy recipient beds. It is best to consider microvascular reconstruction as a method of first choice in appropriate circumstances rather than a method of last resort after failure of more commonly used reconstructive alternatives. Free tissue transfer should be considered for the following problems:

1. Extensive loss of soft tissues where local tissues are unavailable or inappropriate for reconstruction (eg, because of vascular impairment or infection)
2. Extensive segmental bone loss and overlying soft tissue or vascular injury
3. Chronic osteomyelitis
4. Reconstruction of weight-bearing surfaces
5. Treatment of select cases of avascular nonunion fractures
6. Reconstruction and rehabilitation of patients after extensive ablative cancer surgery
7. Salvage of ischemic wound beds (eg, postirradiation necrosis)

Microvascular technique gives the surgeon the ability to select optimal tissues for any given reconstructive requirement; harvest those tissues on a reliable and consistent vascular pedicle; and successfully transfer the tissues to a recipient site, where they are revascularized. The versatility and utility of such flaps make their use for the resolution of difficult reconstructive problems appropriate.

Complications of Wound Healing

Three complications that are encountered in the healing of wounds on non–weight-bearing surfaces are contractural deformities, a fragile epithelial scar, and development of an acral pruritic granuloma (ie, "lick granuloma"). Contractural deformities are generally the result of open-wound healing of a large wound over the flexion surface of a joint (eg, carpometacarpal joint). As wound contraction occurs, it results in joint contracture and inability of joint extension. When open-wound healing occurs in the presence of insufficient full-thickness skin to cover the wound completely, the remaining wound covers with thin delicate epithelium that is subject to trauma or to the development of a nonhealing wound. Acral pruritic granulomas often develop at the site of second-intention wound healing when such areas are not protected during the healing process.

INTERDIGITAL WOUNDS

The interdigital region in dogs, and to a lesser extent in cats, is prone to trauma and chronic infectious or inflammatory disease. Interdigital lacerations are seen with some frequency. Chronic interdigital pyoderma or bacterial pododermatitis is problematic in dogs.

Techniques

Suturing

Most interdigital lacerations are easily managed by initial debridement and lavage, a period of open-wound management if mandated by the extent of initial contamination, and delayed primary wound closure. Blood supply to the interdigital region is excellent, and healing is generally uncomplicated. It is essential to protect the wound from the environment during healing, however. A well-padded bandage with a half-splint is placed, and owners are instructed to maintain the bandage in a clean and dry environment. If the bandage becomes wet or soiled, immediate reassessment and bandage change are indicated to prevent maceration of underlying tissues. Bearing in mind that dogs sweat from their pads, more frequent bandage changes than on other areas of the body may be indicated to maintain an optimal wound healing environment.

Fusion podoplasty

Bacterial pododermatitis is a problematic disease, usually secondary to underlying causes, such as trauma, fungal infection, or immune-mediated disease, and it often responds poorly to medical management [19]. Excision of all hirsute interdigital tissue, although surgically aggressive, is usually curative in cases that fail to respond to medical intervention [20]. This technique is termed *fusion podoplasty* (Fig. 14). Fusion podoplasty is performed by first identifying all involved tissue. Partial podoplasty can be performed if disease is limited to a confined region of the paw, whereas total fusion podoplasty is required for generalized disease. The paw is clipped and prepared for aseptic surgery. A sterile marking pen is used to outline all affected interdigital skin and interpad skin on the palmar or plantar paw surface as well as on the opposing surface of the metacarpal or metatarsal paw pad. Skin is incised along all marked lines,

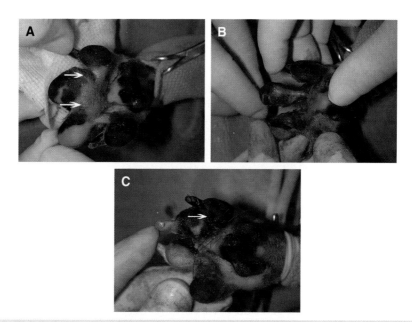

Fig. 14. (A) Partial fusion podoplasty is used to treat chronic nonresponsive interdigital podo-dermatitis (*arrows*). (B) Affected regions of haired skin are resected. (C) Pad tissue is apposed and sutured (*arrow*).

and all interposing skin is excised. Bipolar cautery, radiosurgery, or laser dissection is helpful to control hemorrhage during dissection. Digital pads are sutured to one another; as a unit, they are sutured to the metacarpal or metatarsal paw pad. Excised skin is submitted for histopathologic confirmation of disease. The paw is bandaged and placed in a non–weight-bearing clamshell splint (see article 6 in this issue). The bandage is changed daily during the first week when drainage is maximal. This is followed by changes every other day on week 2 and once- or twice-weekly changes on week 3. Sutures are removed in approximately 14 days. Splints can usually be removed after week 3, with gradual reintroduction of weight-bearing stresses.

Fusion podoplasty can also be used for the management of chronic digital flexor tendon disruption, with subsequent digital hyperextension and ulceration of digital pads. Fusion podoplasty prevents digital hyperextension, facilitates healing of eroded weight-bearing surfaces, and improves long-term function in these cases [21].

WEIGHT-BEARING PAW INJURIES
Evaluation of Wounds
The paw pads are highly specialized structures designed to withstand the rigors of weight bearing. They consist of a highly specialized stratum corneum as well as a fibrovascular paw pad cushion that anchors the dermis to underlying bone.

The paw pad cushion acts as a "shock absorber" and also serves to dissipate shear stresses during weight bearing. Reconstructive techniques for weight-bearing surfaces include digit amputation, local paw pad transposition, paw pad grafts, and microvascular paw pad transfer.

Before embarking on extensive reconstruction of weight-bearing surfaces, the surgeon must carefully evaluate the extent of injury. Injuries limited to the soft tissues of the paw are appropriate for aggressive reconstruction and paw salvage. Injuries complicated by extensive injury to bone, tendons, and joints may be more appropriately managed by amputation, however.

Techniques

Paw pad abrasions

Superficial lesions of the pads include blister-like lesions where the stratum corneum is lost, generally as the result of stress on unconditioned pad epithelium. The deeper layers of epithelium remain. With topical application of wound healing stimulants (see article by Krahwinkel and Booth elsewhere in this issue) under a bandage, new stratum corneum usually forms within a few days. Deep-abrasion lesions may have deeper epithelial damage or loss of all the epidermis. If there is intact pad skin at the edges of such lesions, wound healing stimulants under a bandage can result in healing by contraction and epithelialization with a dense keratinized epithelium [3].

Paw pad lacerations

An important procedure with pad lacerations is assessing the depth of the laceration, (ie, full or partial thickness). Debridement, lavage, and suturing are indicated, and with full-thickness wounds, a Penrose drain under the pad is often indicated. Bandaging and splinting are important after surgery to prevent sutures from tearing through pad skin (see article 6 in this issue) [3].

Phalangeal fillet

Local paw pad transposition mandates the availability of a suitable volume of paw pad tissue that can be raised on a vascular or neurovascular pedicle and transposed into the recipient site [3,22]. This technique is most useful for reconstruction of the metacarpal or metatarsal paw pad using a fillet of the second or fifth digital paw pad with excision of the respective phalanges. The phalanges are approached through a dorsal midline incision, dissected circumferentially staying adjacent to periosteum, and amputated. The soft tissues of the digit are thereby preserved on their neurovascular pedicle. A bridging incision is then made on the palmar or plantar surface of the digit between its pad and the edge of the metacarpal or metatarsal pad defect. The bridging incision is performed carefully, extending only through the dermis, to protect the underlying soft tissues carrying the neurovascular supply to the flap. The digital fillet flap is then transposed into position after debriding the metacarpal or metatarsal pad defect. The digital pad is sutured in a central weight-bearing position, and skin edges are apposed along the bridging incision (Fig. 15). The flap is protected in a well-padded bandage and non–weight-bearing splint (see article 6 in this issue). Delayed

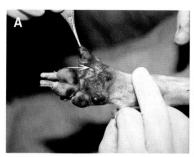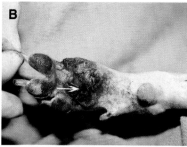

Fig. 15. Phalangeal fillet of the fifth digit is shown for reconstruction of the metacarpal paw pad. (A) Phalanges have been excised via periosteal dissection through a dorsal midline incision (note flaccid fifth digit). A bridging incision has been made between the fifth digital pad and the metacarpal pad defect (*arrow*). (B) Digital pad has been transposed to the metacarpal pad defect via the bridging incision (*arrow*).

transposition of fillet flaps has been recommended, with direct closure of the incision used for the phalangeal fillet initially, followed by transposition through a bridging incision in 5 to 7 days. This technique may reduce the risk of failure attributable to vascular embarrassment but is not necessary in the author's experience.

Paw pad grafts

Full-thickness paw pad grafts, as with skin grafts, require a healthy vascularized recipient site. They are useful for resurfacing areas of extensive paw pad loss [23,24]. Paw pad grafts are harvested from healthy paw pads on the same dog using a 4- or 6-mm skin biopsy punch or by excision of rectangular sections of paw pad tissue from distant sites. Multiple punch grafts are harvested, with the number being determined by the availability of donor tissue and the area of the wound to be reconstructed. Donor sites are closed using cruciate or mattress sutures and are protected with padded bandages for 7 to 10 days, or they can be allowed to heal as open wounds under the influence of a wound healing stimulant. The subcutaneous paw pad cushion is excised from the deep surface of the paw pad graft to the level of the deep surface of the dermis using a number 11 scalpel blade or fine scissors. An area of the recipient granulation bed matching the size of the pad graft is partially excised. Grafts are placed into these depressions in the granulation tissue bed and are stabilized with one or two through-and-through mattress sutures (Fig. 16). Paw pad grafts are arranged around the perimeter of the defect so that re-epithelialization from grafted paw pads progresses toward the center of the wound with tough keratinized epithelium from the grafts and the grafts block re-epithelialization by thin delicate epithelium from surrounding skin margins.

Paw pad grafts are bandaged, splinted, and protected as described for skin grafts, with particular attention to keeping pressure off them. The stratum corneum of the pad grafts typically sloughs in 5 to 7 days, leaving a pinkish graft

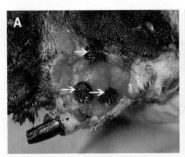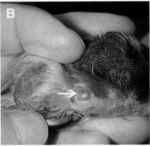

Fig. 16. Paw pad grafts are shown for reconstruction of the weight-bearing surface of a digit in this dog. (A) Paw pad grafts have been harvested using a 6-mm dermal biopsy punch and are secured into granulation tissue at the recipient site using mattress sutures (arrows). (B) Appearance of reconstructed site at day 20. Early reformation of cornified paw pad epithelium is evident (arrow).

from which epithelialization and generation of a new stratum corneum proceed over several weeks. Although paw pad grafts have been used successfully, their functionality may be limited by the inability to transfer the specialized subcutaneous paw pad cushion with the graft. To compensate for this, they have been noted to become extremely tough and hard with time.

Microvascular paw pad transfer
Microvascular, or microneurovascular, free transfer of paw pads allows transfer of the entire paw pad structure. A "dispensable" paw pad is dissected, usually with an area of surrounding skin, based on its neurovascular pedicle and is transferred to a central weight-bearing location at the recipient site, where it is then revascularized by microvascular anastomosis to a recipient artery and vein. Flattening and hypertrophy of the transferred paw pad occur with time, providing a functional weight-bearing surface. Several minor revision operations are often required to recentralize the footpad as it migrates subsequent to initiation of weight bearing. The reader is referred elsewhere for details on microvascular paw pad transfer [17].

AMPUTATION INJURIES
Amputation and partial amputation injuries of the digits or paw are quite common secondary to degloving, strangulation, crush, bandaging, or gunshot injuries. The functional consequences and required treatment depend on the extent of injury and the digits involved.

The third and fourth digits are the primary weight-bearing digits of the paw. The second or fifth digit can be amputated with few functional sequelae, assuming that the remaining digits are intact. Loss of the third or fourth digit is well tolerated but causes more functional disturbance than does loss of the second or fifth digit. Injuries involving the second and fifth digits and sparing the central digits are uncommon. In such cases, amputation of the medial and lateral digits is tolerated; however, in the author's experience, this does lead to a modest loss of function. Amputation of the second and third digits or the fourth and fifth digits causes a more severe functional disturbance in ambulation. In these cases, the paw tends to roll toward the amputation site, causing increased weight-bearing stress, ulceration, and pain (Fig. 17). Loss of the third and fourth digits causes a similar functional disturbance because of splaying of the second and fifth digits, causing increased weight-bearing stress on the interposing tissues (Fig. 18). In addition, in working and field dogs, the digits tend to snag on vegetation. Ulceration of tissue interposed between the second and fifth digits can be treated by resection of the ulcer, development of a granulation bed, and subsequent paw pad grafting of the area. Unfortunately, this technique does not address the biomechanical stress placed on eccentrically located digits during weight bearing. Centralization of the second and fifth digits by middiaphyseal osteotomy of all metacarpal or metatarsal bones, removal of the distal segments of the third and fourth metacarpal or metatarsal bones, transposition of the second and fifth digits onto the central metacarpal or metatarsal bones, and plate fixation functionally convert this type of amputation injury to one characterized by loss of the second and fifth digits. Experience with centralization of digits, to the author's knowledge, is extremely limited, with incomplete follow-up. This technique could be considered, however, particularly for animals that have developed compromised ambulatory function subsequent to loss of the third and fourth digits or other partial amputation injury.

Loss of all digits (ie, pandigital amputation) causes an obvious functional disturbance but does not necessarily mandate amputation. Such losses are often secondary to some thromboembolic abnormality. If the metacarpal or metatarsal paw pad remains intact, all digits can be amputated at the metacarpophalangeal articulation and the weight-bearing surface of the stump can be reconstructed by advancement of the metacarpal or metatarsal paw pad (Fig. 19). If tension precludes advancement of the weight-bearing paw pad over the stump, shortening the third and fourth metacarpal or metatarsal bones

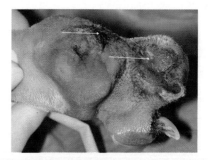

Fig. 17. Loss of second and third digits causes pronation of the foot and ulceration secondary to abnormal weight-bearing stresses (*arrows*).

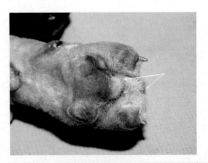

Fig. 18. Loss of third and fourth digits causes splaying of the second and fifth digits, resulting in weight-bearing stress, ulceration (*arrows*), and pain of interdigital skin.

may allow positioning of the metacarpal or metatarsal pad more directly under the bones.

Amputation of the front paw at the level of the carpus can be managed by advancement of the carpal paw pad over the weight-bearing surface. This technique has been described as a single pedicle or bipedicle advancement flap (Fig. 20) [25]. Partial function is preserved but is limited because of the length discrepancy between the limbs. Although correction of limb length in cases of paw amputation has not been described, distraction osteogenesis at the level of the distal radius could be considered. Amputation of the rear paw at the level of the tarsus is more problematic. Paw pad grafting after establishing a granulation tissue bed or microvascular paw pad transfer can be considered for a weight-bearing surface reconstruction. Long-term function is limited, however, because of limb length discrepancy. Clear guidelines as to the functional outcome of limb amputation versus limb salvage are not well established for dogs and cats with complete loss of a paw; however, in patients with no orthopedic injury involving other extremities, the value of extensive reconstruction after loss of a paw must be carefully weighed against the more rapid recovery

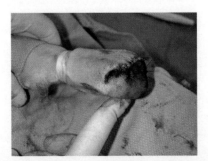

Fig. 19. Advancement of the metacarpal paw pad was used for weight-bearing surface reconstruction after paw amputation at the metacarpophalangeal articulation.

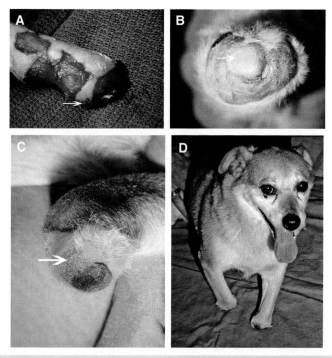

Fig. 20. Carpal paw pad advancement can be used to salvage weight-bearing function after amputation at the level of the carpus. (A) Carpal pad was elevated as a bipedicle flap in this cat (*arrow*). (B) Final appearance of the weight-bearing surface several weeks after reconstruction. (C) Carpal paw pad was advanced as a single pedicle advancement flap (*arrow*) (performed bilaterally on this dog). (D) Weight-bearing function was successfully restored.

and expected function after limb amputation. The potential consequences of limb amputation versus paw or limb salvage on large- and giant-breed dogs must be considered from the standpoint of orthopedic stress and breakdown in other limbs subsequent to the added stress placed on them after amputation.

SUMMARY

Distal limb reconstruction is complicated by the paucity of local tissues and the frequent association of orthopedic injury with cutaneous loss. Second-intention healing or skin stretching techniques are used for wounds involving less than a 30% circumference of the limb. Skin grafts are recommended for reconstruction of larger superficial wounds after establishing a bed of granulation tissue or for immediate reconstruction of clean wounds overlying healthy muscle. Wounds complicated by orthopedic injury benefit from early reconstruction using vascularized tissue. The reverse saphenous conduit flap has proven utility for resurfacing wounds of the tarsus and metatarsus, whereas microvascular free tissue transfer can be used for one-stage reconstruction of more difficult wounds.

Weight-bearing surface reconstruction and management of partial amputation injuries are functionally difficult because of the environmental stress placed on the paw pads. Paw pad grafts, paw pad transposition techniques, centralization of digits, and microvascular free tissue transfer of paw pads can be considered for weight-bearing surface reconstruction. Definitive guidelines describing when each of these techniques should be used have not been established.

References

[1] Richards RR, Schemitsch EH. Effect of muscle flap coverage on bone blood flow following devascularization of a segment of tibia: an experimental investigation in the dog. J Orthop Res 1989;7:550–8.

[2] Pavletic MM. Use of an external skin-stretching device for wound closure in dogs and cats. J Am Vet Med Assoc 2000;217(3):350–4.

[3] Swaim SF, Henderson RA. Small animal wound management. 2nd edition. Baltimore: Lippincott Williams & Wilkins; 1997.

[4] Scardino MS, Swaim SF, Henderson RA, et al. Enhancing wound closure on the limbs. Compend Contin Educ Pract Vet 1996;18:919–51.

[5] Hedlund DS. Surgery of the integument. In: Fossum TW, Hedlund CS, Julse DA, et al, editors. Small animal surgery. 2nd edition. St. Louis (MO): Mosby; 2002. p.134–228.

[6] Keller WG, Aron DN, Rakich PM, et al. Rapid tissue expansion for the development of rotational skin flaps in the distal portion of the hindlimb of dogs: an experimental study. Vet Surg 1994;23:31–9.

[7] Spodnick GJ, Pavletic MM, Clark GN, et al. Controlled tissue expansion in the distal extremities of dogs. Vet Surg 1993;22(6):436–43.

[8] White RAS. Skin grafting. In: Fowler JD, Williams JM, editors. Manual of canine and feline wound management and reconstruction. Cheltenham (UK): British Small Animal Veterinary Association; 1999. p. 83–94.

[9] Pavletic MM, Watter J, Henry RW, et al. Reverse saphenous conduit flap in the dog. J Am Vet Med Assoc 1983;182(4):380–9.

[10] Cornell K, Salisbury K, Jakovlievic S, et al. Reverse saphenous conduit flap in cats: an anatomic study. Vet Surg 1995;24(3):202–6.

[11] Fowler JD, Degner DA, Walshaw R, et al. Microvascular free tissue transfer: results in 57 consecutive cases. Vet Surg 1998;27(5):406–12.

[12] Degner DA, Walshaw R. Medial saphenous fasciocutaneous and myocutaneous free flap transfer in eight dogs. Vet Surg 1997;26(1):20–5.

[13] Philibert D, Fowler JD, Clapson JB. The anatomic basis for a trapezius muscle flap in dogs. Vet Surg 1992;21(6):429–34.

[14] Bebchuk RN, Degner DA, Walshaw R, et al. Evaluation of a free vascularized medial tibial bone graft in dogs. Vet Surg 2000;29(2):128–44.

[15] Philibert D, Fowler JD. The trapezius osteomusculocutaneous flap in dogs. Vet Surg 1993;22(6):444–50.

[16] Szentimrey D, Fowler D, Johnston G, et al. Transplantation of the canine distal ulna as a free vascularized bone graft. Vet Surg 1995;24(3):215–25.

[17] Basher AW, Fowler JD, Bowen CV, et al. Microneurovascular free digital pad transfer in the dog. Vet Surg 1990;19(3):226–31.

[18] Moens NMM, Fowler JD. The microvascular carpal foot pad flap: vascular anatomy and surgical technique. Vet Comp Orthop Traumatol 1997;10:183–6.

[19] Medleau L, Hnilica KA. Bacterial skin diseases. In: Small animal dermatology. Philadelphia: WB Saunders; 2001. p. 20–3.

[20] Swaim SF, Lee AH, MacDonald JM, et al. Fusion podoplasty for the treatment of chronic fibrosing interdigital pyoderma in the dog. J Am Anim Hosp Assoc 1994;30:137–44.

[21] Swaim SF, Milton JL. Fusion podoplasty to treat abnormalities associated with severed digital flexor tendons. J Am Anim Hosp Assoc 1994;30:137–44.

[22] Olsen D, Straw RC, Withrow SJ, et al. Digital pad transposition for replacement of the metacarpal or metatarsal pad in dogs. J Am Anim Hosp Assoc 1997;33(4):337–41.

[23] Swaim SF, Riddell KP, Powers RD. Healing of segmental grafts of pad skin in dogs. Am J Vet Res 1992;53(3):406–10.

[24] Swaim SF, Bradley DM, Steiss JF, et al. Free segmental paw pad grafts in dogs. Am J Vet Res 1993;54(12):2161–70.

[25] Barclay CG, Fowler JD, Basher AWP. Use of the carpal pad to salvage the forelimb in a dog and cat: an alternative to total limb amputation. J Am Anim Hosp Assoc 1987;23:527–32.

Vet Clin Small Anim 36 (2006) 847–872

VETERINARY CLINICS
SMALL ANIMAL PRACTICE

ELSEVIER
SAUNDERS

Large Trunk Wounds

Cheryl S. Hedlund, DVM, MS

Veterinary Clinical Sciences, School of Veterinary Medicine, Louisiana State University,
Skip Bertman Drive, Baton Rouge, LA 70803, USA

L arge trunk wounds may occur as a result of trauma or excision of tumors or infectious lesions, or they may be associated with thermal or chemical burns. A variety of reconstructive procedures are available. It is important to select the appropriate technique or techniques to prevent complications and avoid unnecessary cost. The character of the wound influences the choice of reconstructive technique. Although large trunk lesions can heal by contraction and epithelialization (see article by Hosgood elsewhere in this issue), wound closure may be preferred. Advancing adjacent tissue can be used to close large defects over the trunk because of the abundance of skin. Large or irregular defects sometimes can be closed using relaxing incisions or "plasty" techniques (eg, V-to-Y plasty, Z plasty). Large defects may require that tissue be stretched or mobilized from other sites. Pedicle flaps are tissues that are partly detached from the donor site and mobilized to cover a defect, whereas grafts involve the transfer of a segment of skin to a distant (recipient) site. Careful planning and meticulous atraumatic surgical technique are necessary to prevent excessive tension and circulatory compromise. The amount of skin available for transfer varies between sites on the same animal and between breeds.

PRINCIPLES OF TRAUMATIC WOUND CARE

Initial wound care should facilitate the goals of rapid and uncomplicated wound healing, which results in good cosmesis with minimal labor [1]. Animals presented with wounds should first be assessed for life-threatening injuries. While these are being treated, the wounds should be temporarily covered to prevent further contamination and injury. After initiation of the life-saving therapy, the wound(s) should be promptly addressed.

Assess and classify the wound to determine appropriate therapy (see article by Dernell elsewhere in this issue) [1]. The wound should be cultured when indicated and then covered while aseptically preparing the surrounding area. The wound cover is then removed, and a cleanser is applied. Lavage the wound thoroughly. Ideally, use a balanced electrolyte solution. Cautiously debride necrotic

E-mail address: chedlund@vetmed.lsu.edu

0195-5616/06/$ – see front matter
doi:10.1016/j.cvsm.2006.02.003

tissue, and remove foreign materials. Evaluation of tissue viability in the acute period is difficult. Lavage and staged debridement during the first 3 to 5 days allow the tissues to declare their viability. Bandaging during and after debridement is important in promoting tissue viability until the wound is closed (see articles by Dernell, Krahwinkel and Booth, and Campbell elsewhere in this issue for details on wound management, medication, and bandaging).

PRINCIPLES OF WOUND CLOSURE

Improper primary wound closure is one of the biggest mistakes made in the early management of traumatic wounds. The unclosed wound is the unmet challenge; wounds are often closed too soon, only to result in complications. Surgical manipulation of recently traumatized skin should be minimized until circulation improves. Resolution of contusions, edema, and infection indicates improved skin circulation, which can come with wound management and delayed closure. During the first 6 to 8 hours after injury, only wounds classified as clean or clean contaminated should be considered for immediate closure (see article by Dernell elsewhere in this issue).

Wounds managed for 1 to 3 days with appropriate management, medications, and bandages should be less contaminated and the surrounding tissue should be less compromised; thus, such wounds are better candidates for closure. This delayed primary closure before the appearance of granulation tissue is more successful and healing is more rapid when the wound is healthy and tissue viability has been established. Those closures delayed until after the appearance of healthy granulation tissue are classified as secondary closures, and healing that occurs by contraction and epithelialization without surgical closure is termed *second-intention healing*. Second-intention healing results in normal-appearing skin if contraction is complete. Trunk wounds are more likely than leg wounds to close completely by second intention (see articles by Hosgood and Dernell elsewhere in this issue).

Incision Orientation

Before closing a large trunk wound or excising a lesion, the lines of skin tension should be assessed [1,2]. The location of the wound or lesion, the elasticity of surrounding tissue, the regional blood supply, and the character of the wound bed should be considered when planning reconstructive surgery. Grasping and lifting the skin surrounding the wound or lesion and allowing it to retract spontaneously help to assess skin tension and elasticity and help to determine if primary closure can be accomplished.

General lines of tension have been mapped in animals. Most tension lines on the lateral aspect of the trunk are oriented dorsoventrally, paralleling the ribs. Incisions should be made parallel to tension lines if possible to avoid tension, and manipulation of wound edges should be used to plan closure with minimal tension on traumatic wounds. The direction of closure should avoid or minimize the creation of "dog ears," or puckers, at the ends of the suture line if possible (see article by Amalsadvala elsewhere in this issue).

Undermining

Undermining the skin edges around a wound or excision site before attempted closure most easily relieves wound tension [1,2]. It is the simplest tension-relieving procedure. Undermining skin by using scissors to separate the skin or skin and panniculus muscle from underlying tissue releases skin from underlying attachments so that its full elastic potential can be used as it is stretched over the wound. Skin should be undermined deep to any panniculus muscle layer to preserve the subdermal plexus and direct cutaneous vessels that run parallel to the skin surface (Fig. 1). Where there is no panniculus muscle layer (middle and distal portion of the extremities), the skin should be undermined in the loose areolar fascia deep to the dermis to preserve the subdermal plexus. Elevated skin should include a portion of the superficial fascia with the dermis to preserve the direct cutaneous arteries. In areas in which skin is closely associated with an underlying muscle, (eg, over the sternum and biceps femoris areas) a portion of the outer muscle fascia should be elevated with the dermis by sharp dissection rather than dissecting between these structures. Avoid injury to the subdermal plexus by using atraumatic surgical technique, including cutting skin with a sharp scalpel blade instead of scissors and avoiding crushing instruments (eg, Allis tissue forceps). Brown-Adson thumb forceps, skin hooks,

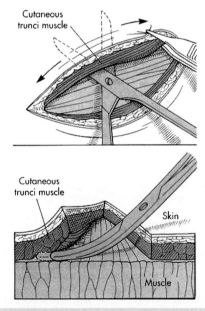

Fig. 1. Eliminate tension before wound closure by using scissors to undermine skin and subcutaneous tissue or skin and panniculus muscle from the underlying tissue. Repeatedly insert Metzenbaum scissors beneath the subcutaneous tissue or panniculus muscle layer with the blades closed, open the blades, and then withdraw the scissors in an open position to separate the tissue layers. (*From* Fossum TW. Small animal surgery. 2nd edition. St. Louis (MO): Mosby Publishing; 2002. p. 156; with permission.)

or stay sutures should be used to manipulate skin. Blunt undermining involves separating tissue layers by repeatedly inserting Metzenbaum scissors with the blades closed, opening the blades, and then withdrawing the scissors in an open position (see Fig. 1). Tissue is cut with the scissors as necessary with sharp undermining. As an alternative, orient the scissors parallel to the cleavage plane and advance the partly opened scissors along the cleavage plane without cutting. While undermining, determine if tension relief is adequate by periodically attempting to approximate the skin edges. Undermining should be kept to a minimum. It is often necessary but not desirable.

Undermining areas associated with delayed wound closure requires that the epithelialized skin edge be separated from the granulation tissue. The skin should be excised with a scalpel blade at the junction of normal skin and new epithelium. The incision should be continued through the granulation tissue edge to the normal cleavage line of subcutaneous fascia, deep to the subdermal plexus.

Bleeding usually is minimal during undermining. Skin tension and bandaging are generally adequate to control hemorrhage and prevent hematomas and seromas. Excessive bleeding may be controlled with electrocoagulation or ligation. Hematomas, seromas, wound closure under excessive tension, rough surgical technique, and division of direct cutaneous arteries interfere with cutaneous circulation and may cause skin necrosis, wound dehiscence, or infection.

Suture Patterns

Sutures are used to approximate tissue edges, reduce tension, and reduce dead space [1]. Tension-reducing suture patterns are described in detail elsewhere in this issue (see article by Amalsadvala). External tension-relieving sutures help to prevent sutures from cutting through skin, which occurs when the pressure on skin within the suture loop exceeds the pressure that allows blood flow. Pressure is reduced by spreading it over a larger area of skin (eg, placing sutures farther from the skin edge, using mattress or cruciate sutures, or placing buttons or rubber tubing under sutures). When external tension-relieving sutures are used with apposition sutures, they can usually be removed by the third or fourth day after surgery.

Drainage

Provision of adequate drainage is important in wound management (see article by Dernell elsewhere in this issue) [1]. Leaving the wound open provides optimal drainage. Other forms of drains allow evacuation of potentially harmful fluids (eg, blood, exudate, serum) from wounds and help to eliminate dead space. They often are necessary for the treatment of bite wounds, lacerations, skin avulsions or separations, tumor excision sites, seromas, and abscesses. Drains may also be used to help maintain contact between a flap or graft and its bed. Drains used at the time of wound closure are beneficial to minimize dead space and provide an outlet for continued removal of debris and tissue fluids. The use of a controlled subatmospheric pressure vacuum dressing has been shown to help remove interstitial fluid (allowing tissue decompression), to help remove tissue debris, and to promote wound healing in open wounds [3].

CLOSURE TECHNIQUES
Closure of large trunk wounds may use a variety of techniques to facilitate closure and prevent complications. In addition to incision orientation, undermining, and appropriate suture patterns, other closure techniques may include tension-relieving incisions, skin stretching and expansion, and the creation of a variety of flaps to close large defects and appose skin edges.

Tension Relief
Incisions
Relaxing incisions or incisions made near a defect are beneficial in allowing skin closure around fibrotic wounds or important structures or after extensive tumor excision [1]. They are rarely needed on the trunk. During closure after routine undermining, one or more (multiple punctuate) tension-relieving incisions are made at points of maximum skin tension as the skin edges are being apposed (Fig. 2A, B). One incision actually creates a bipedicle advancement flap. Simple relaxing incisions heal by contraction and epithelialization in 25 to 30 days. Some relaxing incisions surrounded by loose elastic tissue can be closed primarily after the wound is approximated. Multiple punctate relaxing incisions are more cosmetic than single relaxing incisions but provide less relaxation and have a higher risk of causing significant circulatory compromise if there are too many or they are too large (see article by Fowler elsewhere in this issue).

Other tension-relieving incisions occasionally used to close difficult trunk defects include the V-to-Y plasty and Z-plasty techniques [1]. A V-to-Y plasty is a type of relaxing incision that provides an advancement flap to cover a wound. It is used to close chronic inelastic wounds or wounds that would distort adjacent structures if closed under tension. An initial V-shaped incision is made with the open end of the "V" approximately 3 cm from the wound, and it is closed in the shape of a "Y" (see Fig. 2C–F).

A Z-plasty is a form of relaxing incision. The Z-shaped incision is made adjacent to the wound to facilitate closure with less tension. The central limb is made in the direction in which relaxation is needed. The two arms of the "Z" are made the same length as the central limb. The angles of the Z can vary between 30° and 90°, but 60° is advised. Length is gained in the direction of the Z when the flaps of the Z are transposed (see Fig. 2G, H) (see article by Fowler elsewhere in this issue).

Skin stretching
Skin stretching is a technique used in reconstructive surgery that takes advantage of the skin's ability to stretch beyond its natural or inherent elasticity, by the processes of mechanical creep and stress relaxation, when continuous tension is applied [1]. During this process, dermal collagen fibers are stretched and tissue fluid is slowly displaced from around the collagen fibers, which are

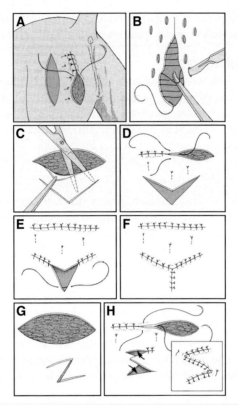

Fig. 2. Relaxing incisions made near defects facilitate skin apposition. (*A*) After undermining the skin, a simple relaxing incision is made adjacent to the wound to allow its closure. (*B*) After preplacing a continuous subcuticular suture pattern, multiple punctuate incisions where excess tension is noted are made parallel to the wound as the suture is tightened. (*C–F*) V-to-Y plasty provides an advancement flap to cover the wound. (*G, H*) Z-plasty can be made adjacent to the wound to allow relaxation for wound closure. (*From* Fossum TW. Small animal surgery. 2nd edition. St. Louis (MO): Mosby Publishing; 2002. p. 161; with permission.)

straightening and compacting longitudinally in the direction of the stretching force. Skin can be prestretched hours to days before surgery to allow the skin to be closed with less tension at the time of the procedure. Presuturing, adjustable sutures, skin stretchers, and skin expanders are used in this technique (see article by Fowler elsewhere in this issue).

X-Banders. The skin stretcher (X-Banders; X-Bander Corporation, Woodville, Massachussetts) is a noninvasive device capable of stretching skin adjacent and distant to the wound or proposed excision site [1,4]. More skin can be stretched or recruited using this technique than by using presuturing or tissue expanders [4]. Skin stretchers are most effective on the neck and trunk. Self-adherent skin pads with Velcro (Velcro; Velcro USA Inc, Manchester, NH) material are applied to clipped, clean, dry skin adjacent to and at a variable distance from the surgical site, depending on the amount of stretching needed. A thin coat of additional cyanoacrylate adhesive is used to help ensure pad adhesion. Pads are placed 1 to 2 cm from the wound margin, with their long axis perpendicular to the direction of skin tension (Fig. 3). Elastic connecting cables with the other portion of the Velcro material are attached to pads on one side of the wound and stretched before they are attached to the pads on the opposite side of the wound. An additional row or tier of pads and cables can be placed more distant from the wound if further skin recruitment is required. The cables are adjusted every 6 to 8 hours to generate an optimum high-tension load to accelerate skin stretching or deformation. Sufficient skin may be recruited within 24 to 48 hours, although 96 hours may be required. Pads are peeled from the skin or removed with glue solvent before surgery. Little or no undermining is generally required after skin stretching, and the creation of more complicated skin flaps can be avoided. Skin stretchers can also be used after surgery when incisions are closed under excessive tension. Skin stretchers generally are removed 3 to 5 days after surgery.

Sutures. Subdermal fascia is strong and tolerates tension better than subcutaneous tissue or skin. Sutures placed in subdermal or subcuticular tissue reduce tension on skin sutures and bring skin edges into apposition. These sutures also reduce scarring. For subdermal and subcuticular sutures, 3-0 or 4-0 monofilament absorbable suture with a buried knot is used.

   "Walking" sutures move skin across a defect, obliterate dead space, and distribute tension around the wound surface [1,2]. Skin is advanced toward the center of the wound by placing staggered rows of interrupted subdermal sutures beginning at the depths of undermined skin around the wound. The suture should be placed through fascia of the body wall at a distance closer to the center of the wound than the bites through the subdermal fascia or deep dermis (Fig. 4). Walking sutures do not penetrate the skin surface. The sutures are placed perpendicular to the direction of advancement to minimize

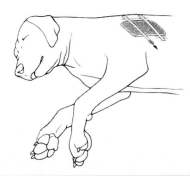

Fig. 3. Skin stretchers (X-Banders) apply tension across a wound (*arrow*) to stretch skin before closure. (*From* Fossum TW. Small animal surgery. 2nd edition. St. Louis (MO): Mosby Publishing; 2002. p. 157; with permission.)

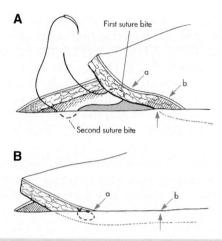

Fig. 4. Walking sutures are used to advance skin toward the center of the wound. (A) Place the second suture bite through the fascia of the body wall at a distance closer to the center of the wound than the first bite, which is placed through the subdermal fascia or deep dermis (a). (B) Note that the distance from a to b increases because of skin stretching when the suture is tied. (*From* Fossum TW. Small animal surgery. 2nd edition. St. Louis (MO): Mosby Publishing; 2002. p. 158; with permission.)

the damage to the subdermal plexus. Tying the suture advances skin toward the wound center. Walking sutures are placed no closer than 2 to 3 cm apart. Successive rows of walking sutures further advance the skin toward the center of the wound. Sutures are placed on both sides of the defect to advance undermined skin toward the center. The number of walking sutures should be minimized to avoid creating subcutaneous loculi or compromising circulation. Subdermal and skin sutures are used to complete wound closure.

When a wound is too large to be closed completely with walking sutures immediately, partial wound closure allows the remaining wound to be treated as an open wound to heal by second intention or to be stretched. In the latter case, elastic skin stretchers can be placed when a wound is surgically debrided. Later, when wound debridement is completed and infection is controlled, additional walking sutures can be placed to advance the skin further toward the center of the wound before final closure. Other options for large trunk wound closure are (1) walking sutures with closure of the remaining wound by mesh grafts made from dog ears that develop during closure or (2) using a second walking suture technique 14 to 21 days after the first one.

Adjustable horizontal mattress sutures can be used to stretch skin over a wound gradually (see article by Fowler elsewhere in this issue) [5]. This is a continuous intradermal suture (2-0 monofilament nonabsorbable) anchored at one or both ends, with a button secured on the skin surface with a split-shot fishing weight or hemoclip (Fig. 5). On succeeding days, traction on the suture advances the wound edges over the wound and new weights or hemoclips are applied to maintain tension. These sutures are used primarily on limb

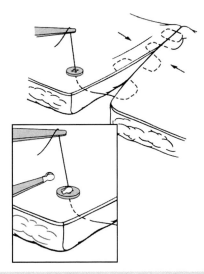

Fig. 5. Adjustable horizontal mattress suture. Upward tension on the suture advances the wound edges toward each other. (*Inset*) Split-shots placed on the suture adjacent to a button hold tension on the suture. (*From* Fossum TW. Small animal surgery. 2nd edition. St. Louis (MO): Mosby Publishing; 2002. p. 157; with permission.)

wounds in which the wound edges cannot be apposed initially. If the dermis is compromised, sutures may pull through.

X or Double-Y Closure

Large square or rectangular trunk wounds may be closed completely or partially using the X or double-Y closure technique [1,2]. This technique should be used when skin is available on all four sides of the defect. Centripetal closure begins with suture closure at each corner of the defect and advances toward the center to form an X-shaped suture line for square wounds or a double-Y–shaped suture line for rectangular wounds (Figs. 6 and 7).

Trunk Flaps

Pedicle flaps are "tongues" of epidermis and dermis that are partly detached from donor sites and used to cover defects [1]. The base or pedicle of the flap contains the blood supply essential for flap survival. Pedicle flaps often allow immediate coverage of a wound bed and avoid the prolonged healing, excessive scarring, and contracture that may be associated with second-intention healing. They can be classified in various ways based on location, blood supply, and geometric shape. A specific flap may be classified in more than one way. Most flaps are called subdermal plexus flaps; however, those with direct cutaneous vessels are called axial pattern flaps [6]. Flaps that remain attached to the donor bed by only the direct cutaneous vessels and subcutaneous tissues are called island flaps [6]. Flaps created immediately adjacent to the defect in loose elastic skin are called local flaps. Interpolation flaps are rectangular flaps

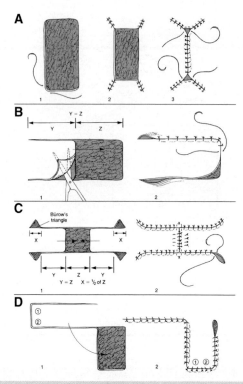

Fig. 6. Closure of large square or rectangular defects. (*A*) Centripetal closure beginning at the corners advances skin toward the wound center for a double-Y–shaped suture line for a rectangular wound. (*B*) Single pedicle advancement flap. (*C*) Bilateral single pedicle advancement flaps (H-plasty). (*D*) Transposition flap. (*From* Fossum TW. Small animal surgery. 2nd edition. St. Louis (MO): Mosby Publishing; 2002. p. 164; with permission.)

that are rotated into a nearby rather than adjacent defect. The pedicle passes over intact skin and can be sutured into a tube [6]. Flaps created at a distance from the defect are called distant flaps and usually require multiple-stage reconstruction and transfer. Flaps that include tissue other than skin and subcutaneous tissue are called compound or composite flaps and may include muscle (myocutaneous), cartilage, or bone.

Increasing the width of a pedicle flap does not necessarily increase the surviving length of the flap. Narrowing the base of the pedicle by back-cut techniques to increase its mobility increases the possibility of necrosis because of the decreasing flap vascular supply, however. The base of a single pedicle advancement flap should be slightly wider than the width of the flap body. Multiple small flaps may be preferable to a large flap if circulation is questionable. Delaying flap transfer 18 to 21 days after initial creation may improve circulation and survival (delay phenomenon). Donor sites should have sufficient skin to permit primary closure after skin transfer to the recipient site. Donor sites

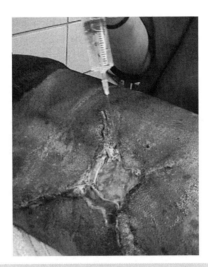

Fig. 7. A large tumor was excised from the trunk in a square. Centripetal closure was performed under tension with subsequent partial dehiscence and central necrosis.

with excessive motion and stress should be avoided. If possible, reconstruction should be planned so that the color and direction of hair growth after transfer of flaps to the recipient site are similar to those of the donor site.

The part of the flap that fails is the part that is needed most—the end of the flap. Failure is generally attributable to venous congestion. Venous congestion in a flap may be suspected if the flap becomes dusky or cyanotic in color, if capillary refill time is quicker than normal, or if rapid or dark bleeding occurs in response to a needle prick.

Advancement flaps
Advancement flaps are local subdermal plexus flaps. They include single pedicle (see Fig. 6B), bipedicle (see Fig. 2A), H-plasty (see Fig. 6C), and V-Y advancement (see Fig. 2C–F) flaps [1,2]. Single pedicle advancement flaps are formed incrementally in adjacent, loose, elastic skin that can be slid over the defect. The flap is developed parallel to lines of least tension to facilitate its forward stretch over a wound. These incisions should diverge slightly as they approach the flap's base, and small back cuts can be made into the flap's base to facilitate its advancement. Advancement flaps do not bring additional loose skin to the wound but allow closure because of the skin's elasticity. Advancement flap stretching is opposed by retractive forces that may lead to dehiscence. Dog ears can be removed from the area adjacent to the flap's base if necessary. An H-plasty consists of two single pedicle advancement flaps created on opposite sides of the wound. It is often appropriate for trunk wounds.

Rotational flaps
Rotation flaps. Rotation flaps are local flaps that are pivoted over a defect with which they share a common border. They move like the hands of a clock to

cover the defect. They are semicircular and may be paired or single. They may be used to close triangular defects on the trunk. Paired flaps are used to close wide triangular defects or rectangular defects. A curved incision is created, and the skin is undermined in a stepwise fashion until it covers the defect with little or no tension (Fig. 8). If excessive tension develops, a small stab incision perpendicular to the line of greatest tension can be made. A small back cut at its base could facilitate flap rotation (see Fig. 8).

Transposition flaps. Transposition flaps are rectangular local flaps that bring additional skin into defects when transposed. One edge of the flap is a portion of the defect. Most are created within 90° of the long axis of the defect. To obtain the bulk of the flap required to cover the defect, 90° transposition flaps are aligned parallel to the lines of greatest tension. The donor site is easily closed, because minimal tension lines are perpendicular to the suture line. The width of the flap equals the width of the defect. The length of the flap is determined by measuring from the pivot point of the flap to the most distant point of the defect. This compensates for the loss of functional length that occurs as the flap is rotated. Dog ears at the base of the flap may flatten with time (see Fig. 6D).

Forelimb and flank fold flaps. Forelimb and flank fold flaps are useful transposition flaps for trunk wounds [1,7,8]. These skin fold flaps can be harvested bilaterally to close large axillary, sternal, inguinal or lateral body wall wounds. The size and length of skin fold flaps vary with body conformation. Creation of these flaps begins by grasping the loose skin extending from the elbow or flank to the body wall to determine the amount of skin that can be harvested. Symmetric lateral and medial incisions are first outlined and then made. These incisions are connected with a curved incision made proximal to the elbow (forelimb) or stifle (hind limb). The flap is elevated from the triceps (forelimb) or quadriceps (hind limb), transposed, and sutured to the prepared wound bed on the trunk (Figs. 9 and 10). The donor site is closed after flap transposition. Bilateral flaps can be used to close large trunk wounds (see Figs. 9 and 10). The flank fold flap

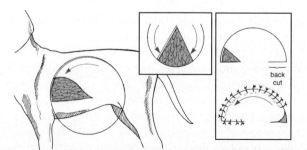

Fig. 8. A large triangular defect can be closed by creating one or two (*small inset*) rotation flaps at the defect edge. A back cut (*large inset*) may be needed to relieve tension at the base of the flap but may risk damage to the blood supply. (*From* Fossum TW. Small animal surgery. 2nd edition. St. Louis (MO): Mosby Publishing; 2002. p. 163; with permission.)

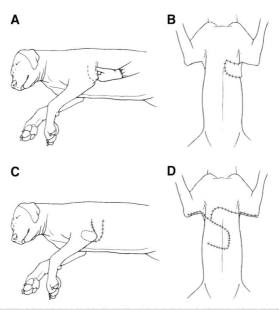

Fig. 9. The forelimb skin fold is harvested to close axillary, sternal, or lateral thoracic wounds. (A) Grasp loose skin from the elbow to the body wall to determine the amount of skin that can be harvested. Create lateral and medial skin incisions (*broken lines*) to define the width of the flap, and then connect these incisions with a curved incision proximal to the elbow (*broken line*). (B, C) Elevate, transpose, and suture the flap into the wound, and then close the donor site. (D) Create and transpose bilateral flaps to close larger sternal wounds. (*From* Fossum TW. Small animal surgery. 2nd edition. St. Louis (MO): Mosby Publishing; 2002. p. 167; with permission.)

supplied by the lower branches of the ventral branch of the deep circumflex iliac artery can be considered an axial pattern flap.

Axial pattern flaps

Axial pattern flaps are pedicle flaps that include a direct cutaneous artery and vein at the base of the flap [1,6,9]. The terminal branches of these vessels supply the subdermal plexus. They have better perfusion than pedicle flaps with random subdermal plexus circulation. Axial pattern flaps are elevated and transferred to cutaneous defects within their radius similar to random pattern flaps. They usually are rectangular or L-shaped flaps. Axial pattern flaps using the caudal auricular artery branches, the superficial temporal artery, the omocervical artery, the thoracodorsal artery, the superficial brachial artery, the cranial superficial epigastric and caudal superficial epigastric arteries, the deep circumflex iliac artery, the genicular artery, and the lateral caudal arteries as direct cutaneous arteries in dogs have been described (Fig. 11) [6–13]. Although similar flaps can be created in cats, only thoracodorsal, caudal superficial epigastric, caudal auricular, and superficial temporal artery axial pattern flaps

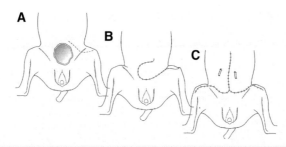

Fig. 10. The flank skin fold is harvested to close an inguinal wound. (A) Determine the amount of skin that can be harvested, and outline the flap (*broken line*). (B) After creating the flap, transpose it, suture it into the defect, and then close the donor site. (C) Create bilateral flaps to close larger wounds. (*From* Fossum TW. Small animal surgery. 2nd edition. St. Louis (MO): Mosby Publishing; 2002. p. 167; with permission.)

and reverse saphenous conduit flaps have been evaluated [7,8,10,11,13]. Of these axial pattern flaps, those most useful for trunk wounds include flaps based on the thoracodorsal, caudal superficial epigastric, deep circumflex iliac, and superficial lateral caudal arteries.

Axial pattern flaps require careful planning, measuring, and mapping on the skin surface to minimize errors. Positioning is important to ensure that the skin and underlying landmarks are in a normal anatomic position. Except for epigastric flaps, the animal is positioned in lateral recumbency and the limbs are placed in relaxed extension; the thoracoabdominal skin is then grasped, lifted, and allowed to retract spontaneously to a normal position before the flaps are outlined. Axial pattern flaps can be modified to create island arterial flaps by severing the cutaneous pedicle but preserving the direct cutaneous artery and vein. Island flaps have the potential for use as free flaps for transfer and microvascular anastomosis [6].

Axial pattern flaps are used most commonly to facilitate wound closure after tumor resection or trauma. The survival rate for axial pattern flaps is approximately twice that for subdermal plexus flaps of comparable size. Axial pattern flaps also provide durable full-thickness skin that can be transposed primarily without the need for a vascular bed or postoperative immobilization. Complications include wound drainage, partial dehiscence, distal flap necrosis, infections, and seroma formation. The cosmetic results are good.

Thoracodorsal axial pattern flaps. Thoracodorsal axial pattern flaps are used to cover defects involving the shoulder, forelimb, elbow, axilla, and thorax [6,10,11]. The flap is based on a cutaneous branch of the thoracodorsal artery and associated vein. The origin of these flaps is at the caudal shoulder depression at a level parallel to the dorsal border of the acromion. These flaps are preferred to omocervical flaps because they are more robust. In cats, the thoracodorsal flap extends to the carpus. In dogs, distal limb coverage depends on body conformation and limb length. Flaps extending ventral to the contralateral scapulohumeral joint usually survive. Development of long thoracodorsal axial pattern flaps may require staging and division of the opposite cutaneous branches of the thoracodorsal artery and vein.

Outline the flap by drawing a line over the scapular spine to mark the cranial incision (see Fig. 11). Draw the caudal incision line parallel to the scapular spine at a distance approximately twice the distance from the acromion to the caudal shoulder depression. Extend these parallel lines to and continue along the dorsal midline. If necessary, an L-shaped flap extension can be made by extending the cranial incision across the midline by 50%, making a caudally directed incision at its end and a parallel incision to this incision along the dorsal midline. These latter incisions are connected to create the L-shaped extension. Incise the outlined flap, and undermine deep to the cutaneous trunci muscle. For distant transposition, the pedicle can be tubed or its edges sutured to a bridging incision. Eliminate dead space with Penrose or closed-suction drains, and close the defects.

Caudal superficial epigastric axial pattern flap. The caudal superficial epigastric axial pattern flap is a versatile flap that is used to cover defects involving the caudal abdomen, flank, prepuce, perineum, thigh, and hind leg. In cats, the flap can extend over the metatarsal area [10]. In dogs with long bodies and short limbs, it may extend to or below the level of the tibiotarsal joint. The flap includes three to four caudal mammary glands and is supplied by the caudal superficial

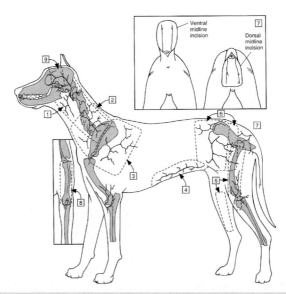

Fig. 11. Direct cutaneous vessels and their respective axial pattern flaps are outlined by broken lines: 1, caudal auricular; 2, omocervical; 3, thoracodorsal; 4, caudal superficial epigastric; 5, medial genicular; 6, deep circumflex iliac; 7, superficial lateral caudal (*inset*); 8, superficial brachial (*inset*); 9, superficial temporal. (*From* Fossum TW. Small animal surgery. 2nd edition. St. Louis (MO): Mosby Publishing; 2002. p. 170; with permission.)

epigastric artery and associated vein, which pass through the inguinal ring (see Fig. 11).

Position the patient in dorsal recumbency. Outline the flap with the ventral midline as the location of the medial incision. In male dogs, the incision is at the base of the prepuce. Mark a parallel lateral incision at a distance equal to the distance from the teats to the midline. Determine the number of mammary glands to include in the flap based on the size and location of the defect. Create the flap by connecting the two parallel lines between the first and second or second and third glands with a curved incision. Undermine the flap at the level of the external abdominal oblique aponeurosis, deep to the supramammarius muscle. Make the flap wider as needed to cover the defect if abundant loose elastic skin is available for closure of the donor site. Transpose the flap, place the drains, and appose the skin edges. An island flap is created by making a curved incision just caudal to the last teat. Caution is used during flap dissection and transposition to avoid trauma to or kinking or stretching of the caudal superficial epigastric vessels. A concurrent ovariohysterectomy is recommended, because transposed glands remain functional. Mammae may be resected later if their appearance is objectionable.

Cranial superficial epigastric axial pattern flap. The cranial superficial epigastric flap is smaller and less versatile than the caudal superficial epigastric axial pattern flap; however, it can be quite useful for closure of large skin defects overlying the sternum [1,12]. The flap is kept small, because these vessels are short and less developed than the caudal vessels and some flap necrosis is expected. The flap may include the third, fourth, and possibly fifth mammary glands. In male animals, the flap ends cranial to the prepuce. Although there is some variability, the cranial superficial artery penetrates the medial aspect of the rectus abdominis muscle at the junction between the second and third mammary glands. Cranial and caudal superficial epigastric arteries anastomose between or near the third and fourth mammary glands. The positioning and creation of the flap are similar to those for the caudal superficial epigastric flap. The base of the flap is located in the hypogastric region, where the cranial epigastric vessel enters the skin lateral to the abdominal midline, and a few centimeters caudal to the cartilaginous border of the ventral thorax (xiphoid process).

With the flap based just lateral to the xiphoid process, outline the flap with the ventral midline as the location of the medial incision. Mark a parallel lateral incision at a distance equal to the distance from the teats to the midline. Determine the number of mammary glands to include in the flap based on the length of flap required to reach and cover the defect. Create the flap by connecting the two parallel lines between the fourth and fifth mammary glands or caudal to the fifth gland with a curved incision. Undermine the flap at the level of the external abdominal oblique aponeurosis, deep to the supramammarius muscle. Ligate branches of the caudal superficial epigastric artery as necessary. Transpose the flap, place the drains, and appose the skin edges. An island flap is created by making a curved incision between the second and third mammary glands. Use caution during dissection and flap transposition to prevent trauma to and kinking or stretching of the cranial superficial epigastric vessels. A concurrent ovariohysterectomy and later mammae resection are performed as indicated with the caudal superficial epigastric axial pattern flap.

Deep circumflex iliac axial pattern flap. The dorsal branch of the deep circumflex iliac vessel is used in flaps to cover defects involving the caudal thorax, lateral abdominal wall, ipsilateral flank, lateral lumbar area, medial or lateral thigh, greater trochanter, and pelvic area [1,6,13]. The ventral branch of the deep circumflex iliac artery supplies the flank fold used to cover caudolateral abdominal wall, inguinal, pelvic, or sacral defects. The dorsal and ventral branches of the deep circumflex iliac artery originate at a point cranioventral to the wing of the ilium (see Fig. 11).

Position the patient in lateral recumbency with the hind limb in relaxed extension perpendicular to the body. Outline the flap by first drawing its caudal border midway between the cranial border of the wing of the ilium and the greater trochanter. For the cranial incision, draw a second line parallel to the first line and equal to the distance from the iliac border to the caudal line. Extend the lines to the dorsal midline, and create an L-shaped extension, if needed, to cover the defect. Incise the outlined flap. Elevate the flap below the level of the cutaneous trunci muscle. Transpose the flap, place the drains, and appose the skin edges.

The ventral branch of the deep circumflex iliac artery is used in flaps to cover defects of the lateral abdominal wall and as an island flap for pelvic and sacral defects. Make the reference lines as for the previous flap. Draw the caudal incision line extending distally cranial to the border of the femoral shaft. Extend the cranial incision line down the flank and thigh region parallel to the caudal flap border. Connect the two lines above the patella. Elevate the flap below the level of the cutaneous trunci muscle. Incise the outlined flap. Transpose the flap, place the drains, and appose the skin edges.

Superficial lateral caudal axial pattern flap. The lateral caudal arteries of the tail may be used to reconstruct areas involving perineum and caudodorsal trunk defects [1,14]. The largest source of skin is from the proximal third of the tail. The tail skin may also be used as a tube flap to cover defects on the hind leg. The lateral caudal vessels are bilateral and are located in the subcutaneous tissue of the tail. The lateral caudal arteries arise from the caudal gluteal arteries and have several anastomotic branches with the median caudal artery. Use of this flap requires tail amputation.

Make a dorsal midline incision along the length of the tail to cover dorsocaudal defects (see Fig. 11). Make a ventral midline skin incision to cover defects of the perineal and upper hind limb areas (see article by Bellah elsewhere in this issue). Dissect the subcutaneous tissues from the deep caudal fascia, preserving the right and left lateral caudal arteries and veins. Amputate the tail at the third or fourth caudal (coccygeal) intervertebral space. Transpose the skin flap over the defect, place the drains, and appose the skin edges.

Omental flaps

Omental flaps may be used to cover soft tissue defects, to contribute to circulation and drainage, to enhance healing, to control adhesion, and to combat infection, similar to muscle flaps. Although less durable than muscle flaps, they stimulate the formation of granulation tissue to allow earlier wound closure with skin flaps or grafts [11,15–17]. Omental flaps are useful over nonhealing wounds covered by a skin flap. They are especially useful for chronic nonhealing wounds involving the thorax, abdomen, and inguinal and axillary areas and can be used for facial and distal extremity wounds if omental lengthening or microvascular transfer is employed. In dogs and cats, the omentum is a thin double sheet of mesothelium that folds on itself in the caudal abdomen. It attaches ventrally to the greater curvature of the stomach and dorsally to the pancreas and spleen. The omental blood supply is from peripheral vessels of the right and left gastroepiploic arteries.

Two methods may be used to mobilize the omentum. One involves creating a vascular pedicle of the entire omentum based on the right or left gastroepiploic artery by releasing the dorsal leaf of the omentum. The other involves releasing the omentum from the pancreas and then lengthening it with an inverted L-shaped incision. Both methods require a ventral midline celiotomy. Possible complications after omental transposition include seroma formation, herniation through the omental exit hole, and omental necrosis.

Create a vascular pedicle based on the right or left gastroepiploic artery by ligating the segmental gastric arteries as they leave the gastroepiploic artery and enter the greater curvature of the stomach. Ligate the right or left gastroepiploic artery, depending on which side of the body the omentum is needed, ligating on the side opposite where it is needed. Incise additional attachments to the pancreas and spleen, and ligate vessels as necessary to mobilize an appropriate length of omentum for transposition. The multiple vessel ligations required for this technique increase the risk of hematoma formation, which may affect omental flap viability.

Using the lengthening technique, retract the dorsal omental leaf cranially and exteriorize the spleen. Release the dorsal leaf from the pancreas using sharp dissection, and ligate or cauterize vessels as encountered. Ligate and transect the one or two vessels originating from the splenic artery close to the spleen. Extend the dorsal leaf caudally, unfolding the omentum. Begin the inverted L-shaped incision on the left side just caudal to the gastrosplenic ligament (Fig. 12). Double-ligate and transect omental vessels when encountered as the incision is extended across one half to two thirds of the omentum's width. Continue the incision caudally, parallel to the remaining omental vessels, along two thirds of the length of the omentum. Ligate or cauterize vascular branches as encountered. Rotate the omentum caudally to extend the pedicle fully. After the omentum has been mobilized, make a small incision (2–3 cm) through the lateral abdominal wall near the wound or several centimeters lateral to the celiotomy for distant wounds. Create a subcutaneous tunnel to the wound, gently drag the omentum through this tunnel, and secure it to the wound with

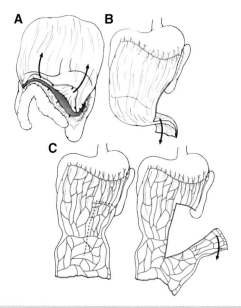

Fig. 12. Harvesting omental flaps. (A) Exteriorize the omentum and spleen, and then retract the dorsal omental leaf cranially (*arrows*) and free it from its pancreatic attachments. (B) Extend the dorsal leaf of the omentum caudally (*arrow*). (C) Make an inverted L-shaped incision just caudal to the gastrosplenic ligament, and rotate the left side caudally to achieve full extension. (*From* Fossum TW. Small animal surgery. 2nd edition. St. Louis (MO): Mosby Publishing; 2002. p. 181; with permission.)

interrupted absorbable sutures. Take care when handling and transposing the omentum to keep it warm and moist and to prevent occlusion of remaining omental vessels to maintain its viability. If desired, a skin flap can be placed over the omental flap.

Full-Thickness Wall Defects

Body wall injuries with tissue necrosis or body wall excisions (en bloc resections) for removal of neoplastic lesions, chronic infections, and congenital defects may require reconstruction of the body wall [18–25]. Full-thickness body wall defects may be reconstructed using one or more of the following techniques: direct reapposition of tissues, diaphragmatic advancement, prosthesis implantation, omental flaps, muscle flaps, or myocutaneous flaps. The goal of reconstruction is to provide a functional strong replacement for the missing tissue. Reconstruction of the thoracic wall is more difficult than that of the abdominal wall, because the rigidity of the ribs often necessitates replacement with prosthetic material. Repair after traumatic injuries should include debridement of necrotic tissue, exploration for concurrent visceral damage, and postoperative body cavity drainage.

Direct tissue reapposition

Small defects in the thoracic (one or two ribs) or abdominal wall are directly apposed by stretching or rotating surrounding tissue. Defects involving the loss of one or two ribs can usually be repaired by placing circumcostal sutures (polydioxanone, polypropylene, or nylon) or hemicerclage sutures (stainless steel) through intact adjacent ribs to narrow the defect and bring soft tissues into closer apposition. Closure of the intercostal muscles may then be possible. Alternatively, more superficial muscles of the thoracic wall (serratus ventralis, latissimus dorsi, pectoral, external abdominal oblique, and rectus abdominis muscles) are pulled or rotated and sutured over the defect. Fractured ribs are stabilized with suture, hemicerclage wires, pins, scaffold sutures, or external splints as needed [24]. Small defects in the abdominal wall are closed by apposing muscles adjacent to the defect. Use of postoperative drains is essential in many of the larger wounds. Skin is then advanced over the wound.

Diaphragmatic advancement

Complex rigid reconstruction of the thoracic wall with prostheses and tissue flaps can be avoided when wounds involve the caudal thorax and the diaphragm is advanced cranially [25]. If necessary, the block of ribs is resected. This maneuver converts the thoracic defect to an abdominal defect. Injury or resection involving the thoracic wall supported by the ninth through 13th ribs is most amenable to this technique, although the diaphragm can be advanced further if necessary. The diaphragm is incised near its peripheral attachments, advanced forward, and sutured to the epaxial musculature, intercostal muscles, or the most caudal intact rib. The diaphragm can be advanced to the level of the eighth intercostal space in dogs without significantly compromising lung expansion or protection of underlying viscera. More rostral advancement might require caudal lung lobectomy.

Reconstruction with prostheses

More complex techniques for repair of thoracic wall defects include use of polypropylene mesh or similar synthetic materials combined with muscle, omental, or myocutaneous flaps and, sometimes, spinal plates [19–23]. Mesh closure is more often needed for thoracic wall defects than for abdominal wall defects. Paradoxic motion of the chest wall may be apparent immediately after surgery but resolves within 48 to 72 hours with moderate resections (four or fewer ribs). Thoracic wall reconstruction may be unstable and viscera poorly protected when more than six ribs are removed. Complications associated with prostheses and flaps include dehiscence, seromas, infection, forelimb edema, pleural effusion, pneumothorax, subcutaneous emphysema, and flail chest.

After excision of diseased or traumatized tissue, sterile polypropylene mesh (Marlex mesh; Davol, Providence, Rhode Island) is cut slightly larger than the defect so that the edges of the mesh can be folded to create a double thickness 1 to 1.5 cm in width around the periphery. This adds strength and minimizes fraying. Position the folded mesh in the defect so that the folded free edges face exteriorly. The mesh is ideally placed intrapleurally during thoracic wall reconstruction. Secure the folded mesh edge to the margins of the defect encircling the ribs when possible with polypropylene suture (0-0 or 2-0). After securing one border, continue placing sutures around the periphery with the edge of the mesh folded and the sheet kept taut (Fig. 13). Cover the mesh by apposing adjacent muscles or by transposing a muscle flap. If there is insufficient muscle to provide a soft tissue covering over the mesh, harvest and transpose omentum over the mesh before skin closure. To avoid lung adhesions to the mesh, omentum can also be mobilized and advanced through the diaphragm and used to line the mesh. Place a closed-suction subcutaneous drain and a thoracic drain. Close skin over the reconstruction using skin flaps as needed. Finally, support the reconstruction and protect the drains with a comfortable padded bandage for 7 to 10 days.

Mesh alone may not be sufficient to provide thoracic wall stability when four or more ribs are excised, resulting in paradoxic movement. In these cases, reinforcement using flexible spinal plates, methylmethacrylate polypropylene composites, or bone grafts to support the mesh and maintain thoracic wall conformation may be beneficial [19–23]. Flexible spinal plates are secured to remaining rib segments with wire before placement of the mesh over the plates. The mesh is secured to the margins of the defect and the plates using the plates' holes.

Muscle flaps and myocutaneous flaps

Muscle flaps with overlying skin (myocutaneous flaps) or without skin (muscle flaps) may be created to facilitate herniorrhaphy, cover soft tissue defects, contribute circulation to ischemic areas, and combat infection [1]. They may also provide support, facilitate return of function, improve cosmesis, and reduce wound contamination. Use of muscle in reconstruction is limited by tissue availability and the surgeon's ability. The muscle flap may be used over mesh or other implants that provide support, and it is sutured to adjacent

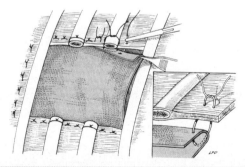

Fig. 13. Thoracic wall reconstruction after removal of ribs may require a mesh implant. Fold the edges of a piece of mesh over, and suture the double thickness of mesh to the pleural side of the defect, keeping the mesh taunt. Circumferential sutures attach mesh to rib ends. (*From* Fossum TW. Small animal surgery. 2nd edition. St. Louis (MO): Mosby Publishing; 2002. p. 785; with permission.)

muscle or fascial planes. Myocutaneous flaps should be used when reconstruction with local flaps, axial pattern flaps, or free grafts is not feasible. These flaps must be sufficiently large to cover the defect and have an easily accessible and constant dominant vascular supply. Donor sites should be easily closed. Muscles in dogs and cats that may be sacrificed in the repair of thoracic and abdominal wall defects without loss of function include portions of the latissimus dorsi, external abdominal oblique, and rectus abdominus. A vascular pedicle sufficient to maintain circulation is required to facilitate flap rotation into defects. Increased rotation may impair circulation and require that the flap length be reduced. Seromas are common after muscle or myocutaneous flap procedures; other potential complications include herniation, infection, dehiscence, and omental adhesions.

Latissimus dorsi flaps. The latissimus dorsi muscle is a flat triangular muscle overlying the dorsal half of the lateral thoracic wall. It originates from thoracolumbar fascia of the thoracic and lumbar spinous processes and from muscular attachments to the last two or three ribs. The aponeurosis of the latissimus dorsi inserts on the major teres tuberosity of the humerus. The ventral portion of the muscle is supplied by branches of the thoracodorsal artery (dorsal and lateral thoracic arteries), which penetrate the muscle and supply the overlying cutaneous trunci muscle and skin. Intercostal arteries supply segmental branches to the dorsal portion of the latissimus dorsi muscle and overlying cutaneous trunci muscle. Latissimus dorsi myocutaneous flaps are bulky because they contain the cutaneous trunci muscle and skin, subcutaneous fat, and latissimus dorsi muscle [26,27]. The latissimus dorsi muscle may be used alone as a muscle flap (Fig. 14).

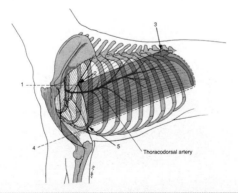

Fig. 14. Landmarks for the latissimus dorsi and cutaneous trunci myocutaneous flaps: 1, ventral border of the acromion; 2, adjacent caudal border of the triceps muscle; 3, vertebral attachment of the last rib; 4, distal third of the humerus; 5, axillary skin fold. To construct flaps, draw a line from 2 to 3 and a second parallel line from 5. Incise skin and muscle, connecting the two parallel lines dorsally. (*From* Fossum TW. Small animal surgery. 2nd edition. St. Louis (MO): Mosby Publishing; 2002. p. 175; with permission.)

With the patient in lateral recumbency and the forelimb in relaxed extension perpendicular to the trunk, plan and outline the flap with a marking pen. Draw a line from the caudal border of the triceps muscle to the vertebral attachment of the last rib. Draw a parallel line caudodorsally from the axillary skin fold, and connect the two lines to outline the flap (see Fig. 14). Incise the skin and extend the incision to the underlying latissimus dorsi muscle. The muscle flap equals the size of the skin flap. Elevate the latissimus dorsi and skin as a unit. Isolate, ligate, and divide the lateral intercostal vessels deep to the latissimus muscle. Identify and preserve the thoracodorsal artery and vein located at the caudal shoulder depression at a level parallel to the dorsal border of the acromion. Transpose the flap to the desired location without occluding the thoracodorsal vessels. If necessary, make a bridging incision or partial tube of the flap for transposition. Place Penrose or closed-suction drains at the donor site and beneath the flap at the recipient site. Secure the flap in position, suturing the muscle border and the skin flap, and close the donor site.

External abdominal oblique muscle flap. The external abdominal oblique muscle is elastic and mobile and may be used to facilitate the repair of defects in the abdominal wall or caudal thoracic wall. This flap may be used to fill defects larger than 10 cm × 10 cm in medium-sized dogs [18]. The external abdominal oblique muscle is a long flat muscle covering the ventral half of the lateral thoracic wall and lateral abdominal wall. Its fibers are directed caudoventrally.

Make a paracostal skin incision from the level of the epaxial muscles to the ventral midline, beginning 5 cm caudal to the 13th rib. Identify and divide the lumbar fascial edge of the external abdominal oblique muscle ventrally and caudally, leaving a 0.5- to 1-cm margin of fascia along the muscular edge (Fig. 15). Undermine the lumbar external abdominal oblique muscle from a ventral-to-dorsal direction. Identify and preserve the neurovascular pedicle (branches of the cranial abdominal artery and cranial hypogastric nerve and satellite vein) located in a craniodorsal position just caudal to the 13th rib. Divide the dorsal fascial attachment of the lumbar external abdominal oblique muscle, and then sever the muscle at the level of the 13th rib. Transpose the flap to an adjacent defect. Overlap the defect with the flap, and suture the inner fascial surface with 2-0 polydioxanone or polyglyconate using a simple interrupted pattern. Place closed-suction drains, and appose the defect edges.

Second-Intention Healing

Healing by contraction and epithelialization may be appropriate for large trunk wounds with resistant infections or after reconstruction and dehiscence (see article 1 in this issue). Management of these wounds can be labor-intensive and costly because of frequent bandage changes and the need for hospitalization or frequent veterinary visits, which may be necessary for weeks to months. Wounds healing by second intention near the flank or elbow may result in contracture and loss of mobility (see article by Amalsadvala elsewhere in this issue).

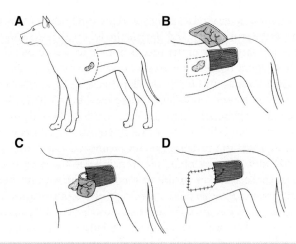

Fig. 15. An external abdominal oblique flap is created. (*A*) Make a paracostal skin incision (*broken line*) from the epaxial muscles toward the ventral midline, beginning 5 cm caudal to the 13th rib. (*B*) Create the muscle flap by severing the fascial attachments of the lumbar portion of the external abdominal oblique muscle, first at its ventral and caudal aspects. After undermining to identify and protect the neurovascular pedicle located in a craniodorsal position just caudal to the 13th rib, incise the muscle's dorsal fascial attachment and sever the muscle at the 13th rib. (*C, D*) Transpose and suture the muscle over an adjacent defect. (*From* Fossum TW. Small animal surgery. 2nd edition. St. Louis (MO): Mosby Publishing; 2002. p. 177; with permission.)

POSTOPERATIVE CARE

Postoperative care of trunk wounds includes bandaging, topical medications for open wounds, systemic antibiotics for contaminated and implant wounds, provision of appropriate analgesia and nutrition, and assessing for complications and healing (see articles 3–6 in this issue). Wounds should be evaluated frequently for infection, tension, fluid accumulation, dehiscence, and necrosis. They may be evaluated visually and with the aid of ultrasonography, which helps to detect and localize fluid accumulation [15]. Remove sutures from wounds in 7 to 14 days.

Most large trunk wounds benefit from bandaging during the first few days after surgery (see article by Campbell elsewhere in this issue). Closed healing wounds become increasingly resistant to bacterial penetration. Thus, prolonged bandaging is not necessary. Bandages are applied to large wounds of the trunk to absorb fluid from a drain or incision line, support the incision, apply pressure to compress dead space, or prevent trauma or contamination. These bandages improve the patient's comfort by supporting wounds. Bandages should be applied firmly but without constricting the thorax or abdomen. The intermediate layer of the bandage should be thick enough to prevent strikethrough when drainage is expected. The primary and secondary bandage layers are held in place with elastic or adhesive tape. Assess the character and amount of drainage with each bandage change, which may be daily for the first few changes and then only as needed. Frequently, a figure-of-eight type bandage crisscrossing between the forelegs or hind legs is necessary to keep the bandage from slipping. Areas inaccessible to standard bandaging techniques (eg, hip, shoulder, axilla) may be covered with island or tie-over bandages.

Most complications are prevented by using good surgical and wound management techniques. Potential complications include inflammation, edema, seroma and hematoma formation, drainage, infection, dehiscence, necrosis, granulomas, and contracture, all of which result in failure to heal. Seromas are caused by excessive dead space or motion. Dehiscence may occur when tissues necrose, if sutures are placed too close to the margin, if tension exceeds suture strength, if sutures absorb too quickly, or if sutures strangulate and cut through tissue. Dehiscence may also occur secondary to self-trauma, infection, severe cough, hypoproteinemia, hypovolemia, or administration of drugs that interfere with healing. Wounds that dehisce should be assessed as to the cause of dehiscence and be treated accordingly. Management by second-intention healing or debridement and reconstruction should then be considered. There are numerous other causes for nonhealing or abnormal healing wounds (see article by Amalsadvala elsewhere in this issue).

SUMMARY
Management of large trunk wounds begins with good wound management and bandaging. When a healthy wound bed exits and adequate tissue is present, the wound is closed. Fortunately, there is an abundance of loose trunk skin in most animals, and wound closure can be accomplished by simple reconstructive techniques, such as undermining and tension or walking sutures. Nevertheless, some wounds and areas of the torso may require more advanced tension-relieving techniques, skin stretching, and tissue implants or flaps to achieve tension-free closure and successful wound healing. Use of these techniques allows wound closure and good cosmetic results for even those wounds that initially may seem foreboding.

References
[1] Hedlund CS. Surgery of the integument. In: Fossum TW, Hedlund CS, Hulse DA, et al, editors. Small animal surgery. 2nd edition. St. Louis (MO): Mosby; 2002. p. 134–228.
[2] Swaim SF, Henderson RA. Small animal wound management. 2nd edition. Philadelphia: Williams & Wilkins; 1997. p. 143–275.
[3] Argenta LC, Morykwas MJ. Vacuum-assisted closure: a new method for wound control and treatment: clinical experience. Ann Plast Surg 1997;38(6):563–77.
[4] Pavletic MM. Use of an external skin-stretching device for wound closure in dogs and cats. J Am Vet Med Assoc 2000;217(3):350–4.
[5] Swaim SF. Advances in wound healing in small animal practice: current status and lines of development. Vet Dermatol 1997;8:249–57.
[6] Pavletic MM. Canine axial pattern flaps, using the omocervical, thoracodorsal, and deep circumflex iliac direct cutaneous arteries. Am J Vet Res 1981;42:391–406.
[7] Hunt GB. Skin fold advancement flaps for closing large sternal and inguinal wounds in cats and dogs. Vet Surg 1995;24:172–5.

[8] Hunt GB, Tisdall PLC, Liptak JM, et al. Skin-fold advancement flaps for closing large proximal limb and trunk defects in dogs and cats. Vet Surg 2001;30:440–8.

[9] Pavletic MM. Caudal superficial epigastric arterial pedicle grafts in the dogs. Vet Surg 1980;9(3):103–7.

[10] Remedios AM, Bauer MS, Bowen CV. Thoracodorsal and caudal superficial epigastric axial pattern skin flaps in cats. Vet Surg 1989;18(5):380–5.

[11] Lascelles BDX, White RAS. Combined omental pedicle grafts and thoracodorsal axial pattern flaps for the reconstruction of chronic, non healing axillary wounds in cats. Vet Surg 2001;30:380–5.

[12] Degner DA, Bauer MS, Steyn PE, et al. The cranial superficial epigastric skin flap in the dog. Vet Comp Orthop Traumatol 1994;7:18–20.

[13] Jackson AH, Degner DA, Jackson IT, et al. Deep circumflex iliac cutaneous free flap in cats. Vet Surg 2003;32:341–9.

[14] Smith MM, Carrig CB, Waldron DR, et al. Direct cutaneous arterial supply to the tail in dogs. Am J Vet Res 1992;53(1):145–8.

[15] Brockman DJ, Pardo AD, Conzemius MG, et al. Omentum-enhanced reconstruction of chronic nonhealing wounds in cats: techniques and clinical use. Vet Surg 1996;25:99–104.

[16] Ross WE, Pardo AD. Evaluation of an omental pedicle extension technique in the dog. Vet Surg 1993;22(1):37–43.

[17] Smith BA, Hosgood G, Hedlund CS. Omental pedicle used to manage a large dorsal wound in a dog. J Small Anim Pract 1995;36:267–70.

[18] Alexander LG, Pavletic MM, Engler SJ. Abdominal wall reconstruction with a vascular external abdominal oblique myofascial flap. Vet Surg 1991;20(6):379–84.

[19] Bright RM. Reconstruction of thoracic wall defects using Marlex mesh. J Am Anim Hosp Assoc 1981;17:415–20.

[20] Bright RM, Birchard SJ, Long GG. Repair of thoracic wall defects in the dog with an omental pedicle flap. J Am Anim Hosp Assoc 1982;18:277–82.

[21] Ellison GW, Trotter GW, Lumb WV. Reconstruction thoracoplasty using spinal fixation plates and polypropylene mesh. J Am Anim Hosp Assoc 1981;17:613–6.

[22] Johnson RP, Steiss JE, Sorjonen DC. Thermoplastic materials for orthotic design. Compend Contin Educ Pract Vet 2003;25(1):20–8.

[23] Lidbetter DA, Krahwinkel DJ, Williams FAJ, et al. Radical lateral body-wall resection for fibrosarcoma with reconstruction using polypropylene mesh and a caudal superficial epigastric axial pattern flap: a prospective clinical study of the technique and results in 6 cats. Vet Surg 2002;31:57–4.

[24] Shahar R, Shamir M, Johnston DE. A technique for management of bite wounds of the thoracic wall in small dogs. Vet Surg 1997;26:45–50.

[25] Arohnsohn M. Diaphragmatic advancement for defects of the caudal thoracic wall in the dog. Vet Surg 1984;13(1):26–8.

[26] Gregory CR, Gourley IM, Koblik PD, et al. Experimental definition of latissimus dorsi, gracilis, and rectus abdominus musculocutaneous flaps in the dog. Am J Vet Res 1988;49(6):878–84.

[27] Pavletic MM, Kostolich M, Koblick P, et al. A comparison of the cutaneous trunci myocutaneous flap and latissimus dorsi myocutaneous flap in the dog. Vet Surg 1987;16(4):283–93.

Vet Clin Small Anim 36 (2006) 873–893

VETERINARY CLINICS
SMALL ANIMAL PRACTICE
ELSEVIER
SAUNDERS

Bullet, Bite, and Burn Wounds in Dogs and Cats

Michael M. Pavletic, DVM*, Nicholas J. Trout, VetMB

Angell Animal Medical Center, 350 South Huntington Avenue, Boston, MA 02130, USA

GUNSHOT WOUNDS

In veterinary medicine, the number of gunshot wounds seen varies with the location of the practice. Veterinary hospitals located in major cities or in rural areas regularly see gunshot wounds. The weapon used varies to some degree according to location. Handguns are more prevalent in metropolitan areas, whereas rifles and shotguns are more common in rural areas [1]. Air-powered BB and pellet gunshot wounds are most likely the result of shootings by adolescents. Gunshot wounds can be associated with criminal, accidental, or self-defense activity, or they may simply represent a malicious act. There are legal issues that attending veterinarians must be aware of when dealing with evidence gathered in these cases.

Weapons

There are a variety of handguns, rifles, shotguns, and air-powered weapons available to the public. The projectiles or bullets (rounds) discharged can vary in diameter (caliber), mass (weight), material composition, shape, design, and velocity. The ballistics of a given projectile, or its flight characteristics from its course through the barrel to its final passage through "target," also differ based on these variables. As a result, the severity of tissue injury varies according to the characteristics of the projectile, the kinetic energy absorbed on impact, and the tissues struck by the projectile. These variables must be considered when assessing a patient's injuries and determining the appropriate treatment for a given projectile wound [2–6].

Projectile Characteristics

Bullets typically have a lead core; antimony is added to increase the hardness or malleability of lead. Lead bullets may be manufactured with an outer sleeve or jacket to control bullet deformation. Jackets are commonly composed of copper, cupronickel, brass, or soft steel. Military bullets are required to have full metal jackets, whereas hunting bullets typically are partially jacketed. Partially

*Corresponding author. *E-mail address*: mpavletic@angell.org (M.M. Pavletic).

0195-5616/06/$ – see front matter
doi:10.1016/j.cvsm.2006.02.005

jacketed bullets have a portion of the lead core exposed; the shape and design of the exposed lead tip can be altered to enhance bullet deformation or fragmentation on impact. For example, hollow points or grooved (scored) bullets enhance the ability of the bullet to mushroom or flatten, thereby slowing its path through a target and increasing the absorption of the projectile's kinetic energy, resulting in more tissue damage. A hunting bullet designed to mushroom on impact can create wounds up to 40 times the volume of a military bullet of similar mass and velocity. Fragmentation of the bullet also enhances tissue destruction on its passage into or through the tissues in its path. Some nonjacketed bullets (typically 0.22-caliber rim fire) have metallic plating (copper or copper-zinc) applied to the lead surface along with a lubricant; this thin metallic veneer does not restrict bullet deformation [2,3,5].

Shotguns are designed to fire a variety of round pellet sizes depending on the game hunted. Lead pellets are now used less commonly as a result of primary and secondary lead poisoning in waterfowl and predators from consumption of this heavy metal. Shotgun pellets are basically available in steel or lead [2,4,5]. The potential corrosive effects of tissue fluids on retained steel shot, and subsequent tissue irritation in animals, are unknown at this time.

Air-powered weapons rely on compressed air rather than gunpowder to impart velocity on the projectile. BB and pellet guns are typically low-mass and low-velocity weapons used for target practice or killing small game. The common calibers include 0.177 caliber (steel circular BB) as well as 0.177, 0.20, and 0.22 caliber (lead pellets). Pellets are typically shaped like an hour glass (diablo pellet) or like a cone or silo (Sheridan pellet). Although these projectiles have a relatively modest mass and velocity compared with conventional guns, they are capable of seriously injuring or killing larger animals, especially at close range. They rapidly decelerate after exiting the muzzle, however [4,5].

Ballistics and Destructive Capacity

The kinetic energy of a projectile explains the destructive potential of a projectile. This is best understood by reviewing the formula for kinetic energy:

$$\text{Kinetic Energy (KE)} = \text{Mass} \times \text{Velocity}^2/2$$

Doubling the mass of a projectile doubles its kinetic energy, whereas doubling the velocity quadruples its kinetic energy. As a result, a smaller caliber and lower mass projectile with a high velocity may have greater kinetic energy compared with a slow projectile of greater mass at impact with a target [3–6].

For descriptive purposes, projectiles can be classified according to their velocity:

Low velocity: less than 1000 ft/s
Medium velocity: 1000 to 2000 ft/s
High velocity: greater than 2000 ft/s

Most handguns are in the low- to medium-velocity range, whereas most rifled bullets are in the medium- to high-velocity range. As velocity increases, the destructive capacity of the bullet increases. At higher velocities, the phenomenon of "cavitation" is a significant factor in causing tissue destruction. Cavitation is the transient rapid expansion or ballooning of the tissues adjacent to the course of the bullet, which can be up to 30 times the diameter of the bullet. Shock waves released during passage of the projectile compress and stretch tissues lateral and ahead of the bullet. This transient event also creates a vacuum effect that is capable of sucking contaminants deep into the wound. Tissues are disrupted, regional circulation is compromised, and soft tissues outside the path of the bullet can be severely disrupted [4,5].

The bullet's ballistic properties and its ability to deform on impact influence tissue destruction. Modern bullets are fired from barrels containing helical grooves (rifling) that impart gyroscopic spin on the projectile, improving its flight characteristics and accuracy to the target. Bullets can become unstable during flight and deviate from their longitudinal axis, however. As a result, the bullet may yaw or tumble before impacting a body region, thereby increasing its profile of contact during passage through the tissues. Tumbling of a high-velocity projectile increases tissue destruction and may facilitate fragmentation of the bullet, further enhancing tissue injury. Bullets that deflect off a hard surface (ricochet) can distort and tumble, potentially causing a more serious wound, despite variable loss of velocity. From an "offensive" standpoint, the "ideal" projectile has the following characteristics: good ballistic shape (needle-like design), high sectional density (ratio of projectile mass to area of presentation), high velocity, and the capability of deep penetration with controlled expansion (eg, flattening, fragmentation). Tissue destruction is greater when the entire kinetic energy of the projectile is absorbed compared with a projectile that passes through a body region and exits largely intact [3–6].

Exploding bullets are rarely encountered today and are illegal to purchase. Detonation from impact results in the fragmentation of the bullet to enhance local tissue destruction. Care must be taken in the removal of intact exploding bullets. There are frangible bullets specifically designed to fragment on impact without the use of an explosive charge, however [4,5].

Shotguns are capable of firing round pellets that vary in size and number. Shotguns also are capable of firing single large "deer slugs." Shotguns were primarily designed to shoot small moving targets, especially game fowl. Dispersion of a pattern of pellets increases the likelihood of striking an elusive target. Shotgun patterns can be varied by modification of the barrel length and terminal diameter (choke). Shot patterns typically expand from the muzzle in a cone-like configuration. The effective hunting range for the average shotgun is 30 to 40 yd; within 20 yd, the pattern is too destructive; and beyond 40 yd, the shot pattern scatters with a significant loss of velocity. At close range and compared with a single bullet, the shotgun is capable of generating tremendous kinetic energy and massive tissue destruction as a result of the concentrated density of pellets and the surface area presented to the target.

The Sherman and Parrish classification of gunshot wounds is divided into three types:

Type I: subcutaneous and deep fascia penetration
Type II: penetrating tissues below the deep fascia
Type III: deep central zone of tissue destruction usually surrounded by a "halo" of pellets

Type I wounds are typical of scattered pellets noted incidentally on radiographs of hunting dogs. Type II and III wounds are the result of closer range impact, with a greater concentration of pellets [3–6].

Tissue Response to Projectiles

The specific gravity and relative cohesive properties of tissues influence the severity of tissue injury. Dense tissues, such as bone, absorb a greater amount of the kinetic energy of the projectile; bone fragments, in turn, can be driven into the adjacent tissues as secondary projectiles, enhancing local soft tissue injury. Skin and lung have greater elastic properties and are better able to absorb a portion of the kinetic energy of a projectile. Although skeletal muscle and hepatic tissue have a similar specific gravity, the liver is less cohesive and resilient. The liver is prone to fracturing or splitting, especially from the cavitation effects of high-velocity projectiles. As a result, elastic tissues that are capable of stretching are better able to sustain projectile trauma compared with less-cohesive tissues [3–6].

Diagnostic and Immediate Management Considerations

In many cases, an owner has no idea that a pet has been shot. Most injuries occur when a pet escapes or is allowed to roam unsupervised. Without an accurate history, the injuries may be mistaken for bite wounds or vehicular trauma. An owner, witness, or police officer may provide information confirming that the dog or cat was shot and identifying the weapon used. This information should be written in the record in the event that legal action occurs. Knowledge of the weapon, in turn, can help the veterinarian to determine the potential tissue damage and appropriate surgical management of the injuries.

High-velocity projectiles (especially jacketed bullets) are more likely to exit through most soft tissues, without leaving obvious metallic debris on radiographs in many cases. Lower velocity handgun rounds also may exit soft tissues in a similar fashion. Without a history or physical evidence, it can be difficult to prove that the injuries were the result of a gunshot. Wounds presenting on opposing sides of the patient or appearing visually aligned (entry and exit wounds) would raise the index of suspicion [4–6].

Impact with dense cortical bone often results in significant absorption of a projectile's kinetic energy. Lower velocity projectiles may strike and fracture bone without exiting the body region. Nonjacketed or partially jacketed bullets may flatten or fragment on impact. Higher velocity projectiles may shatter cortical bone on impact, with fragmentation of the projectile. Despite direct impact with bone, high-velocity projectiles may exit the body region, depending on the characteristics of the projectile (Fig. 1).

In general, retained projectiles that have not impacted bone can be considered low-velocity projectiles. It also must be kept in mind that high-velocity projectiles decelerate and may strike a distant target with a velocity comparable to that of a handgun [3–6].

In known cases of gunshot injury, the patient is closely examined for entry and exit wounds. Small wounds are easily overlooked, especially in long-haired breeds. Clippers are used to remove fur, and the wounds are inspected for definitive management. In general, entry wounds are smaller than exit wounds. As noted, the surface area and shape of the projectile can alter the size of the entry wound. Deformation of the bullet during passage can result in a larger exit wound as it emerges. The more powerful projectiles can shatter bone, enhancing the size of the exit wound as the projectile fragments and bone fragments are driven outward. In contrast, bullets may enter the skin at an irregular angle (tumbling) and exit with a smaller silhouette. With close or direct contact with the muzzle, the hot gases released may stretch and distort the skin [3–6].

Projectiles may deviate from a linear path through the body. Bullets may rotate or tumble, creating an irregular pathway through the soft tissues, or ricochet off the surface of the bone and deviate from the original pathway. Similarly, bullets may collapse and fragment, creating secondary paths from the original trajectory to the targeted area. Although uncommon, bullets can enter vessels and embolize. Cases have been documented of human beings sustaining a thoracic gunshot wound with the projectile entering a bronchus, only to be coughed up and swallowed. Projectiles also can move by motion of the patient or gravitate distal or ventral from their initial resting point within the body [4,5].

A complete set of radiographs should be taken of the body region involved. If the passage of one or more projectiles is noted, additional radiographs of the

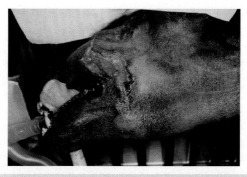

Fig. 1. High-velocity rifle round, exit wound. The high-velocity hunting round shattered both rami of the mandible and the hard palate. The deformed bullet fragments exited the left facial area, creating this large jagged skin wound.

regions cranial and caudal to the entry and exit sites also should be taken. Through and through wounds, without a history to accompany them, make definitive diagnosis of a gunshot injury difficult unless metallic fragments are retained in the tissues traversed by the projectile. Moreover, it is difficult to distinguish a low-velocity handgun round from a high-velocity rifle round under these circumstances. The radiographic presence of a retained projectile without an identifiable entry wound would suggest that the injury occurred in the distant past. Depending on the location and nature of the wounds, ultrasonography, pulse oximetry, electrocardiography, and blood gas analysis can be used to assess the critically injured patient. Myelography, CT, intravenous pyelography, and endoscopy may be advisable depending on the wound location and clinical findings. A baseline complete blood cell count and a serum chemistry profile are advisable in the seriously injured patient to help determine the patient's status and delineate organs that may have been injured by the projectile [4–6].

Treatment Recommendations

Most animals with gunshot wounds are presented through the emergency service. Supportive treatment is dictated by the status of the patient and severity of the wounds. A complete physical examination is used to assess the patient. Vital signs should be assessed immediately (eg, airway, breathing, circulatory status, and emergency measures should be instituted as needed in an unstable patient. When treating gunshot wounds, the general principles of assessing tissue viability and initial treatment should be observed (see the article by Dernell elsewhere in this issue). This includes the use of topical medications and bandages (see the articles by Krahwinkel and Booth and Campbell elsewhere in this issue). Specific factors come into play when dealing with gunshot wounds based on the type of weapon, tissues involved, and body region [4,5]. For principles involved in definitive wound management and reconstruction of wounded tissue, the reader is referred to other articles in this issue dealing with the various body areas.

Low- and high-velocity soft tissue wounds: skin and muscle

Low-velocity injuries usually have limited soft tissue trauma. Management normally is limited to clipping fur around the entry and exit wounds, followed by a surgical scrub of the area. The wounds may be flushed with sterile saline or povidone iodine (1:9 dilution) or chlorhexidine (1:40 dilution) solution with a 35-mL syringe and 18-gauge needle. Small mosquito hemostats may be used to spread the wound gently to facilitate flushing and drainage of the area. A sterile dressing should be applied to the wounds if possible. The frequency of bandage changes varies with the amount and type of discharge. Systemic broad-spectrum antibiotics are frequently administered as a cautionary measure. Wound closure is not recommended, thus allowing for drainage as the wound heals.

High-velocity rounds usually create entry and exit wounds when the course of the projectile is limited to soft tissues. Because of the elasticity of the tissue, some of the missile's kinetic energy is absorbed. Unless there is significant vascular damage, tissue trauma is limited and the wound is managed as a low-velocity gunshot wound as described previously.

Lead poisoning is rarely noted with retained bullets. Retained projectiles are normally encased in connective tissue over time. Removal of projectiles should be considered if they are easily accessible and their removal poses no additional risk to the patient. A bullet fragment or shot within a joint should be removed [4,5].

Shotgun: skin and muscle

Type I shotgun wounds require minimal management because this low-grade injury is often noted as an incidental radiographic finding. Pellet patterns normally are diffuse, and individual shot is primarily limited to the subcutaneous space and underlying skeletal muscle layer. Type II and III wounds may result in significant injury to the skin, underlying muscle, and deeper tissues. At close range, the wadding of the shotgun shell used to separate the shot from the gunpowder may be propelled into the wound. Debridement of the skin and muscle may be necessary because of the trauma to these tissues. Sterile dressings are used to protect the wound after surgery. Serial bandage changes and wound inspection are advisable, because muscle damage may be more severe than initially determined. Serial debridement may be necessary until a healthy granulation bed forms and wound closure options can be determined [4,5].

Orthopedic trauma

Most projectiles are capable of fracturing bone, depending on the mass and velocity of the projectile, the amount of muscle surrounding the bone, and the area of impact (cortical versus cancellous bone). Low-mass and low-velocity projectiles (air-powered projectiles) may have a large portion of their kinetic energy expended from penetrating thick skin and dense underlying muscle or connective tissue. Handgun, shotgun, and rifle rounds may shatter cortical bone, whereas softer cancellous bone normally is less susceptible to fragmentation. The weight-bearing position of a limb on direct or tangential impact by the projectile influences the nature of the fracture. The more powerful projectiles are capable of shattering bone, sending fragments into the adjacent soft tissues, and enhancing tissue destruction.

Joint penetration requires an arthrotomy to remove metallic debris and fragments of cartilage and bone. It must be kept in mind that lead is slowly dissolved in joint fluid and absorbed systemically over time.

In a stable patient, radiography is normally followed by wound exploration, debridement, and copious lavage. Fracture stabilization varies with the individual fracture. Preserving circulation to the local tissues and bone segments is critical to a positive outcome. Extensive dead space is normally managed with a closed-suction drainage system. Amputation may be advisable in patients with extensive extremity trauma [4,5].

Penetrating or perforating abdominal wounds
Exploratory laparotomy is always recommended for penetrating or perforating abdominal wounds. The risk of peritonitis, secondary to visceral trauma, is simply too great to justify a "wait and reassess" approach to the patient: the best time to prevent peritonitis is "as soon as possible." The surgeon works in concert with the anesthesiologist and critical care staff to establish an optimal treatment plan for the patient. The surgeon must be prepared for dealing with a variety of soft tissue injuries, abdominal contamination, and peritonitis during exploration. Visceral wounds with questionable tissue viability normally require a resection and repair approach. Severe peritonitis cases require copious lavage and establishment of effective drainage. Drains or the more demanding "open-abdomen technique" is commonly used for these cases after surgical repair and copious abdominal lavage are completed [4,5].

Thoracic cavity
Radiographs are invaluable in assessing projectile wounds to the thoracic cavity. Pneumothorax and hemothorax are commonly associated with gunshot wounds. Thoracocentesis can be used for diagnostic and therapeutic purposes. In the face of significant air or blood accumulation, thoracostomy tube placement followed by continuous suction is advisable. Exploratory thoracotomy is advisable for the more serious cases and for those cases of unstable hemothorax. Similarly, cardiac tamponade may require pericardiocentesis or surgically opening the pericardium for persistent cases. Endoscopic examination of the esophagus should be considered if the pathway of the projectile could have impacted this structure. Care is taken during insufflation of a perforated esophagus during examination because of the risk of creating a tension pneumothorax or pneumomediastinum [4,5].

Brain and spinal trauma
Exploration of gunshot wounds to the brain is commonly performed in human patients; removal of necrotic tissue and debris is essential to reduce the risk of infection. In dogs and cats, brain surgery is rarely performed. CT can assist in determining the severity of trauma and whether surgical exploration is a reasonable option. Most patients sustaining serious gunshot wounds to the brain are usually euthanized. Exploration of the brain, however, may not be necessary for many brain wounds. In many patients with minimal neurologic deficits, supportive care and broad-spectrum antibiotic therapy may be sufficient [4,5].

Patients with suspected spinal trauma should be restrained to discourage movement. A complete neurologic examination is advisable before the patient is sedated. Radiography and CT are used to assess the severity of the injuries and to determine whether fracture stabilization or spinal cord decompression is advisable [4,5].

Cervical wounds
The cervical area has a concentration of vital structures located in a comparatively narrow area of the body, including the spinal cord, esophagus, larynx,

trachea, and major blood vessels. Massive hemorrhage would necessitate exploratory surgery. Endoscopy may be advisable to rule out perforation of the esophagus and trachea. Of particular concern is compromise to the respiratory tract. An emergency tracheostomy is advisable if respiratory distress secondary to oral trauma or injury to the larynx and cervical trachea has occurred. Open wounds of the trachea may be used for insertion of an endotracheal or tracheostomy tube in an emergency. Holes in the trachea can result in massive subcutaneous emphysema and pneumomediastinum. This should resolve within a few days after successful closure of the defect(s) [4,5].

Penetrating ocular wounds
Low-velocity pellets and BBs may penetrate the eye, necessitating their removal. Left in place, a severe inflammatory response may result in loss of the eye and increase the risk of infection. Trauma to the eye, with severe intraocular damage, is likely to require enucleation [4,5].

It is beyond the scope of this article to cover the detailed surgical management of deeper structures damaged by gunshot wounds. The reader is referred to other texts for this information.

Legal Considerations
Unlike the case in people, gunshot wounds in dogs and cats normally are not reported to law enforcement officers. In some states, anticruelty statutes may require reporting cases to law enforcement officials. Dogs and cats are shot for a variety of reasons, and a portion of these cases may result in legal action. Evidence must be properly collected and handled by the veterinarian. The records should be complete, and all conversations should be documented.

In deceased animals, a complete necropsy by a board-certified veterinary pathologist is advisable. Gastric contents also should be examined; on occasion, the consumed materials may link the perpetrator to the animal. It is useful to photograph the patient and the wounds, including 15 cm around the entry and exit wounds and the pathway of the projectiles. A metric ruler should be included for reference. Photographs taken should be labeled, dated, numbered, and initialed [4,5].

All portions of the projectile collected should be saved. They should be handled gently, preferably avoiding contact with metallic instruments, which may leave unwanted marks on the projectiles. Some textbooks have recommended that the collector place a mark on the base of the bullet for identification purposes. Close-up photographs also are useful to assist in bullet identification. The bullets are rinsed with water and alcohol and allowed to air-dry before being placed in a storage container. They are wrapped in facial tissues and inserted into a vial or container that can be sealed with tape. The container (not the container lid) is labeled with the date and time of collection; file or case number; and names of the owner, patient, and individuals present at the necropsy. Indelible marking pens should be used to mark the container surface or nonremovable label [4,5].

It is important to keep the projectiles in a secure area to prevent tampering or access by other individuals. Projectiles should never be given to pet owners. The container is turned over to a qualified law enforcement officer, who should mark the label with his or her initials and the date and time of transfer [4,5].

BITE WOUNDS

Bite wounds in cats and dogs account for 10% to 15% of all veterinary trauma cases [7,8], although the exact incidence remains unknown. All bite wounds should be considered contaminated [9] whether they are open (skin penetration) or closed (skin crushed) and contain a polymicrobial flora that reflects the aerobic and anaerobic florae of the oral cavity of the biter, skin of the victim, and environment [10]. In cats and dogs, *Pasteurella multocida* is the most common pathogen cultured [11,12].

Although cat bites are more likely to become contaminated than dog bites [11,13] by virtue of the sharp-pointed teeth of cats producing puncture wounds that can inoculate bacteria into underlying tissue, dog bites tend to be more problematic for the veterinarian because of the combination of crush, tear, and avulsion injury.

Local Tissue Damage

The canine jaw can generate a force of 150 to 450 psi [6,11,14]. In one study, victims of more severe and multiple bite wounds were male intact dogs weighing 10 kg or less, with Miniature Pinchers, Pekinese, and small terrier breeds overrepresented [15]. Incisor and canine teeth can apply shearing forces to the skin when applied perpendicular to the skin surface, sharply dividing tissue as they are drawn through like a scalpel. At angles less than 90°, tensile forces can create avulsion of the skin, together with hernias and devitalization of the underlying tissues. Compression forces generate the classic puncture wounds of canine teeth or crushing wounds of premolars or molars.

The unique pathologic findings of bite wounds stem from the penetration of elastic skin into less elastic tissue underneath, damaging the major direct cutaneous artery and vein with compromise to the collateral vascular supply [4]. The "big dog/little dog" interaction that combines lifting and shaking of the skin often results in an innocuous looking surface lesion with the potential for serious damage to the deeper tissues and organs below (ie, "iceberg effect").

Systemic Effects

Multiple and severe bite wounds can initiate a systemic inflammatory response syndrome (SIRS) in which excessive activation or loss of the local control of inflammation leads to a generalized inflammatory response [16]. A detailed discussion of the cellular and molecular mechanisms of SIRS is beyond the scope of this article; however, the veterinarian should appreciate that wound healing cannot progress beyond the inflammatory phase until dead or infected tissue is removed from the wound. The presence of such tissue serves to potentiate SIRS [16].

Initial Patient and Wound Evaluation

Bite wounds, depending on their severity and anatomic location, can produce a wide variety of life-threatening problems. All patients with bite wounds should be triaged on presentation for cardiovascular and respiratory anomalies. Depending on the severity of the injuries, the clinician should be prepared to provide intubation, ventilation, oxygen supplementation, tracheostomy, thoracocentesis, or placement of a thoracostomy tube.

In some cases, external hemorrhage can be severe; whenever possible, bleeding vessels should be identified and ligated. The degree of hemodynamic compromise must be estimated and corrected with intravenous electrolyte or colloid solutions or whole blood [16]. A consideration of the neurologic and urogenital systems completes the process of initial stabilization [17].

Few reports document the distribution of dog and cat bite wounds, but it seems that the limbs, head, and neck are the most frequent sites, followed by tissue of the thorax or abdomen [7,16,18]. Perineal wounds are least frequent. Patient population can be a major factor influencing wound location, because one study demonstrated that thoracic and abdominal wounds were most prevalent among small breeds of dogs [15].

The viability of a bitten limb can be assessed by the color of the damaged tissue, temperature of the extremities, presence of bleeding from a cut toenail (given adequate systemic blood pressure), peripheral pulse oximetry or Doppler ultrasound, toe web temperature, or selective angiography. The patient should be stabilized before performing an orthopedic or neurologic examination.

Bite wounds to the head require cranial nerve and central nervous system (CNS) evaluation. Neck bite wounds raise concerns about laryngeal, pharyngeal, cervical trachea, and esophageal injury. Endoscopy of the esophagus and trachea is indicated when there are deep wounds of the neck. When loss of tracheal integrity is confirmed, a tracheostomy may be necessary distal to the injury to restore normal ventilation and prevent ongoing air leakage. Trauma may be direct through tear, crush, or avulsion injury; in the case of the larynx, trauma may be indirect through damage to the recurrent laryngeal nerve. Tracheal bites can produce dyspnea, pneumomediastinum, and significant subcutaneous emphysema (Fig. 2).

Thoracic bite wounds may cause pneumothorax, lung contusions or lacerations, hemothorax, or thoracic tracheal trauma [19]. Thoracic radiography can help to define these sequelae [8], but negative findings cannot rule out injury [16]. Wounds over the thorax should be explored, and the surgeon should be prepared and equipped to use artificial ventilation if the pleural space is compromised.

Radiographic evidence of pneumoperitoneum secondary to abdominal bite wounds is not common [20]. Diagnostic peritoneal lavage may be helpful in wounds several hours old; however, the authors recommend thorough exploration of bite wounds over the abdomen with a celiotomy when necessary to define visceral organ damage, body wall hernias, and diaphragmatic hernias [16,21].

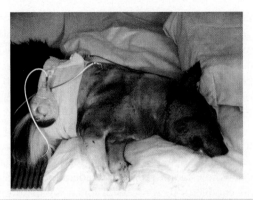

Fig. 2. Severe bruising and subcutaneous emphysema after cervical bite wound trauma to a Sheltie. Note the use of closed-suction drains.

Perineal wounds require careful evaluation for concurrent injury to colorectal and urinary structures. Surgical exploration is indicated once the patient is stable.

Based on the wide range of potential injuries to deeper structures, it can be seen that management of numerous medical situations beyond superficial wounds may be necessary. The reader is referred to other texts for detailed information on these procedures.

Treatment

Bite wounds must be explored to discover the degree of underlying trauma. The hair around the bite wound should be liberally clipped, prepared, and draped for aseptic surgery. The surgical field should be large enough for wounds over the thorax and abdomen so that a thoracotomy or exploratory laparotomy can be performed if indicated. Puncture wounds can be sharply excised, creating an opening into which a sterile hemostat or gloved finger can be inserted to spread apart the underlying tissue so as to assess the hypodermis, fascia, and muscle. Wounds with little or minimal tissue trauma may be left open to drain and heal by second intention or closed with skin sutures after thorough lavage. In more contaminated wounds, hair and foreign debris are removed. Shredded or necrotic muscle, fat, and fascia are excised. Ideally, debridement is accomplished in one stage. When loose skin is available over the neck and trunk, more aggressive debridement is possible. Over the extremities, a more conservative approach is necessary. The surgeon must decide whether wounds to the extremities are likely to leave viable limbs or necessitate amputation [5].

Lavage reduces bacterial inoculum in the wound and removes debris, foreign material, and clots. Use of a 35-mL syringe and 18-gauge needle to generate a lavage pressure of 8 psi has been well reported [7,8,11]. Certain wounds benefit from bactericidal lavage solutions of chlorhexidine diacetate, chlorhexidine gluconate, or povidone iodine. Chlorhexidine is more effective than povidone iodine in reducing bacterial numbers and allows for more rapid healing [22].

Each bite wound should be considered on an individual basis in terms of how long it has been since the trauma was inflicted, severity, single versus multiple wounds, degree of contamination, and quality of blood supply. When in doubt, delay wound closure. Some bite wounds deserve primary closure. A wide local excision of all contaminated and traumatized tissue should allow for a routine closure without dead space, without excessive tension and with minimal use of absorbable suture material. If there is doubt about the condition of the tissue, a drain should be placed. An alternative would be delayed primary closure with wet-to-dry dressing changes for 3 to 5 days to make use of natural wound healing and declaration of viable from nonviable tissue. Closure would be performed before a granulation bed develops but after infection has resolved [5,23].

Managing the wound by second-intention healing must favor the benefits of granulation, contraction, and epithelialization with optimal wound drainage versus the time and expense of wound care, risk of scar contracture over a joint causing impaired joint function, and potential for poor cosmesis. In cases in which this approach gives less than optimal results, use of flaps or free skin grafts may be necessary [5,23].

Drainage is essential to prevent dead space and seroma formation. Simple dependent stab incisions, passive drains, or active drainage systems should be used depending on the wound [5,23].

Surgical repair of bite wounds related to fractures may take place at the time of initial wound exploration or may be delayed to allow wound management and development of healing tissue in which to perform definitive repair. The authors know of no report in the veterinary literature suggesting that one approach is preferable in comparison to the other.

Body wall defects are common in small dogs after fights with larger dogs. Defects, depending on their exact location, can be repaired with a wide variety of techniques, such as diaphragmatic advancement, local muscle flaps, surgical mesh, suture scaffold technique [24], and omental pedicle flaps (see the article by Hedlund elsewhere in this issue).

Antibiotic Considerations

Selection and use of antibiotics in bite wound management remain controversial. Prompt intravenous administration of antibiotics within an hour or so of wounding is indicated to prevent infection in severely injured or compromised bite patients when used in combination with appropriate wound management. There is no indication for systemic antibiotics in uncomplicated low-risk bite injuries [5].

In human beings, antimicrobial therapy for bite wounds is considered therapeutic and not prophylactic [25]. Antibiotics are recommended for all deep bite wounds, including puncture wounds and wounds over tendons or bone.

In the presence of infection, aerobic and anaerobic wound cultures are recommended so as to select appropriate antibiotics. Culturing acute uninfected bite wounds is useless in determining the "potential" infectious organism. When taken, culture samples need to be obtained from deep within the wound to avoid growth of contaminants. Broad-spectrum bactericidal antibiotics are best selected. Intravenous penicillin or penicillin derivatives are the antibiotics of choice for bite wounds. Cephalosporins, including cephalexin, are generally effective against *Pasteurella* spp and a variety of other organisms. Amoxicillin or clavulanate potassium can be useful against *P multocida* resistant to penicillins and β-lactamase *Staphylococcus*. Fluoroquinolones are useful for resistant gram-positive and gram-negative infections.

The clinician should be prepared to change the antibiotic used based on culture and sensitivity results, lack of wound healing after 2 to 3 days, or a decline in the patient's condition [26]. Antibiotics are not a substitute for appropriate surgical management of bite wounds.

Bites and Transmission of Infectious Disease

Rabies can be transmitted in dog and cat bites. Unvaccinated pets bitten by a wild mammal that is not available for testing should be euthanized unless the owner refuses, in which case, the pet should be isolated for 6 months and vaccinated 1 month before release. Vaccinated pets should be revaccinated immediately, confined by the owner, and monitored carefully for 45 days. For more specific details, the clinician should consult with local and state regulations [27].

Cat bites can transmit feline leukemia virus and feline immunodeficiency virus. Assessment of transmission should be evaluated by serologic testing of bitten cats 6 months after the bite. Such infections can also result in nonhealing wounds (see the article by Amalsadvala elsewhere in this issue).

BURNS INVOLVING THE SKIN

Overview

Thermal wounds are relatively uncommon in veterinary practice. Causes include flame burns (accidental or deliberate), scalds (accidental or deliberate), automobile mufflers, hot stove surfaces, radiators, hot air dryers, electrical heating pads, hot water bottles, chemical (exothermic) hot packs, heat lamps, electrical cords, and improperly grounded electrocautery units. With the increasing use of radiation therapy in veterinary oncology, radiation burns present a problem in wound healing. Most burns referred to the authors are the result of accidental burns occurring at veterinary practices, and most are associated with application of supplemental heat to treat or prevent hypothermia in patients under or recovering from general anesthesia. Burns are generally classified according to the depth of the burn and the body surface area involved.

Depth of Burn

   Superficial: first degree, involving the outermost epidermis
   Partial thickness: second degree, involving the epidermis and a portion of the dermis
   Full thickness: third degree, involving full-thickness epidermis and dermis

Burn depth is an important prognostic factor, because superficial and partial-thickness burns have the potential to heal without implementation of skin flaps and skin grafts. Re-epithelization can occur from surviving germinal epidermal cells in superficial burns, whereas the external root sheath of compound hair follicles is the most important source of epithelial cells in partial-thickness burns. In contrast, full-thickness burns result in complete loss of the skin. Contraction and epithelization or interventional surgical management is required depending on the surface area of the body involvement [5,28,29].

Most burns seen by veterinarians do not involve more than 20% of the body surface area. As a result, major metabolic derangements, including fluid and electrolyte imbalances, red blood cell destruction, and increased susceptibility to systemic infection, are not likely to be noted. Pulmonary injury also may be noted in animals trapped in enclosures in which toxic irritating smoke accumulates.

Burn Wound Assessment

Early assessment of the depth of a burn wound can be problematic in the initial phase of injury. Occult burns (most commonly, heating pad burns) are easily overlooked by the veterinarian or owner because of fur coverage until the injury is evident several days later. Advanced full-thickness skin necrosis is often distinguishable as a brown to black leathery eschar. Marginal fissures eventually form as the eschar begins to separate from the adjacent viable skin [29].

Skin with third-degree flame burns may appear to be scorched, with hair burned off the area. The patients frequently have a smoky or "burnt hair" odor. Occasionally, full-thickness burned skin presents as bloodless and pearl white, depending, in part, on skin pigmentation. In full-thickness burns, hair may pluck out easily with tissue forceps [5].

Superficial and partial-thickness burns of the exposed skin may appear reddened or inflamed, with a variable degree of edema. The surface may appear relatively dry or moist depending on the integrity of the epidermis. With the exception of the inner pinna, skin in the dog and cat normally does not blister, unlike superficial burns in human beings. Scabbing may be noted, however. Over several days, partial-thickness burns may form an outer leathery eschar. Until this outer partial-thickness eschar separates, deep partial-thickness burns may not be easily differentiated from full-thickness burns. As the outer necrotic skin of a partial-thickness burn delaminates, one often sees areas of epithelialization. In full-thickness burns, the underlying tissues may have variable amounts of hypodermal fat and areas of granulation tissue. Epithelialization is usually confined to the viable skin margins surrounding the full-thickness burn. Occasionally, the deeper compound hair follicles located in the hypodermal tissues form small epithelial islands as the eschar is elevated [5]. These islands provide the epithelial cells that are responsible for second-intention healing.

When in doubt as to the depth of a burn, conservative management and a wait-and-reassess approach are usually indicated. This is particularly true for large burns, especially those involving the extremities and head. The cost of reconstructive surgery can be sizeable, and preservation of potentially viable skin can reduce or eliminate the need for subsequent surgical closure. Smaller and more manageable burns may be handled in the same fashion or simply excised and closed depending on their location [5].

The surface area of the burns in human beings is estimated by the "Rule of 9s": the head and neck account for 9% of the body surface area, each arm is 9%, each leg is 18%, the thorax is 18%, and the abdomen is 18%. Adapting this rule to dogs and cats is not accurate but can give the veterinarian a "ball park" estimate of the surface area burned. Considering the elastic redundant skin covering many dogs and cats, there is a tendency to overestimate the surface area involved. In general, patients with burns involving greater than 20% of the body surface area have the potential of developing significant life-threatening metabolic derangements. The veterinarian should be aware of this potential and monitor the patient closely. Supportive therapy can be initiated, and the therapy can be adjusted according to the patient's needs. Large areas of full-thickness burns can be challenging to manage, especially when multiple extremities are involved (Fig. 3) [5,28].

The cost of managing extensively burned animals is measured in thousands of dollars. It is important to discuss this issue clearly with the client and to maintain close communication with the owner as the patient's condition evolves. Massive burned areas approaching 50% of the body surface area may warrant euthanasia, based on humane considerations and a poor prognosis for recovery.

Burn Management
Medical management
The severity of the burn, based on depth, body surface area, age of the injury, and location, dictates the most appropriate treatment options. After 1 week, the

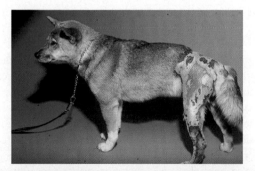

Fig. 3. Extensive burn in a Sheba, deep partial- and full-thickness burns. (*From* Pavletic MM. Dressings, bandages, external support, and protective devices. In: Atlas of small animal reconstructive surgery. 2nd edition. Philadelphia: WB Saunders; 1999. p. 115; with permission.)

depth and extent of the burn are normally easier to determine in the dog and cat. Burns also may vary in depth in various locations.

Many animals with burns are not presented to the veterinarian immediately after the time of injury, often because of the fact that the owner not may know the burn occurred or may be uncertain as to the extent of the wounds. If an animal is seen within 2 hours after injury, the hair can be clipped from the area and chilled saline or water (3°C–17°C) can be applied to the wound for at least 30 minutes. Analgesics are an integral part of burn wound management. Topical contaminants can be removed by rinsing the area and carefully removing the fur with clippers or scissors [5].

Topical silver sulfadiazine is the broad-spectrum water-miscible ointment of choice for application to burn wounds. The ointment is applied liberally after the fur has been clipped from the area and the skin has been gently cleansed with warm sterile saline. A 1:40 dilution of chlorhexidine or 1:9 dilution of povidone iodine solution may be used in conjunction with sterile saline before ointment application. Depending on the wound location(s), a nonadherent dressing and protective bandage can be used to help reduce contamination and maintain the local integrity of the ointment. Triple-antibiotic ointment may be considered for the early treatment of relatively small minor burns after basic skin preparation [5,28].

Partial-thickness burns normally heal within 2 to 3 weeks after injury with proper support. In some cases, the outer necrotic skin surface may adhere to the viable dermal layer of partial-thickness burns. As epithelization occurs beneath this superficial eschar, the borders of the dead skin begin to separate. These "delaminated" folds of necrotic tissue can be trimmed with scissors in a staged fashion [5].

Full-thickness burns often heal slowly. Without surgical intervention, the wounds necessarily heal by contraction and epithelialization. Necrotic skin is prone to infection, although prompt and continuous use of silver sulfadiazine can reduce this risk. Local infections may expand into areas of multiple abscessation; systemic infection can be life threatening in the extensively burned patient (see section on surgical management).

Systemic antibiotics are normally not indicated for burn wound management unless the patient is considered to be septic. Topical silver sulfadiazine is considered to be the ointment of choice to control infection. Analgesics are an essential component of burn therapy. Morphine, oxymorphone, butorphanol, ketamine hydrochloride, and fentanyl transdermal patches are commonly used analgesics depending on the extent of the burn and the individual needs of the patient [5,28,29].

As a general rule, fluid therapy is considered for the burn patient with greater than 20% of the body surface area involved. As noted previously, veterinarians tend to overestimate the surface area burned, because it is difficult to account for the additional loose elastic skin available over the neck and trunk. On a number of occasions, patients are presented several days after incurring an extensive burn but are remarkably stable despite the fact that they received little or no intensive care support. This particular set of patients normally does not require intensive medical support at this late presentation. Treatment is focused on wound management and closure [5].

Fluid loss from burn patients is iso-osmolar as a result of increased capillary permeability at the wound site and throughout the body of extensively burned patients. There is loss of plasma, electrolytes, and plasma proteins. Red blood cells also are destroyed, but the overwhelming loss of fluids can result in a relative rise in the hematocrit initially. Damage to red blood cells also shortens their relative life span. As a result, anemia may be noted in the days after the injury. The hematocrit and total protein level can be used to monitor the relative number of red blood cells and can help to determine if a transfusion is required (ie, hematocrit drops below 25%) [5].

In the first 18 to 24 hours after injury, capillary permeability increases; it subsequently decreases after 24 hours. Adequate fluid replacement in the first 24 hours is directed at restoring cardiac output, patient hydration, and renal perfusion. Lactated Ringer's solution is usually administered at this time. After 24 hours, colloids may be useful in expanding plasma volume and may compensate for the loss of plasma protein [5].

Burn formulas designed for severely burned human patients have been adapted for veterinary use. The percentage of surface area burned is multiplied by 4 mL per kilogram of the body weight of the patient. Half of this estimated volume is given over the first 8 hours, and the remaining half is given over the remaining 16 hours. Colloid, plasma, 5% albumin, or dextrans may be considered in the last 8-hour period as needed. Measuring the patient's body weight, central venous pressure, and urine output (1 mL/kg/h) assists in regulating fluid therapy [5,28,29].

In the second 24 hours, capillary permeability normally improves and less lactated Ringer's solution intravenous fluid support is needed. Five percent dextrose may be used to help offset water lost through large burn surface areas at an administration rate of 1 to 2 mL/kg of body weight times the percentage of the burn surface area. After the initial 48-hour period, mobilization of burn wound edema occurs and the body weight gradually returns to preburn levels in the ensuing days. Intravenous fluid support is progressively decreased as the patient begins to eat and drink after this time. Electrolytes must be closely monitored throughout fluid therapy so as to avoid many of the common fluid, metabolic, and electrolyte problems noted in seriously burned patients, including hypernatremia, hyponatremia, hyperkalemia, hypokalemia, acidosis, anemia, dehydration, and fluid overload [5].

Nutritional support is important in maintaining the health of the extensively burned patient, which is normally in a hypermetabolic state. Nutritious high-calorie and high-protein diets can be introduced provided that renal and hepatic function is adequate. Maintaining the hospital room environment at 31°C can help to reduce calorie expenditure [5,28,29].

The respiratory system can be adversely affected by the metabolic derangements associated with extensive thermal injury. Inhalation of smoke and hot air can cause pulmonary injury and predispose the patient to pneumonia and pulmonary edema. Aggressive intravenous fluid therapy also may result in fluid overload with pulmonary edema. With extensive burns and systemic infection, acute lung injury (ALI) may be noted. Its more severe manifestation, acute respiratory distress syndrome (ARDS), may be noted as a sequela to the SIRS. Close monitoring of the patient's pulmonary function is warranted. Thoracic radiographs (three views), pulse oximetry, and blood gas analysis supplement close monitoring of the patient's respiratory rate and auscultation of the lung fields. Supplemental oxygen may be advisable; severe cases may require positive-pressure ventilation. Appropriate fluid therapy and wound care are essential in the overall management of these conditions, however [28–31].

Surgical management
Debridement options. Debridement of clearly devitalized skin can reduce the risk of infection and facilitate wound healing. Smaller full-thickness burns may heal without surgical intervention; however, surgical resection may be considered to speed wound closure and reduce the likelihood of scarring. In general, the authors favor resection of full-thickness burns, because the natural separation of the burn eschar can be a slow process. Surgical debridement helps to establish a healthy granulation bed. Its establishment enables the surgeon to implement the appropriate methods to close the skin defect(s) [5].

Debridement of the burn eschar can be facilitated with the application of warm sterile water or isotonic saline wraps (wet-to-wet dressings), use of hydrogel or immersion of the body area (20–30-minute sessions two to three times per day). As the mummified skin rehydrates and softens, forceps and scissors are used to excise the detachable segments. This stepwise approach of conservative debridement can be particularly useful for those areas in which aggressive debridement is difficult to perform or is not advisable based on (1) the current health status of the patient, (2) the location of a wound near a vital structure, and (3) the difficulty in differentiating partial- from full-thickness skin loss. Enzymatic debriding agents also may be useful but are usually limited to removal of smaller areas of necrotic tissue in problematic areas. Dakin's solution, dilute sodium hypochlorite (0.25% or 0.125%), can be useful for debridement in human beings, but information regarding its clinical use in small animals is lacking [5].

Aggressive surgical debridement (wound excision) is particularly useful for large areas of dead skin over the trunk, especially in the face of infection. Under general anesthesia, scalpel blades or a grafting knife is used to excise the dead skin tangentially at the level of the hypodermis. A healthy granulation bed normally forms within a week after debridement [5].

Escharotomy. Escharotomy is the surgical incision of a restrictive eschar. Although it is rarely performed in veterinary medicine, circumferential eschars involving the lower extremity have the potential to form a biologic tourniquet, impairing circulation to the lower extremity. Large eschars involving the thorax may impair normal breathing in a patient. Use of an "eschar release" incision(s) can relieve the problem until appropriate debridement and wound closure can be attempted [5,29].

Wound closure options. Permanent wound closure options include the use of undermining and advancement of adjacent skin, local skin flaps, distant skin flaps, axial pattern flaps, skin grafts, and skin stretching techniques (eg, skin stretchers, tissue expanders, walking sutures). Split-thickness skin grafts normally are reserved for large full-thickness thermal wounds. In problematic cases, two or more techniques may be useful depending on the location of the burns and availability of mobile skin [5,29].

Scar revision and contracture management. In the event that problematic epithelialized scars form after open-wound management, selective scar resection can be performed at a later date, once the patient has recovered and the burn has healed. This also allows for inflammation to resolve, facilitating the process of scar resection and subsequent closure of the area. Many pet owners fret over scars, and it is useful to remind the owner that scar resection and revision can be effectively achieved on an elective basis, as needed [5].

Wound contracture, the loss or restriction of movement secondary to extensive scarring and wound contraction, normally is corrected at the time of definitive wound closure with skin flaps and skin grafts. Most problematic contractures involve the extremities. Restrictive fibrotic tissue is carefully incised or resected, and the involved extremity is manipulated during surgery to ensure that reasonable mobility is regained before definitive wound repair. Physical therapy and splinting are useful in the process of improving regional function and reducing the risk of contracture reformation [5].

References

[1] Pavletic MM. A review of 121 gunshot wounds in the dog and cat. Vet Surg 1985;14:61–2.

[2] Heard BJ. Ammunition. In: Handbook of firearms and ballistics. New York: John Wiley and Sons; 1997. p. 33–72.

[3] Heard BJ. Ballistics. In: Handbook of firearms and ballistics. New York: John Wiley and Sons; 1997. p. 73–104.

[4] Pavletic MM. Gunshot wound management. Compend Contin Educ Pract Vet 1996;18: 1285–99.

[5] Pavletic MM. Management of specific wounds. In: Atlas of small animal reconstructive surgery. 2nd edition. Philadelphia: WB Saunders; 1999. p. 66–95.

[6] Pavletic MM. Penetrating wounds. In: Wingfield WE, Raffe MR, editors. The veterinary ICU book. Jackson Hole (WY): Teton New Media; 2002. p. 967–70.

[7] Kolata RJ, Kraut NH, Johnston DE. Patterns of trauma in urban dogs and cats: a study of 1000 cases. J Am Vet Med Assoc 1974;164:499–502.

[8] McKiernan BC, Adams WM, Huse DC. Thoracic bite wounds and associated internal injury in 11 dogs and 1 cat. J Am Vet Med Assoc 1984;184:959–64.

[9] Harari J. Surgical complications and wound healing in the small animal practice. Philadelphia: WB Saunders; 1993. p. 54–5.

[10] Brook I. Management of human and animal bite wounds: an overview. Adv Skin Wound Care 2005;18:197–203.

[11] Goldstein EJ, Richwald GA. Human and animal bite wounds. Am Fam Physician 1987;36: 101–9.

[12] Talan DA, Citron DM, Abrahamian FM, et al. Bacteriologic analysis of infected dog and cat bites. N Engl J Med 1999;340:85–92.
[13] Lewis KT, Stiles M. Management of cat and dog bites. Am Fam Physician 1995;52:479–90.
[14] Swaim SF, Henderson RA. Bite wounds. In: Small animal wound management. 2nd edition. Philadelphia: JB Lippincott; 1992. p. 112–7.
[15] Shamir MH, Leisner S, Klement E, et al. Dog bite wounds in dogs and cats: a retrospective study of 196 cases. J Vet Med 2002;49:107–12.
[16] Holt DE, Griffin G. Bite wounds in dogs and cats. Vet Clin North Am Small Anim Pract 2000;30:669–79.
[17] Syring RS, Drobatz KJ. Preoperative evaluation and management of the emergency surgical small animal patient. Vet Clin North Am Small Anim Pract 2000;30:473–89.
[18] Cowell AK, Penwick RC. Dog bite wounds: a study of 93 cases. Compend Contin Educ Pract Vet 1989;11:313–20.
[19] Davidson EB. Managing bite wounds in dogs and cats. Part I. Compend Contin Educ Pract Vet 1998;20:811–20.
[20] Saunders WB, Tobias KM. Pneumoperitoneum in dogs and cats: 39 cases (1983–2002). J Am Vet Med Assoc 2003;223:462–8.
[21] Shaw SP, Rozanski EA, Rush JE. Traumatic body wall herniation in 36 dogs and cats. J Am Anim Hosp Assoc 2003;39:35–45.
[22] Sanchez IR, Swaim SF, Nusbaum KE, et al. Effects of chlorhexidine diacetate and povidone-iodine on wound healing in dogs. Vet Surg 1988;17:291–5.
[23] Davidson EB. Managing bite wounds in dogs and cats. Part II. Compend Contin Educ Pract Vet 1998;20:974–91.
[24] Shahar R, Shamir M, Johston DE. A technique for management of bite wounds of the thoracic wall in small dogs. Vet Surg 1997;26:45–50.
[25] Smith PF, Meadowcroft AM, May DB. Treating mammalian bite wounds. J Clin Pharm Ther 2000;25:85–99.
[26] Aucoin DP. Rational use of antimicrobial drugs. In: Kirk RW, Bonagura JD, editors. Current veterinary therapy. Philadelphia: WB Saunders; 1992. p. 207–11.
[27] General AVMA policies. Model rabies control ordinance. Available at: http://www.avma.org/issues/policy/rabies_control.asp. Accessed July 10, 2005.
[28] Dhupa N. Burn injury. In: Wingfield WE, Raffe MR, editors. The veterinary ICU book. Jackson Hole (WY): Teton New Media; 2002. p. 973–81.
[29] Pope ER. Thermal, electrical, and chemical burns and cold injuries. In: Slatter D, editor. Textbook of small animal surgery. 3rd edition. Philadelphia: WB Saunders; 2003. p. 356–72.
[30] Drobatz KJ. Smoke inhalation. In: Wingfield WE, Raffe MR, editors. The veterinary ICU book. Jackson Hole (WY): Teton New Media; 2002. p. 982–8.
[31] King LG, Waddell LS. Acute respiratory distress syndrome. In: Wingfield WE, Raffe MR, editors. The veterinary ICU book. Jackson Hole (WY): Teton New Media; 2002. p. 582–90.

Vet Clin Small Anim 36 (2006) 895–912

VETERINARY CLINICS
SMALL ANIMAL PRACTICE

Management of Specific Skin Wounds

Richard A.S. White, BVetMed, PhD, DSAS, DVR, FRCVS

Dick White Referrals, The Six Mile Bottom Veterinary Specialist Centre, London Road,
Six Mile Bottom, Newmarket, CB8 0UH England

INTERTRIGINOUS DISORDERS

Etiopathogenesis

Intertriginous diseases are the result of persistent frictional skin-to-skin contact that arises through the abnormal folding of skin or mucocutaneous surfaces [1]. The most commonly encountered sites for intertriginous disease in small animals include the labial, facial, vulvar, tail, body, head, and leg folds. Such abnormal skin conformations may be the result of congenital anomalies, for example, the spiral configuration of the Bulldog's tail causing infolding of the perineal surface. They may also be acquired through obesity, for example, in the case of vulvar fold disease or through a concurrent chronic inflammatory process (see the article by Bellah elsewhere in this issue). It is also important to recognize the contribution of coexisting, often generalized, dermatoses (eg, atopic diseases), because many patients may have an underlying anatomic predisposition but do not progress to intertriginous disease in the absence of a further inflammatory stimulus. Intertriginous disease itself, however, promotes its own inflammatory process that is often complicated by pyoderma of varying severity.

The normal physiologic processes of the skin, which include secretion and shedding of cells, are dependent on a surface environment that permits evaporative function and unimpaired desquamation. Folding of the skin and constant contact between surfaces alters the skin microclimate and promotes physical abrasion of the surfaces, interfering with skin function. Normal evaporative function is diminished by reduced ventilation within the fold and permits the collection of sebaceous secretions and a focus for accumulation of other materials, such as saliva, feces, urine, lacrimal secretion, or vaginal discharge. Fatty acids contained in normal sebaceous secretions exert a bacteriostatic and fungistatic effect on surface microorganisms. In the presence of excessive accumulation of sebum, this function is lost, with consequent bacterial and fungal overgrowth. This microorganism overgrowth contributes to a localized inflammatory process by absorption of metabolic by-products through impaired

E-mail address: dw@dickwhitereferrals.com

cutaneous permeability. The barrier created by the stratum corneum and other epidermal layers normally controls transcutaneous migration of skin surface materials, with the former preventing most of the transepidermal absorption of materials from the surface of the skin. These layers become damaged through repeated frictional contact and lose their protective function, allowing materials generated by surface bacterial activity to reach the deeper layers of the skin, thus promoting an inflammatory response. The absorption of deleterious surface materials is further favored by the changes in blood flow, temperature, and localized lymphocyte suppression.

It is doubtful if this process is, in fact, true pyoderma in the sense that the inflammatory reaction is not the consequence of cutaneous bacterial invasion. The combination of microorganism overgrowth and inflammation creates a similar pathophysiologic process, however. Among the microorganisms from intertriginous lesions, coagulase-positive *Staphylococcus intermedius* is most common [1]. Surface contamination with coliform organisms is often found in vulvar and tail fold lesions, however. Advanced lesions that undergo significant anatomic change may promote conditions that favor infection with *Pseudomonas* organisms. Yeasts, such as *Malassezia* and *Candida*, may also become established in the inflamed skin [1].

The clinical signs of intertriginous disease are consistent, almost irrespective of the site of the lesion [2]. These include the accumulation of significantly malodorous moist surface exudate and localized erythematous changes associated with the inflammatory process. Lesions are commonly pruritic, and patients often self-traumatize the area by rubbing; the additional impact of this self-trauma promotes further inflammatory changes that supersede the initiating cause in some cases.

Management
Medical
Most patients with intertriginous disease may be successfully managed with appropriate medical management. The principles of management include cleansing the affected areas and removal of hair to reduce the collection of sebum and other secretions. Folds should be cleansed with topical antiseptic solutions (eg, chlorhexidine, povidone iodine); topical and systemic steroids combined with antibiotic therapy may help to limit the progress of lesions to their more chronic condition [1]. Weight loss is beneficial in those patients in which the skin folds are the result of obesity.

Surgical
Lesions that have become refractory to medical management should be managed surgically. The aim of surgery is to revise the skin fold anatomy so as to remove the abnormal microenvironment [2]. Many patients benefit from extended parenteral antibiotic therapy and topical treatment before surgery to limit the potential for bacterial contamination during the procedure and to provide a healthier surgical field.

Wide areas around the lesions should be clipped and prepared aseptically. Such lesions as facial folds or tail folds necessitate repeated cleansing of the accumulated surface exudate. This may need to be undertaken repeatedly over the 24-hour period before surgery. Procedures are normally considered as clean-contaminated or contaminated, and appropriate antibiotic therapy strategies should be instigated (see the article by Krahwinkel and Boothe elsewhere in this issue). Many sites (eg, labial, facial, vulvar folds) do not lend themselves to the application of pressure bandaging after surgery. Hence, every care should be taken to minimize the risk of dead space that may allow seroma or hematoma development. Meticulous closure of subcutaneous layers with interrupted fine (3-0 or 4-0) absorbable sutures should be performed. Active drains should be placed where indicated to help control fluid accumulations. Skin closure is usually best performed as a cutaneous layer of simple-interrupted monofilament nylon sutures (2-0 or 3-0) to minimize the possibility of dehiscence. The absence of protective bandaging amplifies the importance of postoperative analgesia and the provisions for prevention of self-inflicted trauma. Fold ablation involving the facial and tail area should be discussed in some detail with owners before surgery, because the procedure may alter the perceived conformation from a breed requirement aspect.

Labial folds
Labial fold dermatitis is encountered bilaterally in the lower lip normally between the level of the canine and molar teeth and results from congenital excessive skin folds. Affected breeds include Cocker Spaniels, English and Irish Setters, Golden Retrievers, and some of the giant breeds, including Newfoundlands, Bloodhounds, and Saint Bernards. Many dogs may have this anatomic anomaly without becoming clinically affected, and there is often an underlying dermatosis (eg, atopy) responsible for initiating the problem. Salivary overflow combined with the accumulation of food debris in the fold gives rise to a secondary bacterial infection with a typically malodorous smell. Many patients show marked discomfort, and the problem is often exacerbated by repeated self-trauma. Examination of the area may reveal the characteristic diamond-shaped inflammatory response with ulceration (Fig. 1A). In chronic cases, the skin may undergo hyperplastic change with verrucose thickening that is refractory to medical management.

Lip fold disease is often successfully managed by surgical ablation of the skin fold. The patient is positioned in lateral recumbency with the nose elevated to ensure a flat operative surface. The margins of the ulcerated skin and inflammatory change (normally diamond shaped) are easily identified with the upper lip and commissure retracted. The affected area is marked with a surgical pen. The diseased skin is best excised with an elliptic incision to simplify the reconstruction of the wound. The skin incisions and resection should be made as superficially as possible so as to avoid damage to the underlying orbicularis oris muscle. The dorsal aspect of the incision should be positioned well ventral to the mucocutaneous junction to avoid eversion of the lip margin. The area is

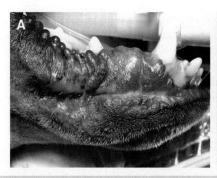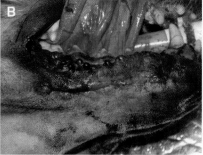

Fig 1. Labial fold intertrigo. (A) Labial fold intertrigo in a Springer Spaniel. (B) Postoperative appearance after ablation of the labial fold.

often quite vascular, and thermocautery should be combined with superficial dissection to control hemorrhage. The wound should be reconstructed with layers of fine (3-0–4-0) multifilament absorbable suture material. The cutaneous layer may be closed with fine simple-interrupted pattern monofilament nylon. A better closure is achieved with an intradermal repair because this avoids suture irritation (see Fig. 1B) and the need for subsequent removal. The condition is consistently bilateral, and both sides should be operated on. Swelling at the surgical sites is common, and patients benefit from appropriate opiate and nonsteroidal analgesia. Provision should be made to protect the wounds from self-trauma, because disruption of the wound can be problematic to manage and revise.

Tail folds

The reader is referred to the article by Bellah in this issue. "Screw," "corkscrew," or "ingrown" tail is a condition encountered frequently in the severely brachycephalic breeds, particularly English and French Bulldogs. Pugs and Boston Terriers are occasionally presented with this problem. Tail fold dermatitis is reported periodically in cats with sacrococcygeal abnormalities, such as the Manx. The condition results from the anatomic tendency of the terminal coccygeal vertebrae to adopt a spiral configuration. The anatomic vertebral configuration results in an intertriginous process with moist dermatitis and possible ulceration of the area. The condition is exacerbated by the patient rubbing the lesion, which potentiates fecal contamination.

Medical management dictates continual cleansing of the fold area and intermittent antibiotic therapy that may palliate the disease for extended periods. The condition is unlikely to be resolved permanently by medical management, however, and lifelong attention is required.

Surgical management is directed toward amputation of the coccygeal vertebrae with or without the associated tail soft tissue "bob." The reader is referred to the article by Bellah in this issue for details of the surgical treatment procedures.

Vulvar folds
The presence of skin folds around the dorsal and lateral aspects of the vulva may be a congenital or acquired condition. Congenital vulvar folds are usually encountered in younger bitches and represent hypoplastic development of the vulva, which then becomes surrounded by folds of otherwise normal skin. The condition is seen more commonly, however, as an acquired problem in spayed bitches that become obese, allowing the excessive skin folds to engulf a normal vulva. The German Shepherd Dog is consistently the most frequently represented breed in the author's clinic, and there is often a concurrent generalized dermatosis that is responsible for initiating the signs. The excessive folds allow the accumulation of urine and vaginal secretions, with inflammation and ulceration seen on the vulvar skin surfaces and the surrounding skin folds. The affected areas are often extremely painful for the bitch, and there may be discomfort during posturing for urination. Medical management is directed toward identifying and managing any underlying dermatosis and/or weight loss and control of any associated urinary tract infection.

In cases of persistent vulvar ulceration that are refractory to medical management, it is often more appropriate to proceed with surgical intervention at an early stage of the disease. Surgery (vulvar fold resection or episioplasty) is intended to remove the excess folds of skin that surround the vulva. The reader is referred to the article by Bellah in this issue for details of the surgical treatment procedures.

Body and leg folds
Excessive skin folding involving the legs and flanks is seen almost exclusively in the Chinese Shar-Pei, whereas leg folding may be encountered in the Basset Hound. The conformation that allows this condition reflects the generalized cutaneous excess in these breeds. The pathologic change involving the skin folds is surprisingly unusual unless there is concurrent generalized dermatosis. Management is thus directed more toward recognition of the underlying generalized problem, and surgery is only occasionally performed. Body folds may also be encountered in particularly obese dogs and are occasionally seen in bitches that have particularly pendulous mammary tissue. Surgical manipulation entails preparation for aseptic surgery, excision of intertriginous skin, and meticulous closure of the resulting defect.

Facial folds
Facial folds are encountered in the more prominently brachycephalic breeds and are located over the dorsum and lateral aspects of the nose (Fig. 2A), where there may be several folds. The condition represents a congenital excess of skin that has developed in combination with the foreshortening of the skeleton generally and the skull in particular. Affected breeds include the English and French Bulldogs, Pekingese, and Pug [1]. The Boston Terrier is less commonly affected. Extreme or "ultra" examples of the Siamese cat breed may also be affected by this condition. The fold is somewhat atypical in that the disease has two "contact" surfaces: the ventral surface of the fold contacts the nose and

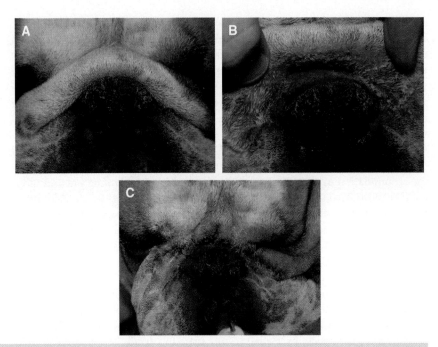

Fig. 2. Facial fold intertrigo. (*A*) Facial fold intertrigo in an English Bulldog. (*B*) Intertriginous changes associated with facial folds (fold elevated). (*C*) Postoperative appearance after fold resection.

permits accumulation of the nasal secretions (see Fig. 2B), whereas the dorsal surface contacts the lower eyelids and promotes lacrimal accumulation. In more advanced cases, the dorsal surface may also contact the corneas, causing direct abrasion and a contact keratitis that may lead to ulceration. This is more commonly encountered in the long-haired breeds.

Medical management involves persistent cleansing of the folds with solutions that do not cause ophthalmic irritation and management of concurrent corneal lesions. Removing hair from the dorsal aspects of the folds also alleviates the corneal irritation. Although surgical resolution is successful in alleviating the condition, it is often regarded as a last-resort option by many owners, who may prioritize facial appearance.

Facial fold resection is performed with the patient positioned in sternal recumbency. The protuberant and often traumatized corneal surfaces should be lubricated with ophthalmic ointment and protected with moist surgical sponges before aseptic preparation of the facial area. The skin fold(s) should be elevated to permit estimation of the amount of tissue to be removed, which is marked with a surgical pen. Complete resection of the entire fold is usually not essential, and removal of excessive amounts of skin may lead to unnecessary tension in the repair. A conservative approach that allows for further excision is therefore advised. After removal of the skin fold, tacking sutures should be placed at quadrants of the two margins to ensure accurate reapproximation of the skin (see Fig. 2C). Care should be taken to avoid damage to nasolacrimal ducts and angularis oculi vessels at the medial canthi. Monofilament nylon sutures may not be an ideal choice for the cutaneous repair because of the proximity of the corneal surfaces, and intradermal repair may thus be a suitable alternative that does not dictate subsequent removal.

Head folds

Head folds are encountered in such breeds as the Chinese Shar-Pei and Bloodhound. The significance of these folds does not lie primarily in the development of intertriginous disease, which is surprisingly uncommon, but in the resulting palpebral deformity (entropion or "diamond eye") attributable to the weight of the excessive folds. Reconstruction of the entropion is often a fruitless task in such severe cases, with recurrent deformity being a common outcome. Resection of the folds from the dorsum of the head that removes some of the "weight" of the excess tissue has a more lasting and effective outcome. Patients are positioned in sternal recumbency with the head elevated on packs. Skin hooks are used to elevate the skin over the dorsum of the head until the surgeon judges that sufficient tissue has been elevated for removal to permit normal palpebral conformation. A sterile surgical marker is used to delineate the margins of what is often a considerable area of skin. The skin is resected, and the subcutaneous tissue is carefully repaired with absorbable sutures to obliterate any potential dead space and then to prevent further advancement of the skin toward the eye. Anchoring this layer of sutures to the underlying fascia of the temporal muscle is thus essential. The cutaneous layer is closed routinely. The application of a pressure bandage after surgery is controversial, and great care should be exercised in bandaging patients to ensure the use of elastic dressings that permit expansion and avoid upper airway compression. When the bandage is applied while the dog is entubated, it should be closely observed after tube removal to ensure that airway compression has not occurred. Active suction drains may sometimes provide an alternative and safer method of managing dead space.

Chronic fibrosing interdigital pyoderma

The development of so-called "cysts" within the interdigital spaces is probably not the consequence of an intertriginous etiology in the strictest sense of the term. The disease shares many similarities with intertriginous disease in other locations, however. Interdigital cysts are most commonly recognized in West Highland White Terriers, Scottish Terriers, and English bulldogs and are thought to be the result of localized trauma that promotes the inoculation of hair fragments and debris into the skin [3]. Once embedded in the skin, they act as a foreign body focus and cause draining sinus tracts to develop. These tracts are usually infected with *Staphylococcus aureus* organisms, and the spaces become pruritic with chronic exudation. More advanced cases may cause the dog to adopt a plantigrade posture at the carpometacarpal, tarsometatarsal, and interphalangeal joints. Medical management is directed toward long-term antibiotic therapy to control the secondary infection and immunosuppressive therapy for the sinus tracts.

Surgical ablation of the abnormal tissue is frequently successful in resolving the condition. It is essential that the surgeon is able to distinguish all the sinus tissue during surgery. Because the region is significantly vascular, the procedure is best performed under tourniquet with the paw exsanguinated. The consequence of this is not only that bleeding is nonexistent, but, more importantly, the brown-tinged sinus tissue is easily recognized and can be completely resected, leaving as much normal tissue as possible. The outcome of this operation is to remove the "web" tissue between the digits. It is normally difficult to place sutures in the subcutaneous tissues, and, often, only a single layer of cutaneous sutures is possible. After removal of the tourniquet, a pressure bandage should be applied to the paw with interdigital packing; this should be changed on a daily basis until the wounds have healed.

DERMAL SINUSES

A sinus can be defined as a congenital or acquired epithelialized tract that opens onto the skin surface.

Pilonidal Sinus

A pilonidal sinus (PS; dermoid sinus) represents the failure of complete separation of ectodermal and neural tissue during embryogenesis. The lesion is congenital and heritable in some breeds. The condition has been linked most frequently with the Rhodesian Ridgeback, in which the mode of inheritance is thought to be simple recessive, and affected dogs should not be bred [4,5]. Breeders and owners of Rhodesian Ridgebacks are usually educated as to the incidence of this condition in the breed; hence, most affected dogs are identified (and eliminated) as pups. The condition has also been documented in other breeds, including the Shih Tzu, Boxer, Yorkshire Terrier, English Bulldog, Siberian Husky, Chow Chow, and Springer Spaniel [3,6–9]. The etiology and mode of inheritance in these breeds are less clear. Sinuses have a tapering tubular structure and extend from the skin surface through varying depths of the dorsal midline soft tissue structures. Most end in a strand of fibrous tissue, whereas the more extensive lesions continue to communicate with the spinal dura mater. The tube is lined with skin, and hence contains all the expected dermal elements, including squamous epithelium, sebaceous glands, and hair follicles. Sinus openings are often small, discrete, and located in the dorsal midline; most are found in the cervical or cranial thoracic region (Fig. 3A), but lesions have also been reported in the lumbosacral area [8]. The sinus can be difficult to identify but is often found to have protruding hair. The opening is usually found in the midst of a whorl of hair in the Rhodesian Ridgeback; however, in other dogs, this can be obscure, and cannulation is necessary for diagnosis. Secondary infection is, however, a common and consistent long-term complication and arises through plugging of the sinus opening with keratin secretions. Perisinus cellulitis and abscessation are commonly encountered

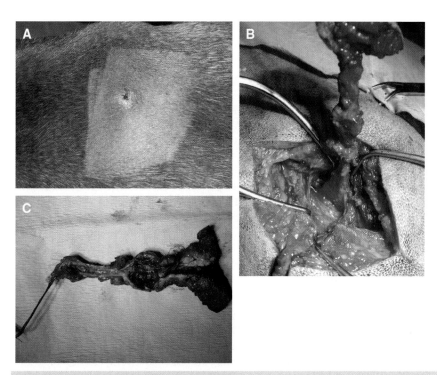

Fig. 3. PS (dermoid sinus). (A) PS in the cervical midline of a Rhodesian Ridgeback. (B) Dissection of PS from dorsal cervical musculature. (C) Excised sinus shows dermal structures lining the sinus and terminal fibrous tissue.

and may become extensive if the infection is unrecognized or unmanaged. Less commonly, in cases that communicate with the dura, the secondary infection may lead to septic meningitis and the onset of neurologic signs. The extent of sinuses is notoriously difficult to assess on clinical examination or cannulation and is commonly underestimated, leading to disastrously inadequate surgical interventions. Imaging studies, including sinography, may be more informative, but contrast may not reach the deeper parts of the tract and does not highlight the fibrous strand that sometimes extends far beyond the obvious limit of the tubular component of the sinus. Spinal and vertebral involvement may be detected on plain radiographs, where there are vertebral anomalies and absent dorsal processes. Neural changes are best assessed with advanced imaging techniques, such as CT or MRI scanning.

Superficial sinuses or lesions that are recognized and managed with a cleansing regimen implemented at an early age can remain asymptomatic for long periods into adulthood. Infected lesions may respond to extended antibiotic therapy with sinus irrigation and cleansing. Once the lesions become symptomatic or if neurologic signs appear, the only long-term solution is surgical resection of the complete sinus structure.

Surgery should be performed by excisional dissection separating the fascial planes from the outer aspects of the sinus. Exploratory operations (incisional dissection) following the sinus lumen are to be discouraged, because failure to remove the sinus in its entirety leads, at best, to the development of a further discharging sinus, whereas disruption of a secondarily infected sinus may lead to serious septic complications. Surgery should only be undertaken once the depth of the sinus has been appropriately imaged and preparations have been made for neurosurgery, when appropriate, including a laminectomy to permit access to the dura.

Perioperative antibiotics should be administered, and a wide area of the dorsum should be prepared aseptically to permit access to what may be the spinal structures. The patient is positioned in sternal recumbency, and intervertebral exposure is maximized by positioning the affected region over packs. A wide circular incision around the sinus is made, and retractors are used to facilitate access through the dorsal cervicothoracic musculature (see Fig. 3B). The sinus tract can be identified with the assistance of a probe within its lumen and dissected by a combination of sharp and blunt dissection with the use of thermocautery. Most sinuses terminate without neural involvement as fibrous bands, and care should be taken to remove all residual tissue. Sinuses that perforate the nuchal or supraspinous ligaments should be dissected by longitudinal separation of the ligamentous fibers. Sinuses involving the vertebrae require removal of the dorsal spinous processes, whereas those attached to the dura necessitate dorsal laminectomy and resection of involved dura mater. Wounds should be closed carefully to eliminate all dead space, because seroma development is a distinct possibility in these dorsal wound sites. The placement of active suction drains is indicated to prevent the development of seromas; likewise, with cellulitis or abscessation, active suction drains and antibiotic therapy are often indicated. The prognosis after resection is generally good, provided that a complete resection of all the dermal tissue has been performed (see Fig. 3C). The prognosis for dogs that have neurologic complications is more guarded; however, complete and early resection is usually curative.

Nasal Dermoid Sinus Cyst

A nasal dermoid sinus cyst (NDSC) is a congenital lesion found in the nasal midline and is thought to represent a similar embryologic failure of neuroectodermal separation as a PS. NDSCs are recognized in Golden Retrievers and spaniels [10]. During embryologic development, the meninges in the frontal bones protrude through the foramen cecum, a canal in the skull base, and contact the somatic ectoderm. This canal normally closes in later embryogenesis but persists in NSDCs, providing for permanent contact between the neural tissue and dermal elements. The persisting elements are located in the dorsal midline caudal to the external nares and perforate through an incomplete suture line in the nasal septum. Communication with the meninges, and consequent meningitis, is recorded in human beings but has not been reported in the dog. NDSCs are histologically similar to PSs and contain a complete range of dermal components. Dogs are usually presented in young adulthood for the management of a sebaceous discharge immediately caudal to the nasal planum. Secondary infection and inflammation are usually less obvious than in the case of a PS. The extent of the lesion can be gauged by insertion of a probe or catheter. Lesions require careful dissection from the dorsal nasal midline, where many terminate in the septum. Placement of a probe within the sinus lumen is helpful to allow recognition of lesion margins. The potential for extension to the cranial vault should always be considered, and MRI is helpful in determining any brain involvement.

There is little potential for dead space during tissue closure, and the development of seromas is an unlikely outcome. The prognosis after resection of lesions is favorable but with the same proviso that all dermal tissue must be completely removed, because once disrupted, residual sinus tissue can provide a focus for cellulitis and ongoing abscessation.

CHRONIC LIMB WOUNDS
Hygroma
A hygroma can be considered as a chronic tissue swelling lined with granulation tissue and containing serous fluid. The lesion develops as the result of repetitive compression trauma to soft tissues between an underlying bony prominence and an extraneous hard surface. Hygromas can be found in the region of the olecranon, carpus, nuchal crest, tuber ischium, and os calcis. The condition occurs primarily in dogs and has only rarely been recorded in cats. Although dogs of any age or large breed can be affected, juvenile giant-breed dogs (especially Great Danes, Irish Wolfhounds, and Newfoundlands) less than 2 years of age seem to be most prone to the condition. The problem is most commonly seen in dogs housed on hard unyielding surfaces but may arise as the result of any persistent trauma. Nuchal crest hygromas, for example, usually arise through repetitive head contact between feeding pups. The condition develops initially as a pressure sore, and as the local vascular supply to the area becomes progressively impaired, localized edema and ischemia become more marked. The combination of the poor vascular supply and the accumulation of edema leads to a marked inflammatory response and the characteristic development of a granulation tissue lining surrounded by a thickened capsule of connective tissue. Serous fluid accumulates within the hygroma as the result of exudation from the chronic inflammatory tissue. The cycle of etiopathogenesis is perpetuated by further episodes of trauma that promote persistence of the chronic granulation tissue.

Management of hygromas is directed toward identifying and removing the underlying etiology, which permits the inflammatory process to recede and the granulation tissue to undergo fibrosis ultimately. This entails bedding patients on yielding surfaces. Most lesions resolve with such conservative management, although the process may be slow in some cases. So-called "conservative" interventions, including aspiration of serous fluid and compressive bandaging, are rarely successful. Instilling long-acting steroidal preparations into the hygroma should be resisted, because this merely promotes and perpetuates the chronic inflammatory changes in most cases. The temptation to yield to owner pressure for early surgical intervention should likewise be resisted until owners have complied with the need for management improvement and this regimen has been given an opportunity to resolve the condition. Investigation of any concurrent orthopedic disease (eg, hip dysplasia) that may cause excessive weight to be taken on the elbows during the process of getting into sternal recumbency should be undertaken. Extension and immobilization of the limb prevent flexion of the affected joint in sternal recumbency and promote healing by preventing pressure on the tissues and immobilizing tissues so they can heal together.

Surgical intervention is rarely a good substitute for adequate medical management and is likely to end in failure, with the possibility of the development of a chronic open wound (Fig. 4A). Lesions that do break down, become secondarily infected through iatrogenic interference, or develop persistent pain may be candidates for surgical intervention. The fundamental principles of such surgical management include removal of all chronic granulation tissue, closure without any dead space, adequate immobilization in the postoperative period, and adequate removal of the underlying etiology. Any surgical

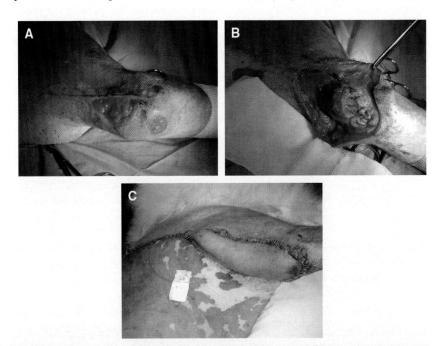

Fig. 4. Chronic elbow wound. (A) Appearance of the elbow after multiple attempts to resect hygromas. (B) Resection of chronic granulation tissue and meticulous dead space closure are essential prerequisites for successful hygroma removal. (C) Closure of elbow dissection without tension using a thoracodorsal axial pattern flap.

intervention that achieves less than this, for example, passive or active drain placement [11,12], fails to address the underlying problem of the residual chronic granulation tissue and runs the real risk of aggravating the problem. Hygromas should thus be dissected in their entirety from the surrounding tissue whenever feasible using a combination of a tourniquet and thermocautery cutting to limit bleeding from what is often extremely vascular tissue. Involvement of the underlying joint is a rare complication, although the lesion may often be attached to the joint capsule. Skin incisions should be sited away from the underlying bony prominence whenever possible, and the residual dead space should be obliterated by careful multilayer repair (see Fig. 4B). Placement of passive drains should be avoided because they may recreate dead space within the wound, although active drains of short duration (24–48 hours) may be helpful. In the case of skin deficit overlying the wound, it may be necessary to recruit skin from an adjacent area by means of a random or axial pattern flap (see Fig. 4C) so as to avoid tension in the skin repair (see the article by Hedlund elsewhere in this issue). Compressive dressings should be used to limit dead space development and movement at the site until the wound has healed. Dressings should be changed on a daily basis.

Pocketing Wounds

These are defined as nonhealing open wounds that become lined with chronic granulation tissue (ie, granulation tissue is found on the wound surface and on the dermal surface of the overlying skin without any adherence of the two surfaces). They can develop in any skin deficit that comes under tension and experiences frequent movement, but "classic" sites include the shoulder in dogs (Fig. 5A) and the axilla in cats. The two problems of tension and movement promote failure of the cutaneous layers to adhere to the underlying tissues. As granulation tissue matures, that on the dermal surface of the wound causes

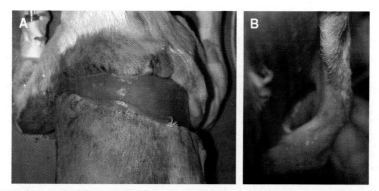

Fig. 5. Chronic pocketing wound in a dog. (A) Chronic pocketing wound over the shoulder and axillary region of a terrier 6 months after a bite injury. Note the smooth quiescent granulation tissue surface. (B) Pocketing wound shows granulation tissue lining the pocket and overlying skin.

contraction of the overlying skin. The consequence of this is that the wound edge begins to "roll in" to the point that, eventually, the dermal edge contacts the bed of chronic granulation tissue within the "pocket" (see Fig. 5B). Once the wound reaches this stage, it is highly unlikely to progress to a satisfactory closure and may remain permanently unhealed. The role and importance of subcutaneous adipose tissue in the healing of open wounds have recently been highlighted [13], and it is likely that wounds that are depleted or devoid of subcutaneous adipose tissue may be more at risk of pocketing complications. Pocketing wounds can be among some of the most frustrating to manage, but successful treatment is predicated initially on recognition of the pocketing process as soon as possible so as to permit early surgical intervention. The principles of intervention should include the following:

- Treatment of any bacterial growth in the wound as determined by culture and sensitivity testing and appropriate antibiotic therapy
- Resection of all granulation tissue: inadequate wound debridement and closure of the wound over chronic granulation tissue is often likely to fail
- Relief of any skin tension before attempting closure; this may dictate undermining of subcutaneous tissues and the creation of skin flaps
- Meticulous closure of all dead space with walking sutures
- Compressive dressing combined, ideally, with active drains to maintain close contact between the skin and deeper layers of tissue

Feline Axillary Wounds

Chronic nonhealing wounds involving the axilla (Fig. 6A) and, less commonly, the inguinal region of cats are well-recognized types of feline pocketing wounds. The original etiology is usually associated with a traumatic injury resulting from a collar or wire "sawing" through the tissues. Microbiologic isolation often isolates sparse growth of *Pasteurella* spp, but this is not thought to be significant, and cats are invariably feline immunodeficiency virus (FIV)- and feline leukemia virus (FeLV)-negative. Although vascular deprivation and continual movement when walking have been postulated as possible underlying etiologies, the consistent failure of these wounds to heal has defied explanation until the recent recognition of the role of adipose tissue in cutaneous healing [13]. Management following the principles outlined previously for pocketing wounds using primary closure or even using tension-relieving techniques, including skin flaps, usually result in failure. The introduction of omental pedicles (see Fig. 6B, C) into the underlying wound before closure significantly improves wound healing rates [14], whereas omentalization combined with tension relief with thoracodorsal flaps (see Fig. 6D, E) provides a consistently successful outcome [15]; axial pattern flaps on their own do not seem to provide an adequate solution, however.

Lick Granuloma

A lick granuloma (lick dermatitis or acral granuloma) is a skin lesion that develops as a behavioral dermatosis, leading to persistent lick trauma to a localized area of skin (see the articles by Amalsadvala and Swaim and Hedlund

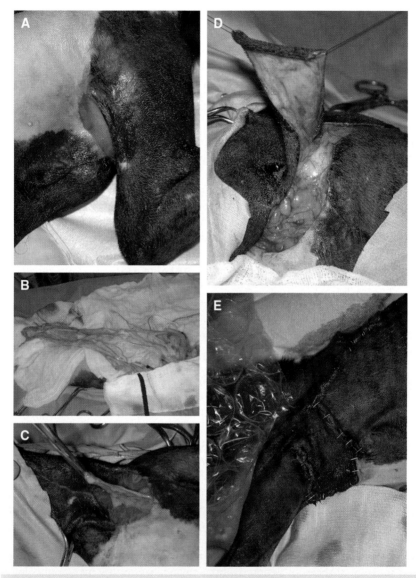

Fig. 6. Chronic axillary wound in a cat. (A) Chronic axillary wound in a cat. (B) Omental lengthening to facilitate omentalization of the axillary wound. (C) Omentum is drawn into the axillary wound. (D) Creation of thoracodorsal axial pattern flap for axillary reconstruction. (E) Thoracodorsal axial pattern flap in situ for axillary reconstruction.

elsewhere in this issue). The underlying etiology of this disease is not well understood. Local sensory neuropathy or pre-existing tissue trauma has been postulated as an initiating factor. It seems, however, that stress factors, such as separation anxiety, home abandonment, household additions, or changes in the household routine, may also be important [16]. In more serious cases, there is evidence of obsessive-compulsive behavior patterns. The condition is most frequently recognized in the Doberman Pinscher, but it is also encountered in the German Shepherd Dog, setters, Golden and Labrador Retrievers, and Great Danes. Common sites for lesions include the cranial aspect of the carpus, forelimb, stifle, hock, and, occasionally, flank. Lesions are often raised and discoid, with alopecia, ulceration, and secondary pyoderma. Steps should be taken to rule out local factors, such as foreign bodies and neoplastic infiltration; microbiologic isolation, including unusual bacterial and fungal organisms, should be performed to investigate the consistent pyoderma (see the article by Amalsadvala and Swaim in this issue) [17].

Lesions should be managed by addressing any identifiable underlying etiologic factors whenever possible. Behavioral modification using a range of drugs, including phenobarbital, diazepam, narcotic antagonists, and the tricyclic antidepressants, has been described. Extended antibiotic therapy based on microbiologic isolation testing often resolves or improves the appearance of lesions. A variety of topical treatments, including corticosteroids, dimethylsulfoxide, cobra venom, radiation therapy, and cryosurgery, have been reported, but none has been shown to be consistently successful.

Surgical resection is indicated in cases in which the lesion fails to resolve completely after medical management. Lesions over the distal limbs may require closure with skin grafting, direct distant flaps, or even microvascular free transfer to accommodate the lack of skin for reconstruction (see the article by Fowler elsewhere in this issue). Recurrence after resection and reconstruction is a possible long-term complication if the underlying etiology remains unidentified or unmanaged.

SPECIFIC WOUND INFECTIONS
Methicillin-Resistant *Staphylococcus aureus*
Although methicillin-resistant *Staphylococcus aureus* (MRSA) infection has been recognized as potential risk in human surgical patients for some time, it is only recently that this organism has been identified in small animal wound infections. It seems that this is also an emerging pathogen for veterinary patients, and at the present time, its importance and impact for veterinary wound care remain unclear. The organism is known to colonize the upper respiratory tract and mucosal surfaces in people without giving rise to any symptomatology. Several studies in veterinary hospitals have now recovered MRSA from staff [18–21], who should be regarded as colonized rather than infected carriers. Despite this, all the current evidence indicates that MRSA wound infections in veterinary patients represent a community-acquired rather than hospital-acquired problem. Health care workers may represent a particular risk to their pets in this respect. Infection can be seen in even the simplest of surgical interventions (eg, minor lacerations, ovariohysterectomy) and are thought to be acquired through subsequent contact with carriers once they are back in the home environment.

Strains of MRSA isolated from human patients require careful selection of antibiotic therapy, such as vancomycin as an alternative for methicillin. MRSA isolates recovered from veterinary patients are often indistinguishable from human strains, and they seem to share similar patterns of antibiotic resistance [18]. Some strains seem to be sensitive to less exotic antibiotic options in some cases, however, including enrofloxacillin, oxytetracycline, clindamycin, and trimethoprim sulfa. Fortunately, however, wounds infected with MRSA do not seem to be particularly difficult to manage, and routine open wound management is often surprisingly successful to bring the problem under control. Presently, we can only speculate on the long-term implications of MRSA infection for wound management as the organism becomes more and more ubiquitous in veterinary hospitals.

Other Organisms

Wound infections that are associated with organisms not commonly implicated in small animal cutaneous contamination, such as *Actinobacillus*, *Actinomyces*, *Mycobacterium*, or *Nocardia*, are periodically encountered in chronic nonhealing lesions. Lesions are typically found to have sinus tracts, pocketing wounds, or fistulae, and underlying etiologies include foreign body migration, intertriginous change, immune-mediated disease, and even tumors. These organisms are often not easily recovered using routine microbiologic isolation techniques, and additional techniques are required in the investigation of chronic wounds. These include the examination of smears made directly from the wound to identify the presence of acid-fast organisms, such as *Mycobacterium* spp and the collection of tissue samples from the wound itself for culture and sensitivity studies. Culture of wound fluid often identifies only superficial contaminants and not the causal organism itself. Management of such infected chronic wounds depends largely on the underlying etiology. Removal of a migrating foreign body, for example, allows such infections to resolve in most cases. In other wounds, however, atypical organisms can indeed play a significant role in the persistence of infection, and appropriate antimicrobial therapy is necessary before definitive wound closure is attempted or the wound heals by second intention (see the article by Amalsadvala and Swaim in this issue).

References

[1] Scott DW, Miller W, Griffin C. Environmental skin diseases. In: Muller & Kirk's veterinary dermatology. 6th edition. Philadelphia: WB Saunders; 2001. p. 1073–111.
[2] White RAS. Surgical treatment of specific skin disorders. In: Slatter D, editor. Textbook of small animal surgery. 3rd edition. Philadelphia: WB Saunders; 2003.
[3] Scott DW. Bacterial skin disease. In: Scott DW, Miller W, Griffin C, editors. Muller & Kirk's veterinary dermatology. 6th edition. Philadelphia: WB Saunders; 2001. p. 274–335.
[4] Mann GE, Stratton J. Dermoid sinus in the Rhodesian ridgeback. J Small Anim Pract 1966;7: 631–42.
[5] Hillbertz NHC. Inheritance of dermoid sinus in the Rhodesian ridgeback. J Small Anim Pract 2005;46(2):71–4.
[6] Booth MJ. Atypical dermoid sinus in a chow chow dog. J S Afr Vet Assoc 1998;69:102–4.
[7] Cornegliani L, Ghibaudo G. A dermoid sinus in a Siberian husky. Vet Dermatol 1999; 10:47–9.

[8] Pratt JN, Knottenbelt CM, Welsh EM. Dermoid sinus at the lumbosacral junction in an English springer spaniel. J Small Anim Pract 2000;41(1):24–6.

[9] Miller L, Tobias K. Dermoid sinuses: description, diagnosis and treatment. Compend Contin Educ Pract Vet 2003;25:295–300.

[10] Anderson DA, White RAS. Nasal dermoid sinus cysts in the dog. Vet Surg 2002;31(4): 303–8.

[11] Hedlund CS. Surgery of the integumentary system. In: Fossum TW, editor. Small animal surgery. 2nd edition. St. Louis (MO): Mosby; 2002. p. 134–95.

[12] Pope ER. Surgical treatment of hygromas in the dog of the elbow. In: Bojrab MJ, Ellison GW, Slocum B, editors. Current techniques in small animal practice. 4th edition. Baltimore (MD): Williams & Wilkins; 1998. p. 622–5.

[13] Bohling MW, Henderson RA, Swaim SF, et al. Comparison of the role of the subcutaneous tissues in cutaneous wound healing in the dog and cat. Vet Surg 2006;35:3–14.

[14] Lascelles BDX, White RAS. Combined omental pedicle grafts and thoracodorsal axial pattern flaps for the reconstruction of chronic, nonhealing axillary wounds in cats. Vet Surg 2001;30:380–5.

[15] Lascelles BDX, Davison L, Dunning M, et al. The use of omental pedicle grafts in the management of non-healing axillary wounds in 10 cats. J Small Anim Pract 1998;39(10):475–80.

[16] Scott DW. Psychogenic skin disease. In: Scott DW, Miller W, Griffin C, editors. Muller & Kirk's veterinary dermatology. 6th edition. Philadelphia: WB Saunders; 2001. p. 1055–72.

[17] McDonald JM, Bradley D. Acral lick dermatitis. In: Bonagura JD, editor. Kirk's current veterinary therapy XIII small animal practice. Philadelphia: WB Saunders; 2000. p. 551–6.

[18] Weese JS, Dick H, Willey BM, et al. Suspected transmission of methicillin-resistant Staphylococcus aureus between domestic pets and humans in veterinary clinics and in the household. Vet Microbiol, in press.

[19] Duquette RA, Nuttall TJ. Methicillin-resistant Staphylococcus aureus in dogs and cats: an emerging problem? J Small Anim Pract 2004;45(12):591–7.

[20] Loeffler A, Boag AK, Sung J, et al. Prevalence of methicillin-resistant Staphylococcus aureus among staff and pets in a small animal referral hospital in the UK. J Antimicrob Chemother 2005;56(4):692–7.

[21] O'Mahony R, Abbott Y, Leonard FC, et al. Methicillin-resistant Staphylococcus aureus (MRSA) isolated from animals and veterinary personnel in Ireland. Vet Microbiol 2005;109(3–4):285–96.

Vet Clin Small Anim 36 (2006) 913–929

VETERINARY CLINICS
SMALL ANIMAL PRACTICE

Tail and Perineal Wounds

Jamie R. Bellah, DVM

Department of Clinical Sciences, College of Veterinary Medicine, Auburn University, Auburn, AL 36849, USA

W ounds, regardless of primary cause, that involve the tail and perineal region can be particularly difficult to manage. There is little mobile skin in the area for reconstructive surgery, with the exception of the skin over the back cranial to the rump and the skin of the tail itself. Wound healing complications in the perineal area can result in adverse effects on function, especially if the anal and vulvar regions are involved. Fecal and urine contamination of the perineum is a significant issue. Bandages and wounds are commonly soiled, requiring frequent bandage changes and cleansing of the area. Bandaging the area is a challenge. Tail bandages tend to slip off as a result of movement. Because of their proximity to the anus, it is difficult to keep bandages in the perineal area from slipping off caudally. In addition, dogs and cats can easily get to this region to chew, lick, and pull at sutures and bandages; thus, restraint from self-mutilation is a must in treatment of injuries in this area.

PREPARING FOR SURGERY IN THE PERINEAL REGION

Surgery in the perineal region requires special planning because of the anus and the fecal contamination that may occur. Purse-string sutures are commonly placed before surgery, but their use depends on the specific procedure. Surgery peripheral to the anus, anal sacculectomy, or perianal mass excisions are examples where a purse-string suture is useful to prevent contamination. Surgical procedures that involve the anus or caudal rectum (anal mass excisions, perianal fistula excision, or anal stricture resection) may benefit by leaving the anus open so that digital palpation within the anus and rectum during surgery may help to orient dissection around these structures. In the latter instance, preparation of the caudal rectal area by multiple enemas is helpful. Sponges appropriate for the size of the rectum can be placed in the rectum and pushed forward to absorb fluid and obstruct residual fecal material to help prevent surgical field contamination. It is good practice to tie sutures to the sponges and

E-mail address: bellahr@auburn.edu

0195-5616/06/$ – see front matter
doi:10.1016/j.cvsm.2006.04.002

leave long ties before placing the sponges in the rectum to serve as a reminder for removal at the end of surgery.

Perioperative antimicrobial use may be appropriate for tail and perineal surgery, and the surgeon's judgment should include factors that affect predicted surgical time, the presence of presurgical contamination or infection, and the potential need for implantation of foreign materials (eg, polypropylene mesh, implants) that may be adversely affected by secondary infection. The perineal region, in general, has an excellent blood supply, which aids in access of the inflammatory response and antimicrobial drug availability in the region.

Positioning for perineal and tail surgery is dependent on the procedure being done, but most procedures place the dog or cat in sternal recumbency with the tail elevated. Certainly, this varies on the basis of surgeon's preferences and the symmetry of the surgical problem. In general, the author tries to position the animal such that the orientation of the perianal anatomy is as normal as possible, which makes decisions during dissection easier and less confusing. If sternal recumbency is used, the author prefers to pad under the pubis and "frog-leg" the rear limbs. If the rear limbs are pulled back off the surgical table, the edge of the table should be well padded, especially if it is tilted, to prevent temporary bilateral femoral nerve problems [1]. Finally, it is good practice to place an indwelling urethral catheter of a size that is easily palpable when surgical dissection is done in the neighborhood of the pelvic urethra. The ability to palpate this catheter within the urethra during surgery helps to orient the surgeon when dissecting within the pelvic cavity or periurethral region and may prevent a serious iatrogenic surgical error.

TRAUMATIC TAIL AND TAIL-PERINEAL INJURIES

Tail injuries are common in dogs and cats and can vary from minor to severe injuries. An example of a minor injury is the chronic wound on a tail tip resulting from the dog wagging its tail and beating it on structures in its environment. Topical medications (see the article by Krahwinkel and Boothe elsewhere in this issue) and secure bandaging are necessary for healing. To place a secure bandage on a tail, a "shingling" technique can be used. As strips of tape are placed circumferentially around the tail, hair is pulled from under a strip and laid on top of the strip. When the next strip is applied, it sandwiches this hair between tape strips. Doing this two to three times secures the bandage so that it cannot be "wagged" off. Once the wound is healed, application of some paw pad toughening agent may help to prevent wound recurrence. Environmental changes may be necessary to prevent recurrence.

More serious tail injuries include degloving, avulsion, and fracture injuries. Tail injuries that result in degloving may, on occasion, result in avulsion of skin surrounding the anal sphincter and may involve a portion of the anal sphincter [2]. Some degloving injuries of the tail are complicated by avulsive force that separates coccygeal vertebrae and soft tissues within or around them. Careful neurologic examination is important, because nerve root injury can result in loss of innervation of the tail and, occasionally, the nerve roots responsible for urinary and fecal continence. Tail sensation and perineal reflexes should be assessed. Damage to the S1, S2, and S3 spinal segments often results in loss of urinary and fecal continence. Although uncommon, rear limb flexor innervation may be affected by the traction injury, resulting in loss of flexor tone and a diminished withdrawal reflex or, more subtly, a hyperreflexive patellar reflex because of loss of the antagonistic muscle group. In the presence of nerve damage with urinary and fecal incontinence, the prognosis and potential problems with the condition should be discussed with the pet owner before any treatment.

Examination of complicated tail injuries usually requires sedation or general anesthesia so that a thorough examination as well as lavage and debridement can be done. In addition, rectal examination to assess the integrity of the rectum and anal area is important. Avulsion of portions of the anal sphincter can occur concomitant with the avulsive skin loss (Fig. 1), and the neighboring perineal diaphragm can be disrupted. The soft tissue damage may be obvious, or it may be recognized when examined digitally. This injury may be asymmetric in that one side may be affected more than the other. The caudal rectal nerves may be damaged such that the remaining anal sphincter muscle is denervated on the side of the injury or bilaterally.

Surgical resolution of degloving and avulsion injuries may be done after lavage and debridement and assessment of the damage. With simple degloving injury and no other soft tissue or nerve damage, amputation at the level of degloving is indicated. If the skin is available, replacing it in the form of a graft

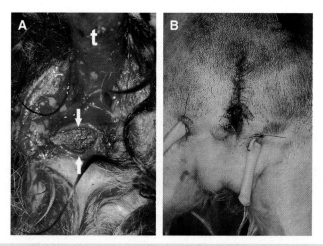

Fig. 1. Tail degloving and anal sphincter avulsion injury. (A) Avulsed anal sphincter (*arrows*) on underside of tail (*t*). (B) Perineal area after caudectomy, perineal diaphragm reconstruction, and creation of anal mucocutaneous junction. (*From* Bellah JR, Williams JM. Wound closure options and decision making. In: Fowler DA, Williams JM, editors. Manual of canine and feline wound management and reconstruction. Shurdington (UK): British Small Animal Veterinary Association Publications; 1999. p. 29; with permission.)

has met with little success because of the tenuous blood supply of the tail. Because the tail is usually degloved completely, it is amputated. A caudectomy high enough to allow cutaneous apposition in the perineal region is done. Remnants of skin of the tail that appear viable near its base are preserved and used in reconstruction. Assessment of the anal sphincter and pelvic diaphragm is made, and if the coccygeus and levator ani muscles are detached, they are sutured in place as for perineal hernia repair. It may be difficult to know if the innervation is intact in some circumstances (and if the patient is sedated or anesthetized), but the associated fascia and muscle, which atrophy if denervated, can still be used to support the herniorrhaphy. Standard techniques for perineal herniorrhaphy apply, and the internal pudendal nerve and vessels, if intact, are preserved. Monofilament absorbable suture material is the author's preference in such a case.

The repair may be augmented using an acellular collagen matrix (BioSISt; SurgiVet, Waukesha, Wisconsin) or a polypropylene mesh (Prolene polypropylene mesh; Ethicon, Somerville, NJ). Once the perineal diaphragm is apposed, closure of the cutaneous wound can be completed. Usually, there is sufficient skin peripheral to the dorsal aspect of the anus to close the wound primarily. Wound closure is done in a manner that reduces tension on final wound closure. A Penrose drain or closed-suction drain may be placed to promote wound drainage if there is dead space that allows wound fluid accumulation or if the wound contamination or infection warrants drainage. If a Penrose drain is used, it must be placed in such a manner so as to avoid fecal contamination. The anal mucosa is identified, and it can be gently moved caudally out of the anal canal and a mucocutaneous junction created. This is done in two layers. Interrupted submucosal sutures are used to adjoin the submucosal, and sometimes the muscular layer of the distal anus, to the subcutaneous tissue, and sometimes to the dermis of the surrounding skin. This is followed by interrupted or cruciate monofilament nonabsorbable sutures to appose the anal mucosa to the peripheral skin edge. Cruciate sutures may be turned 90° to place the knots away from the mucosa, or a figure-of-eight mucocutaneous suture may be used for the same purpose. This lessens irritation to and away from the incision and makes suture removal easier.

Dogs or cats with such injuries may be incontinent after surgery. If the innervation to at least one side of the anal sphincter is intact, continence should return. Urge incontinence may occur after surgery with normal innervation if there is irritation from surgery or perineal soiling (scalding). To prevent the scalding type of irritation to the area, a hexamethyldisiloxane solution (Cavilon No Sting Barrier Film; 3M Health Care; St. Paul, Minnesota) can be sprayed or swabbed on the area.

DORSAL PELVIC HERNIA FROM TAIL AVULSION

Most coccygeal avulsion injuries simply separate the more proximal coccygeal vertebrae, with the resultant loss of tail function and sensation. If the distraction of the coccygeal vertebrae is severe enough, the pelvic fascia located ventral to the coccygeal vertebrae (the inner "roof" of the pelvic canal) may separate, creating a rent and space into which viscera may herniate (Fig. 2). The dog shown in Fig. 2 has small intestine herniated through this dorsal pelvic canal defect. The tail and sacrococcygeal area were prepared for surgery, and the dorsal pelvic defect was identified by sharp and blunt dissection. The hernia was reduced. Fascia strong enough to hold sutures, which was attached to the sacrum and coccygeal vertebra cranial and caudal to the avulsion space, was identified. Monofilament absorbable sutures were used to reappose the fascia and other soft tissues attached to the sacrum and coccygeal vertebra, effectively closing the hernia opening. Skin and subcutaneous tissues were apposed with absorbable sutures in three layers to lessen dead space. A caudectomy was performed to remove the nonfunctional tail. Anal tone was less than normal, but a perineal reflex was intact and urinary continence was normal.

CUTANEOUS WOUNDS AROUND THE TAIL (RUMP)

Large traumatic wounds or wounds created by tumor resection over the sacrococcygeal area of the pelvis often require reconstructive surgery. The tail base and regions of skin at the dorsal aspect of each rear limb typically do not have sufficient redundant skin that can be mobilized toward the rump to cover large defects. A single pedicle advancement flap from the dorsal lumbar area can be

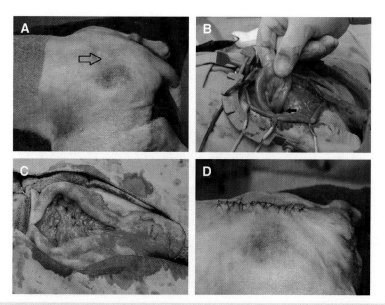

Fig. 2. Tail avulsion injury with sacrococcygeal hernia. (A) Depression over sacrococcygeal area (*arrow*). (B) Small intestine as the hernial content, hernia opening (*arrow*). (C) Sacrococcygeal opening closed with sutures in epaxial fascia. (D) Skin closure after caudectomy.

considered to cover defects over the rump, however, with the advantage that hair growth is in the normal pattern when regrowth occurs (Fig. 3). The flap may be designed with the pedicle based cranial to the rump defect and elevated, thus preserving the cutaneous trunci muscle. Walking sutures may be used to disseminate tension as the flap is advanced caudally. Deep circumflex iliac flaps may also be considered for rotation to cover defects of the sacrococcygeal area or pelvic region. They may be designed as an island flap to allow easier rotation (see the article by Hedlund elsewhere in this issue). The ventral branch of the deep circumflex artery is best used as an island flap and may reach the perineal region in some circumstances, but careful planning is needed for this use [3–5]. Penrose drains or closed-suction drains may be used according to the surgeon's preference.

Free full-thickness grafts are difficult to stabilize in this region, but free full-thickness mesh grafts (see the article by Fowler elsewhere in this issue) or pinch/punch grafts could be considered. Tacking sutures can help to stabilize mesh grafts in place. Placement of pinch/punch grafts in pockets in the granulation tissue helps to stabilize them. Tie-over bandages with both of these graft types provide additional protection. The cosmetic appearance of these grafts is not as good as that of the single-pedicle advancement flap, however, because hair growth is sparse.

Larger wounds that extend to or around the tail base or perineum can be managed using caudal superficial epigastric flaps (Fig. 4) [3,5]. The flap is dissected on the basis of published diagrams (see the article by Hedlund in this issue) and can be rotated back between the legs to the wound. The ability to

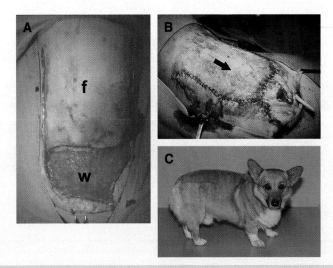

Fig. 3. Flap closure of a dorsal pelvic area wound. (A) Cranially based single pedicle advancement flap (f) and wound (w). (B) Flap moved caudally (arrow) to close wound. (C) Cosmetic appearance of dorsal pelvic area.

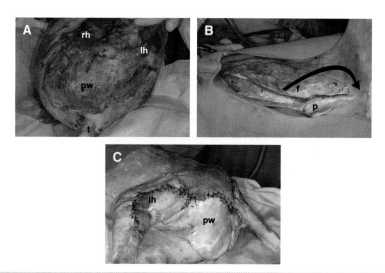

Fig. 4. Caudal superficial epigastric axial pattern flap (cseapf) to correct a wound of the perineum and left hind limb (lh) wound. (*A*) Large wound of the perineum and lh. Tail (t), perineal wound (pw), right hind limb (rh). (*B*) Dissection of axial pattern flap, with prepuce (p) and cseapf (f) rotated caudally (*arrow*). (*C*) Flap sutured in place over pw and lh. (Courtesy of D.J. Krahwinkel, DVM, MS, Knoxville, TN.)

use such a technique may be facilitated in some smaller breeds and in cats, where a long flap can be created with less distance required to reach the tail head or perineum (ie, Dachshunds, cats), whereas careful planning may be required in some of the larger canine breeds. With a peninsular flap, the edges of the flap base can be tubed over intact skin between the donor site and wound or they can be sutured to the edges of a bridging incision [5]. The flap can also be dissected free on all borders, leaving the vascular pedicle intact (an island axial pattern flap), and the flap can be sutured to both sides of a bridging incision that connects to the perineal wound. Once the flap is in position at the wound, it is trimmed to fit in the perineal or tail base defect. When trimming the flap, care is taken not to damage the caudal superficial epigastric vessels. The flap may completely close the wound, or it may decrease the wound area, changing the shape of the defect so that free grafting or second-intention healing may be used for final wound closure.

ANAL SAC ABSCESSES AND SACCULECTOMY

Impaction, anal sacculitis, anal sac abscess, and anal sac rupture are the classifications that describe anal sac disease; however, progression of anal sac disease to rupture and development of a fistulous tract likely represents a continuum or progression of the aforementioned conditions [6]. Anal sac disease is uncommon in cats. Anal sac abscessation may be treated conservatively by promoting drainage from a rupture site, or an incision can be made to allow drainage, irrigation with antiseptics, and antimicrobial therapy. Recurrence of anal sacculitis and abscessation is an indication to remove the offending anal sac. It is best to delay surgical excision of the anal sac until the acute inflammation associated with the abscess is resolved, because this makes surgical dissection easier [1].

Preparation of the perineal region before sacculectomy is done by clipping hair peripheral to the anal region and flushing the anal sacs with an antiseptic solution (ie, chlorhexidine). A purse-string suture is carefully placed around the anal opening just cranial to the anal sac openings so that the anal sac duct can be accessed. There are open and closed methods used to remove anal sacs. The open technique is done by placing a scissors blade into the sac and incising or by placing a probe (fine hemostat) into the anal sac, placing traction caudally, and incising the duct and sac with a scalpel blade. This exposes the edge of the anal sac, which is grasped with forceps; using sharp and blunt dissection, the entire anal sac and duct are then removed. It is important to release muscular and soft tissue attachments close to the surface of the anal sac, because this is the best protection against damaging the caudal rectal nerve that is located cranial to the apex of the sac.

The closed techniques are done by inserting a small-diameter Foley catheter (ie, 3-mL bulb volume) into the anal sac or by injecting paraffin wax or plaster of Paris into the anal sac. Both techniques allow the sac to be slightly distended, which facilitates dissection. After incising the skin over the distended anal sac, it is dissected free using blunt and sharp dissection without entering the sac. The closed techniques provide less anal sphincter muscle damage during the dissection. Once the anal sac is removed, the wound is lavaged and closed using absorbable sutures to appose the deep wound margin and nonabsorbable sutures for skin apposition. A subcuticular closure with absorbable sutures is another option for skin closure.

Chemical cautery (ie, silver nitrate) and cryosurgical techniques used to treat anal sac abscesses are not recommended by the author because both techniques are inconsistent. Any small remnant of anal sac epithelium and adnexa results in recurrent abscessation and sinus tract development. If excision is possible, it is the best therapeutic choice.

Complications of anal sacculectomy are rare but include hemorrhage, temporary or permanent fecal incontinence (caudal rectal nerve damage), tenesmus, and wound infection [7]. Fistulous tracts develop if incomplete excision of the anal sac occurs, because adnexal structures within the sac remnant are a nidus for infection and produce secretions that result in inflammation, secondary infection, abscess, and drainage from a tract. Surgical resolution of this complication is best done when the tract is surrounded by mature scar tissue. A small catheter may be placed into the tract and fixed by a suture or by clamping. Dissection is done sharply and bluntly, staying as close to the tract wall as possible. Fine-tenotomy scissors or Metzenbaum scissors with tenotomy tips aid such fine dissection. Every attempt is made to excise this tissue en bloc.

The wound may be closed as for routine anal sac excision, or the surgeon may choose to leave the wound open to heal by second intention in some cases.

Neoplasms of the anal sac are removed by a closed technique. Placing a probe in the anal sac sometimes helps to guide initial dissection. Dissection around the mass (often, an anal sac adenocarcinoma) is done, trying not to invade the tumor mass but attempting to gain a margin of normal tissue around the tumor. Muscular attachments and fascia are incised around the periphery of the gland and mass. With large masses, the resection margin is often narrow (marginal). Once the mass and associated anal sac are removed, closure is as for routine anal sacculectomy, except that there may be a large amount of dead space, which occasionally benefits from the use of an active or passive drainage technique. Histopathologic examination of the resected tissue is done, and "painting" the surgical margin with India ink labels this surface for the pathologist. Using sutures to label the regions of the mass (ie, cranial, caudal, left right) is also helpful.

PERINEAL SKIN DEFECTS

Defects in the perineal region are often a result of traumatic injury and subsequent skin loss. Extensive skin loss may occur from bite wound complications, anatomic or physiologic degloving injuries, abscessation, or skin loss that occurs secondary to urethral or rectal perforation, with leakage of urine or feces subcutaneously. Accumulations of subcutaneous urine or feces may cause vascular injury and severe skin sloughs. Once diversion of urine or repair of urinary or rectal defects is completed and the wound is debrided thoroughly, reconstruction of the defect may be planned.

Little adjacent skin is available for local mobilization to cover wounds in the perineal region. Thus, it is difficult to create subdermal plexus flaps that are large enough to transpose and cover much surface area. In some breeds, redundant skin is present around the tail base, and small transposition or advancement flaps can be designed to reach the dorsal perineal region (9 o'clock to 3 o'clock position). Redundant tissue below the perineal area, such as scrotal skin in male animals and dorsal vulvar skin in female animals, provides a potential source of skin for local mobilization and transposition.

The tail skin as a flap has recently been described as an axial pattern flap [8]. The skin is incised dorsally along the length of the tail and undermined circumferentially around the tail. Care is taken to preserve the circulation from the lateral caudal arteries that extend parallel and distally on either side of the tail. The muscular and vertebral portions of the tail are amputated at a level that ensures the rump dorsal to the perineum is smooth after closure. Because of a reported incidence of 78% of the flap length surviving, the authors recommended shortening the length of the flap relative to the length of the tail to improve survival [8]. When the skin is flapped cranially, the appearance of hair growth is not completely cosmetic. The tail flap may be transposed to cover defects around the anus and perineal area and cranially over the spine.

The author has used a similar flap to cover wide perineal fistula resection; however, a ventral incision was made so that the tail skin was simply dropped ventrally to cover the wound on each side of the anus (Fig. 5). When the dorsal skin of the tail is preserved by ventral incision after such procedures as tail amputation, the tail skin can be laid ventrally as a flap, and hair growth is cosmetic. Tail amputation is considered an adjunctive method of treatment for perianal fistula disease in German Shepherd Dogs [9].

ANAL STRICTURE AND PERIANAL FISTULAE

Stricture of the anal orifice can be superficial, involving superficial skin, or deep, involving the anal sphincter and/or caudal rectum. Traumatic wounds in the perineal area involving a large circumference around the anal sphincter and circumferential ulceration (ie, from coprostasis) that heal by second intention may result in superficial stricture. Surgical wounds, cryosurgical wounds, and anastomotic sites may also result in stricture that affects the anal sphincter [10]. The author has seen superficial lesions that result in superficial stricture, more commonly in cats (Fig. 6). As wounds circumferential to the anus contract, inelastic scar tissue is produced, resulting in a ring of tissue that progressively narrows. As the opening narrows to a diameter that restricts the exit of fecal material, tenesmus occurs and can progress to constipation or obstipation. In female dogs and cats, this may affect the vestibule as well. The anal sphincter

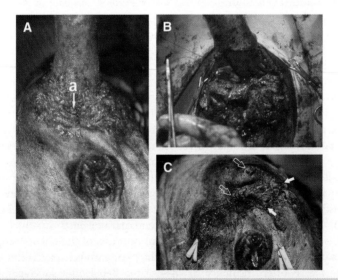

Fig. 5. Tail amputation and use of its skin to close the perianal wound. (A) Perianal fistulae causing anal stricture (*arrow*). Anus, a. (B) Wide excision to resect the fistulae and strictured anal sphincter. (C) Tail has been amputated, and the dorsal skin of the tail has been used as a flap (*open arrows are at tail flap base and solid arrows are at flap apex*) to cover a portion of the perineal wound.

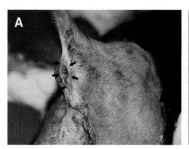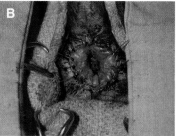

Fig. 6. Relief of superficial cutaneous stricture caudal to the anal sphincter. (A) Cat with superficial anal stricture. Proposed line of incision is around the entire circumference of the inelastic scar (*arrows*). (B) After resection of the ring of inelastic scar, the elastic skin and/or anal mucosa is moved caudally and apposed to peripheral skin edge, which now has a much larger diameter.

is often not involved in superficial scarring and remains functional, although the stricture narrows the anal opening and results in obstruction. If an accurate history of the animal is not available, biopsy of the affected area ensures that the scirrhous tissue is not neoplastic, which may alter resection margins and prognosis.

The goals of surgical resection are to remove the inelastic scar and advance the nonhaired cutaneous zone or anal mucosa out of the anus and suture it to the perianal skin. This opens the anal opening and renews elasticity of the region so that defecation may occur without straining. A circumferential incision is made just peripheral to the inelastic scar, releasing the surrounding skin, which retracts. The scar is elevated and released by sharp and blunt dissection around the entire circumference of the anus until normal skin or mucosa is encountered. Sometimes, the mucosa is not affected, because the stricture can be caudal to the mucocutaneous junction. The ring of scar is removed by resection of the mucosa or the skin just caudal to the mucocutaneous junction in normal tissue. Tissue margins are marked and submitted for histopathologic examination. Closure is started by apposing subcuticular tissues of the skin to submucosal tissues of the anus using fine interrupted absorbable sutures (3-0 to 4-0) with buried knots. Sutures placed at four equidistant sites around the wound help to orient the circumference of the anus, and additional sutures are placed within each quadrant. Nonabsorbable simple interrupted sutures are then placed to appose the skin and anal mucosa.

Strictures that involve deeper structures of the perineum, including the anal sphincter, are managed similarly; however, the additional deep dissection that is required includes varying amounts of the anal sphincter muscle. This situation more commonly results from advanced perianal fistulae, but a similar-appearing problem can occur with neoplasia that rims the anal sphincter. Perianal fistulae that are causing anal stricture are resected by making an incision just peripheral to outer edge of the tracts. Once this boundary is made, dissection by sharp and blunt dissection is performed just underneath the fistulae and toward the anal sphincter. Sharp dissection, electroscalpel technique, and laser excision have been used with success [11,12]. As dissection proceeds closer to the anus, the anal sphincter muscle is identified and an attempt is made to preserve as much of the sphincter diameter as is possible. The dissection next proceeds around the caudal aspect of the anal sphincter, and the mucosa is transected, releasing the inner margin of the fistulous tract tissue from the anus. The anal sacs are removed with the fistulous tracts. Residual tract tissue that remains is removed by blunt or sharp dissection (épluchage) [7,13]. Wound closure is accomplished by interrupted monofilament absorbable sutures to appose the submucosa of the anal mucosa to the subcuticular region of the surrounding skin. Simple interrupted sutures of monofilament nonabsorbable suture material are used to appose the anal mucosa to the surrounding skin. If one side of the anal sphincter muscle and its innervation is left intact, continence should resume, although urge incontinence may be temporary from irritation of the perineal or anal region.

Medical therapy may be used alone or in combination with surgery to attempt resolution of perianal fistulae. In addition to standard cleansing of the perineal area by hair clipping and use of topical antiseptics (ie, chlorhexidine scrub), immunosuppressive and dietary therapies are used [6]. Cyclosporine (5 mg/kg administered orally every 24 hours) has shown the ability to resolve fistulae completely in 85% of dogs within 16 weeks, but there is a 40% recurrence rate [6]. Alternatives to cyclosporine therapy include tacrolimus (0.1% topical ointment) and azathioprine (2 mg/kg administered orally every 24 hours) used with metronidazole to provide a less expensive but less effective alternative, respectively. A 50% remission rate is achieved. Novel protein diets and broad-spectrum antibiotics are palliative and used in conjunction depending on the clinician's preferences [6]. Medical therapy is commonly used initially for perianal fistula disease unless the disease process is causing anal stricture and tenesmus. The latter needs to be treated by surgical resection.

Neoplastic invasion, chronic and progressive fistulae, and wound contraction that affects deep functional structure, such as the anal sphincter muscle, may only be resolved by complete resection of the anal sphincter and associated inelastic scar (see Fig. 6). After removing the strictured area, the transected bowel wall is pulled caudally. The muscular wall of the rectum is sutured to the subcuticular region of the skin with interrupted monofilament absorbable sutures (3-0 or 4-0), burying the knots. Finally, the mucosa is sutured to the skin edge with nonabsorbable monofilament sutures orienting the knots away from the anal canal. Resection of the anal sphincter is done to palliate obstruction, but it leaves the dog or cat subject to fecal accidents in the household. The afferent limb of the defection reflex is still intact; thus, the dog or cat should recognize when fecal material is in the rectum, and this may result in the animal exhibiting behavior that lets the owner know a bowel movement is about to occur. If the animal is an outside pet, this is usually no issue.

VULVAR FOLD EXCISION (EPISIOPLASTY) AND PARTIAL VULVAR RESECTION

Vulvar fold pyoderma and neoplasia involving the vulvar fold and vestibule are treated surgically by episioplasty and partial vulvar excision, respectively. Episioplasty is indicated most commonly when intertriginous dermatitis is associated with the chronic moisture and maceration within the fold [14]. A secondary benefit of episioplasty for vulvar fold pyoderma is elimination of the predisposition to recurrent urinary tract infections. Episioplasty in dogs with vulvar fold pyoderma and chronic recurrent urinary tract infections has resulted in resolution of the latter after surgery [15].

Episioplasty is done by excising the skin fold that drapes over the vulvar cleft (Fig. 7). The procedure is similar to excision of a "dog ear," because the goal of fold excision is to flatten and elevate the surface of the dorsal vulvar region, eliminating the crevice that accumulates moisture. A sterile marking

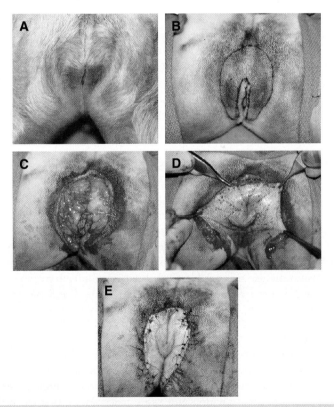

Fig. 7. Episioplasty to correct vulvar fold. (A) Extensive vulvar fold. (B) Lines drawn for proposed fold excision. (C) Fold excised. (D) Trial apposition with forceps to determine if the excision is sufficient. (E) Final apposition for episioplasty.

pen may be used to mark the boundaries of the incision, which is usually in the shape of a horseshoe. The paired incisions are made, and the skin and underlying adipose tissue are removed. Hemostasis is by fine ligature or electrocautery. Trial apposition of the skin edges can be done with forceps to determine if excision is sufficient. If excision is adequate with the vulvar cleft uncovered, absorbable sutures apposing subcuticular tissues are widely spaced across the defect to approximate the skin margins. Skin apposition is completed with absorbable subcuticular sutures and interrupted monofilament nonabsorbable skin sutures. If the excision is inadequate, additional skin is excised from the dorsal border of the wound margin and closure is completed.

Partial vulvar excision is usually done to remove tumors at the mucocutaneous junction or in the perivulvar region. Excision is done with the goal of en bloc resection. It is important to judge the potential for damage to the urethral tubercle. If there is any question, a urethral catheter should be placed to ensure that the urethra is preserved during surgery. After tumor removal, fine absorbable sutures (4-0 monofilament) are used to appose the subcuticular region of the skin to the submucosal tissues of the vestibular mucosa. Fine nonabsorbable sutures are used to complete the apposition of vulvar mucosa to perivulvar skin. A figure-of-eight mucocutaneous suture pattern may be used to prevent knots from irritating the vestibular mucosa and make suture removal easier. When creating new mucocutaneous junctions, it is important that haired skin not be inverted into the vulva. This could lead to inflammation, infection, and dehiscence. To ensure this, skin should be trimmed so that mucosa is everted at closure.

INGROWN TAIL AND TAIL FOLDS

Brachycephalic dogs (and occasionally Manx cats) may be affected by ankylosis of coccygeal vertebrae and tail deformation that may result in tail fold pyoderma [14,16]. The more severe deformities result in a condition called "screw-tail," where the end of the tail is ankylosed in a ventral and cranial direction, resulting in the eventual development of a macerating wound from pressure and secondary bacterial infection. Dogs that have associated generalized skin disease are predisposed to all types of intertriginous dermatitis. Treatment is directed at resection of the skin fold and the tail in most instances.

Tail Fold Excision

Excision of the tail fold to resolve tail fold pyoderma is done in a similar fashion as for vulvar fold excision. After clipping and preparation for surgery, the margins of the fold are incised and the skin is resected to eliminate the crevice that allows moisture accumulation and tissue maceration. Test closure can be done with towel forceps or sutures to determine if resection is adequate. Standard two-layer closure is done. The question that has to be answered before surgical resection is what portion of the problem is caused by tail deviation.

If tail deviation is part of the problem, tail amputation is a necessary step for satisfactory results.

Vertebral Excision and Tail Preservation

Occasionally, pet owners do not allow a caudectomy to treat screw tail. An alternative to caudectomy is to remove the vertebrae and leave the soft tissue portions of the tail (the tail stump) [16]. A U-shaped cranially based incision is made (creating a tail flap) that allows the coccygeal vertebrae to be isolated by sharp and blunt dissection. By elevating the muscular and soft tissue attachments, bone-cutting forceps can be used to transect the coccygeal vertebrae cranially, anterior to the ankylosed vertebrae. The coccygeal vertebrae are further released by incision of the coccygeus and levator ani muscles close to the vertebral bodies and by releasing the most distal vertebrae from the tip of the tail skin. The cranial-based tail flap can then be trimmed to remove most of the tail fold. Dogs with severe cranial deviating ankylosis may not be good candidates for such dissection, because open wounds are common dorsal to the anus. Once this region is removed, apposition of coccygeus and levator ani muscles is done to provide support dorsal to the rectum. Excess skin is removed so that no tail fold occurs but a stub of tail remains after closure is complete. Subcutaneous tissues and skin are apposed routinely. Individual case selection is important when considering a more conservative approach, because residual skin may result in pyoderma that requires long-term management and is not a desired result.

Tail Amputation

Most dogs with tail fold pyoderma and screw-tail need a caudectomy to resolve the secondary pyoderma, especially if the dog has generalized skin disease, such as atopy (Fig. 8). Before surgery, preparation of the surgical site can be difficult because of the ventral tail deviation. Perioperative antimicrobial drugs (ie, cefazolin) are warranted at induction of anesthesia and should be considered after surgery. A purse-string suture is placed to prevent fecal contamination of the surgical site during surgery. Culture of skin removed during surgery (from the skin fold) is advisable so that the necessity for susceptibility testing can be determined.

A skin incision is made around the entire tail base, preserving the dorsal tail base skin to provide a more cosmetic closure. Dissection is performed down to and around the deviated coccygeal vertebrae (at the level that allows the rump to be smooth). Care must be given to the depth of dissection ventral to the coccygeal vertebra, because perineal diaphragm structures and the rectum are immediately ventral to the tail base. Once the coccygeal vertebrae are transected and hemostasis is achieved, a decision is made to insert a passive or active drain. Fine absorbable monofilament sutures are used to appose muscular tissues; however, large deep bites should not be taken, because the rectum and neurovascular structures could be penetrated or entrapped. The remaining tail base skin is trimmed to include any excess tail fold present, and the area

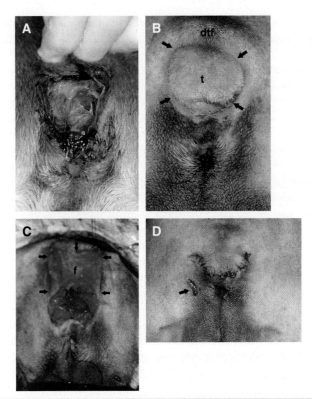

Fig. 8. Ingrown tail amputation. (*A*) Elevation of tail tip from above the anus, revealing exudates and hair underneath. (*B*) Perineal area prepared for surgery with purse-string sutures in the anus. The dorsal tail fold (dtf) extends around the entire circumference of the tail (*arrows*). The dorsal skin of the tail (t) is preserved as a cranially based flap for later closure. (*C*) Tail has been amputated, and a skin flap (f) has been created from the dtf (*arrows*). In focus is the cavity left by excision of the ankylosed tail. (*D*) Skin flap used to close the wound. Penrose drain removal site (*arrow*).

is closed smoothly with two-layer closure. If a drain is used, it is removed 3 to 5 days after surgery.

References
[1] Henderson RA. Anal sacculitis. In: Swaim SF, Henderson RA, editors. Small animal wound management. 2nd edition. Baltimore (MD): Williams & Wilkins; 1997. p. 275–9.
[2] Bellah JR, Williams JM. Wound closure options and decision making. In: Fowler DA, Williams JM, editors. Manual of canine and feline wound management and reconstruction. Shurdington (UK): British Small Animal Veterinary Association Publications; 1999. p. 29–37.
[3] Remedios A. Axial pattern flaps. In: Fowler D, Williams JM, editors. Manual of canine and feline wound management and reconstruction. Shurdington (UK): British Small Animal Veterinary Association Publications; 1999. p. 69–81.

[4] Pavletic MM. Canine axial pattern flaps, using the omocervical, thoracodorsal and deep circumflex iliac direct cutaneous arteries. Am J Vet Res 1981;42:391–406.

[5] Pavletic MM. Pedicle grafts. In: Slatter DH, editor. Textbook of small animal surgery. 3rd edition. Philadelphia: WB Saunders; 2003. p. 292–321.

[6] Sherding RG. Constipation and anorectal disease. In: Birchard SJ, Sherding RG, editors. Saunders manual of small animal practice. 3rd edition. St. Louis (MO): WB Saunders; 2006. p. 831–44.

[7] Lipowitz AJ. Anal sac excision. In: Lipowitz AJ, Caywood DD, Newton CD, et al, editors. Complications in small animal surgery. Baltimore (MD): Williams & Wilkins; 1996. p. 527–9.

[8] Saifzadeh S, Hobbenaghi R, Noorabadi M. Axial pattern flap based on the lateral caudal arteries of the tail in the dog: an experimental study. Vet Surg 2005;34:509–13.

[9] van Ee R, Palminteri A. Tail amputation for the treatment of perianal fistulas in dogs. J Am Anim Hosp Assoc 1987;23:95–100.

[10] Henderson RA. Anal stricture. In: Swaim SF, Henderson RA, editors. Small animal wound management. 2nd edition. Baltimore (MD): Williams & Wilkins; 1997. p. 286–7.

[11] Ellison GW, Bellah JR, Stubbs WP, et al. Treatment of perianal fistulas with ND/YAG laser—results of twenty cases. Vet Surg 1995;24:140–7.

[12] Ellison GW. Excisional techniques for perianal fistulas. In: Bojrab MJ, editor. Current techniques in small animal surgery. 4th edition. Baltimore (MD): Williams & Wilkins; 1998. p. 279–83.

[13] Henderson RA. Perianal sinuses. In: Swaim SF, Henderson RA, editors. Small animal wound management. 2nd edition. Baltimore (MD): Williams & Wilkins; 1997. p. 279–86.

[14] Bellah JR. Surgery of intertriginous dermatoses. In: Birchard SJ, Sherding RG, editors. Saunders manual of small animal practice. 3rd edition. St. Louis (MO): WB Saunders; 2006. p. 537–40.

[15] Lightner BA, McLoughlin MA, Chew DJ, et al. Episioplasty for the treatment of perivulvar dermatitis or recurrent urinary tract infections in dogs with excessive perivulvar skin folds: 31 cases (1983–2000). J Am Vet Med Assoc 2001;219:1557–81.

[16] Henderson RA. Ingrown tail. In: Swaim SF, Henderson RA, editors. Small animal wound management. 2nd edition. Baltimore (MD): Williams & Wilkins; 1997. p. 289–93.

Vet Clin Small Anim 36 (2006) 931–941

VETERINARY CLINICS
SMALL ANIMAL PRACTICE

ELSEVIER SAUNDERS

INDEX

Note: Page numbers of article titles are in **boldface** type.

0195-5616/06/$ – see front matter
doi:10.1016/S0195-5616(06)00066-0

Moving?

Make sure your subscription moves with you!

To notify us of your new address, find your **Clinics Account Number** (located on your mailing label above your name), and contact customer service at:

E-mail: elspcs@elsevier.com

800-654-2452 (subscribers in the U.S. & Canada)
407-345-4000 (subscribers outside of the U.S. & Canada)

Fax number: 407-363-9661

Elsevier Periodicals Customer Service
6277 Sea Harbor Drive
Orlando, FL 32887-4800

*To ensure uninterrupted delivery of your subscription, please notify us at least 4 weeks in advance of move.